PRACTICE MANAGEMENT FOR PHYSICIANS

DONALD L. DONOHUGH, MD, MPH, FACP

1986
W. B. SAUNDERS COMPANY
PHILADELPHIA/LONDON/TORONTO/MEXICO CITY/RIO DE JANEIRO/SYDNEY/TOKYO/HONG KONG

W. B. Saunders Company: West Washington Square
Philadelphia, PA 19105

Library of Congress Cataloging in Publication Data

Donohugh, Donald L., 1924–
Practice management for physicians.

1. Medicine—Practice. 2. Medical offices—Management.
I. Title. [DNLM: 1. Practice Management, Medical. W 80
D687p]

R728.D65 1986 610′.68 85-26153

ISBN 0–7216–1889–8

Editor: John Dyson

Manuscript Editor: Carol Stillman

Production Manager: Frank Polizzano

Practice Management for Physicians ISBN 0-7216-1889-8

Last digit is the print number: 9 8 7 6 5 4 3 2 1

"I swear by Apollo the Physician,
and Aesculapius . . . that, according
to my ability . . . I will impart a
knowledge of the art . . . ."

Preface

Above all, the practice of medicine is a calling, one that is an exhilarating and rewarding blend of science and art. Our education and training prepare us well for this. But in all specialties and all settings it is also a business, and for this part of medical practice we receive no preparation at all. At this writing, there are *no required courses* on practice management in any of the 127 medical schools in the United States, and only 10 irregularly attended electives!

True, there are several books on medical practice management which we can read at the start and as we go along. But these represent every point of view *other than* that of the practicing physician. Books abound on personnel management, legal aspects, financial management, insurance, and so on. Each is written by an expert in his particular subject. But not one book covers all aspects comprehensively from the physician's point of view. We look in vain for one from which we can learn what we should learn during our education and training and which will continue to be of value throughout the years that follow.

During our professional careers, most of us stay somewhere on the periphery of practice management, more concerned with caring for our patients and keeping abreast of medical advances. We hope that the other aspects will somehow fall into place by themselves. In recent years, practice management has become more complicated with the proliferation of governmental regulations, the increasing influence of third-party carriers, emphasis on cost reduction, and greater competition in the medical marketplace. This has edged many of us further out on the periphery when we should be moving toward the center. But during this time, medicine itself has become more demanding with the explosion of knowledge, the proliferation of new procedures and laboratory tests, and increasingly complex relationships with allied health personnel.

What are we going to do? We can't let practice management go by default. If we look closely at it, we find that the problems there are actually simpler to solve than the medical problems we handle well every day. I believe the answer to our present dilemma is to make the solutions just as simple and get the physician involved. That's what this book is all about. The practitioner who becomes actively involved in the management of his practice will find that he has more time to keep up with medical advances, and to care for his patients more competently and compassionately.

This book is the result of taking my own advice. When I first entered private practice, I found little information available to help me set up and run my practice. As with most physicians, it was mostly a process of trial and error. This situation appalled me as much then as it does now. But it did stimulate me to read what articles and books there were then, to attend seminars, and to consult advisors.

As a result of this interest, I taught electives on practice management at the two medical schools where I was on full-time faculty and in the process learned to appreciate the position of the medical student. Then, as director of a residency program at a major teaching institution, I held management seminars for house officers and benefitted immensely from this interchange. More recently, as a consultant for the Joint Commission on Accreditation of Hospitals, I had the opportunity to visit colleagues in all parts of the country and talk with them in their offices and hospitals. This further broadened my understanding. Since then, I have helped many physicians in practice with particular problems.

Then, two years ago, a senior medical editor at the W. B. Saunders Company asked me to write this book. I agreed, because I felt that I could present all aspects of practice management without omitting or overemphasizing any one of them. Unlike other books on the subject, this has only one bias—toward the practicing physician himself. It is written by a physician for physicians.

There *is* a tilt toward those at the start of their careers, and for a reason: it is then that the need for information is greatest. Decisions made in the early years shape all the years ahead. The better these early decisions are, the better the later years will be. I have tried to include all a physician needs to know at the start without leaving out anything an established practitioner might want to improve his practice. This emphasis according to need continues into the various types of practice as well. Advice is more detailed for the physician in solo practice than for one in a group or salaried position. And there is enough for one who is tapering his practice toward retirement.

This design makes the book especially suitable for use as a text in those elective courses on practice management now being conducted in our medical schools. It may encourage the institution of such courses in other schools, and it is my hope that it might even mark the start of required courses in all medical school curricula.

Readers are invited to send comments in care of the publisher. If you have any questions, please ask them by the same route, and I will do my best to answer them.

This book is written with the wish that your professional career will be all that you wanted it to be on the day you first decided to answer the calling.

DONALD L. DONOHUGH

Acknowledgments

Many colleagues, in every type of practice, with experience ranging from three years of residency to three decades in the trenches, have helped with encouragement and critical comments. Among them are Rex A. Adams, M.D., Thomas Badin, M.D., Marlene Coleman, M.D., James R. Seals, M.D., Bernard Virshup, M.D., and Andrew Wilner, M.D. Ruth Donohugh-Moss, M.B.A., reviewed the business portions of the manuscript. Florence Chandler, A.S.I.D., commented on Chapter 11, "Office Design and Decoration." Michael D. Nadler made valuable contributions to Chapters 26 and 27, "Personal Financial Management." William W. Huss, J.D., critiqued various legal points and amended Chapter 32, "Medicolegal Aspects," so extensively that it bears his name. Dr. Virshup, author of *Coping in Medical School,* revised Chapter 33, "Stress and the Physician," so thoroughly that he is listed as co-author. Marlene Coleman, M.D., premedical advisor at the California Institute of Technology, and Diane Wilner, M.P.H., Director of Planning at Hoag Memorial Hospital in Newport Beach, California, contributed to Chapter 35, "What Lies Ahead?" and their names accordingly appear on that chapter. Among the accountants and practice management consultants who were generous with their advice, by far the most helpful was Gary Thompson, C.P.B.C., Vice President of Rocky Mountain Professional Consultants, Inc., Denver, Colorado. The book shows his touches throughout. The Department of Practice Management of the American Medical Association and the American Association of Medical Assistants also deserve acknowledgment, as do several faculty members of the Departments of Medicine and Family Practice, University of California at Irvine School of Medicine. Rosemary Carroll and Arleen Morris patiently typed and retyped the manuscript and met the many deadlines.

Credit for the original concept and continuing support belongs to John Dyson, Medical Editor, W. B. Saunders Company.

To all, my thanks.

Two Notes to the Reader

1. Modern American English provides extraordinary opportunities for precise reporting of scientific data, human feelings, and, I'm glad to say, medical practice management techniques. Still, it has its limitations, one of the most vexing of which I have found to be role-assignment by sex. When a writer wants to refer to *either* a man or a woman, or to *both,* any construction using "one" seems stilted; excessive use of the passive voice wearies the reader; the tortured repetition of "he or she" or "him or her" soon becomes a burden to reader and writer alike. Therefore, while recognizing the risk of being branded sexist, I have taken the time-honored path of assigning sex by majority rule.

Modern medicine has benefitted enormously by the remarkable contributions of women physicians, whose number increases with each year's graduating class. Nevertheless, most physicians are still male, and so I have consistently referred to them as such. Further, most of these men are married and either have or plan to have children. That assumption is also implicit throughout this book, with no bias intended toward my bachelor, divorced, or widowed colleagues.

Similarly, most medical assistants and other ancillary personnel are women, and this fact also is reflected in this text—again with no bias intended toward the dedicated and talented men who hold such positions.

Whenever possible, I have avoided referring to patients by sex. Sometimes it couldn't be avoided, and the reader will find "he" and "she" used about equally. Once again, the intent has been to make the writing easier for me and less tiresome for you.

2. Obviously, there are several shades of opinion on almost every subject in practice management. I have tried to present each topic and list the various conclusions to be drawn and courses of action to be taken as objectively as possible. But it would have been a disservice to the reader to stop there. Whenever my own experience has led me

to believe that one course or conclusion is to be preferred to others, I have said so.

Inevitably, many readers will disagree with me—and on good grounds. This is as it should be. I hardly claim infallibility. If I could sit down and discuss the points at issue with my disagreeing colleagues, learning more about their particular circumstances, chances are that I would take their side. I don't pretend to have all the answers. All I can offer is a distillation of my own experience and the experiences of others whose careers have touched mine. The principles and practices described here have brought me professional and personal satisfaction beyond measure. I hope that they will to you, too.

Contents

1

Professional Goals

This chapter is specifically addressed to those just starting their careers. The discussion of practice management in the succeeding chapters can be of service to you only if you have carefully defined your professional aims. Although your major professional goals were probably clear when you decided to enter premed, they and you have changed during medical school and subsequent training. It is important that you think them through again now, as you set up practice. Bear in mind that you are making decisions at this time that will be binding for many years, and perhaps for your entire career. Therefore, before you decide on such matters as where you would like to practice, the type of office you want, and how you will organize your office, take the time to consider where your professional life will lead. As you formulate your goals, write them down and determine your priorities. This will help you examine choices and make decisions on all the topics in this book.

If you are having trouble putting your goals into words, let me make some suggestions to stimulate your thinking.

First and foremost among physicians is the desire to become as competent as possible in their field, in order to provide the finest care possible to patients.

Second is to care for patients in a humane manner, with courtesy and respect. During our training, we may have seen some patients treated poorly in public institutions. In our careers, we can practice according to the golden rule of medicine: treat your patients as if you were yourself the patient. After all, patients are human beings who are ill or troubled, not just "cases" of something or other.

The third goal of most physicians is to become more skilled in the area of prevention and not to be content with crisis care. Often, as we look around us, we see that modern medicine brings too much care to the patient too late. Preventive medicine is by far the most effective way to relieve anxiety, assuage pain, and lower costs.

The fourth goal is an extension of the third: to broaden one's concern from the patient to the community. Physicians may not have the time or the skill to serve on charity committees, city council, or other community organizations. But they *can* provide service in their own field: to patients in public hospitals, to medical students and house officers in teaching institutions, to the needy in free clinics, and to their own financially pressed patients, all without charge.

And last in this scale of values, although many more might be included, physicians expect to receive fair compensation for their investment of years and dollars and for the exercise of the skills they have acquired.

Think over these suggestions. Adjust or add to them as you will. Something resembling this scale of values is applicable to all physicians. The major problems some physicians encounter in their middle and later years begin at the beginning: they did not sit down quietly and think their values through, set their goals, and chart their course accordingly.

2

Your Curriculum Vitae

A curriculum vitae is a tool you will find surprisingly helpful in many situations: seeking temporary employment, applying for a teaching position, negotiating a bank loan, joining a medical society, giving a newspaper interview, introducing yourself to colleagues, and seeking hospital staff membership and privileges, to name a few. But little or no instruction on its proper preparation is given in medical school or graduate training.

A professionally prepared resume of two or three pages is rarely needed by a physician; a simple, single-page curriculum vitae will almost always suffice, and you can easily compose it yourself. It should be done well, however, because the form as well as the content reflect upon you. The form itself is not cast in concrete. A physician in academic medicine would stress his educational qualifications and professional accomplishments, while a rural solo practitioner would emphasize personal information about himself and family.

Let's outline the standard format. Not every item will be necessary or relevant for every physician, but a discussion of the possible categories will help you to decide what you should or should not include. Do not use letterhead stationery. In the center at the top of the first page, type **CURRICULUM VITAE** in large capital letters. Refer to the example at the end of this chapter as we go along.

The first item, all the way to the left and about four spaces below this heading, is **Name:** Your full name—first, middle, and last—follow the colon, without the M.D. Do not add social security, state license, or Drug Enforcement Agency numbers.

The second item on the left, two spaces below, is **Place and Date of Birth:** after which the appropriate data are entered. Although this information is not required by law, its omission is awkward.

The third item is **Marital Status:** This is also optional, but adds a personal touch to an otherwise formal document. Your spouse's name, the date and place of your marriage, your children's names and their dates of birth are sometimes added for the same reason.

Next is **Home Address and Telephone Number:** followed by that information. Use the two-letter abbreviation for the state, and be sure to give the zip code; include area codes for all telephones numbers. It is followed by **Business Address and Telephone Number:** with that information.

Below that is **Education:** List your schools in reverse chronological order, with your latest educational experience first. The name and location of the university, dates attended, degrees and honors received comprise each entry. Do not include high school, but any outstanding award or honor received then, or elected position held, may be listed under "Awards and Honors." The exact addresses of the institutions need not be given. They are easily found in reference sources.

Then **Graduate Training:** Start with fellowships, then residencies and internships, listed in reverse chronological order. Give names of institutions, types of training, and inclusive dates. Again, no addresses are needed. List unusually complex medical procedures you were trained to perform and any prestigious positions held, such as Chief Resident.

The next item is **Certification and Licensure:** Again, entries are in reverse chronological order. Include type of certification, date, and certification number. List all states in which licensed, with license numbers and dates licensed. The preferred format for certification is "Diplomate, American Board of Internal Medicine, September 1982, Certificate No. 12345." Add the NBME certification if you wish.

Then comes **Faculty Appointments:** if relevant. Give institutions and inclusive dates, in reverse order. Be sure all titles are correct.

Next is **Practice Experience:** with entries once again in reverse order with dates. Start with your present position and describe each briefly.

Below this is **Professional Society Memberships:** These are current ones, with the date you were admitted to each. Past memberships may be included if exceptionally noteworthy. Honorary societies may also be listed here.

Then **Awards and Honors:** Describe each, with the date. Explain briefly, if necessary. Include those for community service and other nonmedical activities. If none, omit this entry.

Following this is **Administrative Experience:** List positions by title with a brief description and include dates. If none, omit the item.

Next is **Scientific Exhibits and Presentations:** Describe briefly, with dates. If you have not had any, omit this item.

Follow with **Personal Data:** Include here anything that would be appropriate, such as pertinent biographical listings, language fluency, unusual skills and hobbies.

Next is **Hospital Appointments:** State whether active, courtesy, or honorary. Add staff positions you have held, such as Chief of Service. Again, inclusive dates are given.

Then **References:** It is advisable to put **Furnished upon Request** after this entry and to submit names of references separately.

The last item in a curriculum vitae is **Bibliography:** List your publications, this time in chronological order, in standard format. If you have none, omit this entry.

Be especially careful to account for all years since graduation from medical school. A careless error causing a gap in chronology may raise questions about your personal or professional history. If you have had military service and your duties were appropriate, these are best included in "Practice Experience" with rank, duties, and dates. Your current Reserve or National Guard status, if applicable, would be under "Personal Data."

Some physicians affix a passport-size photograph of head and shoulders to the right of their name. This can be printed only by a special screening technique, but it does photocopy fairly well. Because a photo may be inappropriate in certain circumstances, you may wish to affix one only when its inclusion is requested.

The appearance of your curriculum vitae is all-important. If you can afford the cost, have 50 to 100 copies reproduced with offset printing by a commercial printer on high-quality 8½ × 11 inch white bond paper. If not, have it typed on similar quality paper, always without letterhead, using a good electric typewriter. This can be photocopied satisfactorily on a high-quality machine. Either way, edit and proofread the galley or typed copy carefully before having it reproduced.

Never send a curriculum vitae without a properly addressed and signed cover letter. Write each letter with the particular recipient in mind and in it expand on any pertinent point in the curriculum vitae. Information not included in the curriculum vitae that would be of interest to that recipient may be added in the letter.

As time goes on, some of the items in your curriculum vitae will change. Rather than make alterations by hand, it is preferable to avoid minor revisions. However, when significant information changes, it is best to have a new curriculum vitae prepared. If you have access to a computer that produces a high-quality printout, you can easily keep your curriculum vitae accurate and up to date.

CURRICULUM VITAE

Name: ______________________

Place and Date of Birth: ______________________

Marital Status: ______________________

Home Address and Telephone Number: ______________________

____

Business Address and Telephone Number: ______________________

____

Education: ______________________

____

____

____

Graduate Training: ______________________

Certification and Licensure: ______________________

____

Faculty Appointments: ______________________

____

Practice Experience: ______________________

____

____

Professional Society Memberships: ______________________

____

Awards and Honors: ______________________

____

Administrative Experience: ______________________

Scientific Exhibits and Presentations: ______________________

Personal Data: ______________________

____

Hospital Appointments: ______________________

____

References: ______________________

____

Bibliography: ______________________

____

____

____

3

The State Medical License

Although ordinarily a physician who is ready to set up his practice already possesses his license, there are exceptions. At last count, 27 states issue temporary permits to allow completion of training without a license. And, sooner or later, up to one-fourth of physicians licensed in one state apply for a license in another. So, even though most who read this book do not need this information, it is worth reviewing the procedure for those who do.

First, write to the **State Board of Medical Examiners** in the state where you intend to practice for an application form and request a copy of their **Medical Practice Act.** Ask if a state narcotics license is required.

Here are the current addresses:

Alabama State Board of Medical Examiners
P.O. Box 946
Montgomery, AL 36102-0946

Alaska Board of Medical Examiners
Division of Occupational Licensing
Pouch D
Juneau, AK 99811

Arizona State Board of Medical Examiners
5060 North 19th Avenue #300
Phoenix, AZ 85015

Arkansas State Medical Board
P.O. Box 102
Harrisburg, AR 72432

California Board of Medical Quality Assurance
1430 Howe Avenue
Sacramento, CA 95825

Colorado Board of Medical Examiners
132 State Services Building
1525 Sherman Street
Denver, CO 80203

Connecticut Medical Examining Board
150 Washington Street
Hartford, CT 06106

Delaware Board of Medical Practice
Margaret O'Neill Building, 3rd Floor
P.O. Box 1401
Dover, DE 19901

District of Columbia Commission on Licensure
to Practice the Healing Art
605 G Street NW
Room 202, Lower Level
Washington, DC 20001

Florida Board of Medical Examiners
130 North Monroe Street
Tallahassee, FL 32301

Georgia Composite Board of Medical Examiners
166 Pryor Street, SW
Atlanta, GA 30303

Hawaii Board of Medical Examiners
Department of Commerce and Consumer Affairs
P.O. Box 541
Honolulu, HI 96809

Idaho State Board of Medicine
700 West State Street
Boise, ID 83720

Illinois Department of Registration and Education
320 West Washington Street
Springfield, IL 62786

Indiana Health Professions Service Bureau
Medical Licensing Board
964 North Pennsylvania
Indianapolis, IN 46204

Iowa State Board of Medical Examiners
State Capitol Complex
Executive Hills West
1209 East Court Avenue
Des Moines, IA 50319

Kansas State Board of Healing Arts
503 Kansas Avenue, #500
Topeka, KS 66603-3449

Kentucky State Board of Medical Licensure
3532 Ephraim McDowell Drive
Louisville, KY 40205

Louisiana State Board of Medical Examiners
830 Union Street, #100
New Orleans, LA 70112

Maine State Board of Registration in Medicine
RFD No. 3, Box 461
Waterville, ME 04901

Maryland Board of Medical Examiners
201 West Preston Street
Baltimore, MD 21201

Massachusetts Board of Registration in Medicine
Leverett Saltonstall Building, Room 1507
100 Cambridge Street
Boston, MA 02202

Michigan Board of Medicine
Department of Licensing and Regulations
611 West Ottawa Street
P.O. Box 30018
Lansing, MI 48909

Minnesota State Board of Medical Examiners
Suite 352
717 Delaware Street SE
Minneapolis, MN 55414

Mississippi State Board of Medical Licensure
P.O. Box 1700
Jackson, MS 39205

Missouri State Board of Registration for the Healing Arts
P.O. Box 4
Jefferson City, MO 65102

Montana State Board of Medical Examiners
1424 Ninth Avenue
Helena, MT 59620

Nebraska Board of Examiners in Medicine and Surgery
P.O. Box 95007
Lincoln, NE 68509

Nevada State Board of Medical Examiners
P.O. Box 7238
1281 Terminal Way, Suite 211
Reno, NV 89510

New Hampshire Board of Registration in Medicine
Health and Welfare Building
Hazen Drive
Concord, NH 03301

New Jersey State Board of Medical Examiners
28 West State Street, Room 914
Trenton, NJ 08608

New Mexico State Board of Medical Examiners
227 East Palace Avenue, Suite O
Santa Fe, NM 87501

New York Board for Medicine
Cultural Education Center, Room 2039
Empire State Plaza
Albany, NY 12230

North Carolina State Board of Medical Examiners
Suite 214
222 North Person Street
Raleigh, NC 27601

North Dakota State Board of Medical Examiners
City Center Plaza
418 East Broadway, No. C-10
Bismark, ND 58501

Ohio State Medical Board
65 South Front Street, No. 510
Columbus, OH 43215

Oklahoma Board of Medical Examiners
P.O. Box 18256
Oklahoma City, OK 73154

Oregon Board of Medical Examiners
1002 Loyalty Building
317 SW Alder Street
Portland, OR 97204

Pennsylvania State Board of Medical Education and Licensure
P.O. Box 2649
Harrisburg, PA 17105-2649

Rhode Island Department of Health
Division of Professional Regulation
104 Cannon Building
75 Davis Street
Providence, RI 02908

South Carolina State Board of Medical Examiners
608 West Avenue North
Sioux Falls, SD 57104

Tennessee State Board of Medical Examiners
3-20 R.S. Gass State Office Building
Ben Allen Road
Nashville, TN 37216

Texas State Board of Medical Examiners
P.O. Box 13562
Capitol Station
Austin, TX 78711

Utah Division of Registration
Haber M. Wells Building, Fourth Floor
160 East 300 South
P.O. Box 5802
Salt Lake City, UT 84110

Vermont Board of Medical Practice
Redstone Building
26 Terrace Street
Montpelier, VT 05602

Virginia State Board of Medicine
517 West Grace Street
P.O. Box 27708
Richmond, VA 23261

Washington Department of Licensing
P.O. Box 9649
Olympia, WA 98504

West Virginia Board of Medicine
3412-B Chesterfield Avenue SE
Charleston, WV 25304

Wisconsin Department of Registration and Licensing
P.O. Box 8936
Madison, WI 53708

Wyoming Board of Medical Examiners
Hathaway Building, Fourth Floor
Cheyenne, WY 82002

Most states regulate the licensing of M.D.s and D.O.s under the same governing body, so this address will do for D.O.s as well. Those that do not will refer D.O.s to the correct address.

Graduates of foreign medical schools, whether U.S. citizens or not, should contact the **Educational Commission for Foreign Medical Graduates,** 3624 Market Street, Philadelphia, PA 19104 and acquire an **ECFMG certificate** before contacting any state board. Many states require this certificate before permitting foreign medical graduates to participate in graduate training programs. Only a few now accept fifth-pathway programs. In fact, the conditions laid down by each state for foreign degree holders change so frequently that each graduate of a foreign medical school would do well to keep current. Nothing further will be said here that applies particularly to them.

Anyone interested in comparing the requirements and procedures of the various states should see the October 1984 issue of **Resident & Staff Physician** (Vol. 30, No. 10) for a recent summary.

As soon as you have sent off your request for an application, if not before, set about assembling the following items. Some may take time to obtain, so start as early as possible. Although not every state wants all of them, most do.

1. **Proof of graduation** from a medical school approved by the Liaison Committee on Medical Education. This can either be a photocopy of the diploma or an original letter signed by the Dean of the Medical School specifying the graduation date.
2. **A transcript.** Some states want to review the curriculum or see your grades. If your state does not request it, you can keep it for your files.
3. **Proof of satisfactory completion** of at least one year of internship/residency in a program approved by the Accreditation Council for Graduate Medical Education. Some states require two years. This may either be a photocopy of the Completion Certificate or an original letter signed by the director of the program confirming dates and satisfactory completion.

4. **Proof of citzenship.** This can be a photocopy of your birth certificate or your certificate of naturalization. First papers are accepted by some states.
5. **Three or four letters of recommendation** from physicians familiar with your professional and ethical qualifications. At least one must be from the supervisor of your internship/residency describing your training. The others can be general character references. Not all states require these, but you will have other uses for them.
6. **Passport-size photographs** (2″ × 2″) of head and shoulders. The number required is usually two, but this varies from state to state. You might as well get a dozen or so to use for other purposes.

This is usually all you will require to complete the application to take the **Federation Licensing Examination** administered in December and June by each State Board. The **Federation of State Medical Boards of the United States,** 2630 West Freeway, Suite 138, Fort Worth, TX 76102 prepares this examination **(FLEX),** which is (as of 1985) a two-part examination. Each state sets its own requirements for its pass–fail level, but most use a minimum FLEX Weighted Average of 75. If you have already passed the FLEX in one state, you may have the test scores sent directly to the State Board of another, but some require that the examination be taken within the last five or ten years.

All states and territories except Louisiana, Texas, and the Virgin Islands accept passage of the three-part examination of the **National Board of Medical Examiners (NBME)** as a substitute for the FLEX. Several states have begun to require NBME certification within a certain period prior to application (California within five years, Florida within ten years, and Arizona within fifteen years). If you are a Diplomate of the NBME, notify the State Board and they will send you a National Board endorsement request card with your application form. Complete this and mail it to the National Board of Medical Examiners, 3930 Chestnut Street, Philadelphia, PA 19104. The NBME will then complete an Endorsement of Certification and mail it with your scores to the State Board. Some states accept a photocopy of your certificate.

Many states still accept a valid license of another state in reciprocity, but with certain qualifications. The first license must originally have been based upon the FLEX or the NBME, not a state-constructed examination; the license has to be current; there must have been no disciplinary action since it was issued; more letters of recommendation may be required; and a personal interview is often necessary.

Your **American Medical Association profile** (a printout from the AMA computer) is sent directly by the AMA to the State Board upon their request, but you may be requested to telephone the AMA at (312) 645-5155 and provide them with information such as your name, medical school attended, year graduated, or the address of the State Board.

When you receive the application form, fill it out carefully and enclose all requested documents. If there is an error and you are counting on taking the FLEX, the registration deadline (6 to 8 weeks before the examination dates) might slip by while you are correcting the error, and then you will have to wait six more months. The completed and signed application has to be notarized and accompanied by a license fee ranging from $100 to $300. Allow at least two months from the time all documents are received by the State Board for your license to be issued.

4

Types of Practice

The three most important decisions of your professional career are (1) deciding to become a physician, (2) selecting your specialty or subspecialty, and (3) choosing the type of practice you will enter—solo, group, or other. The importance of this last decision is somewhere between that of the first two. A shift later from one type of practice to another, though possible, can be difficult. The vast majority of physicians stay with their first selection, so your choice of practice type should receive serious thought.

In theory, the decision process is simple. Find out all you can about the various options available, analyze yourself and your motivations carefully, then make the best match-up. Well, there is a little more to it. The choice you make will affect your spouse and family in terms of financial security, the hours you spend in your practice, the coverage that is available for nights, weekends, and vacations, and the lifestyle you will be able to afford. If you are married, make your decision a joint one.

Before I began writing this chapter, I made a list of all the various types of practice that exist in the United States. I reached 23 and was still going when I realized I was becoming more of a "splitter" than a "lumper." The types of practice can be further subdivided until the resultant categories are without any practical significance.

Let's try to make sense out of the different modes of medical practice today by putting it all into historical perspective. About fifty years ago, the choices were less complicated. Most physicians went into solo private practice. A fraction opted for salaried positions of several descriptions, and another fraction went into what was loosely called an "association," which also consisted of several different arrangements.

So there were really just three major choices. Then practices changed substantially in the forties and fifties. Salaried positions in the military swelled, and shrank again after World War II. The Veterans Administration and Public Health Service steadily increased, as did state and local health services. Academic appointments also multiplied, due to a large influx of federal funds. During the same period, many associations grew in size and began to be called "groups." Lawyers were brought in to change the simple handshake to a legal document, and this began the divergence of the legal definition of an organization from the manner in which the members actually organized their practices. Most groups became partnerships, but there were exceptions. Legally, some remained proprietorships, while others became corporations.

In the sixties and seventies, the threat of malpractice suits contributed to the dissolution of the small, loosely structured associations, after the courts held that any member of an association that was perceived by the public to be operating as a partnership was responsible for the debts and professional actions of all other members, as well as for those of the association itself. Most small associations then became either (1) temporary combinations that developed into larger groups, (2) strictly expense-sharing arrangements, or (3) legal partnerships. The situation became even more complicated during these two decades when prepaid groups (health maintenance organizations), stimulated by federal funds, began to be formed, and when many of the larger groups, until that time simple peer partnerships, incorporated and started to hire salaried physicians. Then the individual professional corporation came on the scene in the 1960s. During the next decade, more than half of the solo practitioners incorporated, so that these physicians then became salaried employees of their own corporations. Many smaller partnerships also evolved into corporations, and some of the corporations themselves became partnerships of corporations!

This is where we are now, and it is quite a maze to sort out. It helps first to set aside legal definitions, because they do not have much effect upon the way medicine is practiced. They matter most to the lawyers. Nonetheless, the four main legal arrangements should be mentioned. They are:

1. Sole proprietorship
2. Salaried employee
3. Partnership
4. Corporation

But for our purposes, a different classification is needed, determined by the manner in which medical care is rendered. Although one or two of the terms are similar to those just listed, it should be emphasized that these four categories have no relationship to the legal entities:

1. Solo private practice
2. Salaried
3. Association
4. Group

Let's look at each in turn. I am going to give the most important characteristics of each in a way that I hope will stimulate you to analyze your own personality and goals and help you see which type of practice would suit you best.

SOLO PRIVATE PRACTICE

A solo practitioner is one who has a direct one-to-one relationship with each patient. He provides professional service to the patient, is personally responsible for that care, and receives a fee in exchange for his service. All assets and liabilities arising out of his practice are his own. This definition describes approximately 60 per cent of the physicians in the United States today. Let's weigh the benefits and drawbacks of this type of practice.

On the positive side, a physician who is in solo private practice is carrying on many of the venerable traditions of the past by his almost constant availability and his dedication to his patients. He is, accordingly, held in high regard by his community. He develops a satisfying relationship with each of his patients as an individual. He is independent in most aspects of his practice: he can determine the location, the office design and decor, its organization, the personnel, the procedures, the fees, the pace, and the professional standards of his practice. He acquires self-discipline and self-reliance, as well as business and managerial skills. His lifetime income is the highest of any type of practice. It starts low, rises to a higher peak than in other types, is sustained over many years, then is reduced somewhat in the years preceding retirement. Within limits, his income can be varied according to his efforts. The data you sometimes see giving group physicians the advantage in income are not age-adjusted and reflect the usual urban-rural difference, since groups occur mainly in population centers, where both cost-of-living and income are high.

For all of these benefits, there is a price to be paid. At the start, the solo practitioner must endure the anxiety of many months of low income. Already heavily in debt for his education and training, he must continue to borrow in order to meet start-up costs and living expenses until his practice gets going. His income is subject to losses due to external factors, such as inflation, recession, government regulation, and competition. Internal or personal factors also affect his income, such as health, stamina, psychological stability, and skill in public relations. He must provide financial protection for himself and his family in case of disability and death. And he alone provides for his retirement.

The solo practitioner works longer hours than most of his colleagues in other types of practice. His time off is less certain and more frequently interrupted. Coverage is usually more difficult, so that vacations are fewer and shorter. Office overhead expense continues during his time off, while income generation stops. The same is true when he is ill. His spouse and family must alter their lives to conform with the limited time he can spend with them.

The business aspects of his practice are a constant concern. From loans, leases, layout and maintenance of his office, scheduling, billing, collections, equipment, supplies and other expenses, insurance, to personnel and payroll—all decisions and supervision are his alone. Factors such as third-party carriers, government regulations, legal problems, and tax tangles all impact upon him directly. He has no business manager to turn to. He is isolated professionally in his office during most of the day. His continuing medical education never seems to be sufficient; journals more often than not are set aside never to be read, and he finds himself slowly slipping behind professionally.

His patients are often more intelligent and expect more than those in other types of practice. He has to consider their ability to pay when making medical decisions. He deals primarily with common maladies and seldom has the chance to observe and treat rare diseases. He must spend added time on patient education and motivation, and in talking to relatives of patients. He must contend with the fact that he is often judged by his patients on superficial characteristics of personality rather than on his skill as a physician. The problems of his patients tend to be more personal than medical, and psychology is one of the tools of his trade that never gets rusty. The stress he feels is more intense, and he often is not able to share the burdens or vent his feelings with close colleagues.

These disadvantages are most frequently experienced by the solo private practitioner in primary care—a specialist or subspecialist can modify or avoid a number of them.

SALARIED

A salaried position offers relief from many of these drawbacks. Positions may range from employment in hospitals, clinics, emergency centers, state and local health departments, public health service, health maintenance organizations, large groups, offices of other physicians, academic institutions, industries, pharmaceutical firms, the military, and the Veterans Administration, to name a few. In general, salaried positions offer greater security in return for some loss of independence and income.

There are certain advantages to a salaried position. It offers a smoother transition from a training program than any other form of practice. Its pace is less demanding and more leisure time is available. Income is assured (only by violating the original agreement of employment do you risk its loss); better benefits are available than in solo practice; and start-up costs are essentially zero. Mobility is greater than in most other types of practice.

The disadvantages are equally compelling, if not more so. Personal and professional independence are curtailed, and income is lower. When personality conflicts with other physicians and staff occur, they cannot be resolved as easily as in solo practice or small groups: you must accept organizational and professional standards as you find them. You may be associated with physicians who are more security than quality-of-care minded. Innovation and imagination are seldom encouraged, and productivity is rarely rewarded. In fact, the hard worker is often frowned upon by his peers.

Although the situation may be changing now, it has always been a truism that most physicians who take salaried positions are not satisfied in them for long. They are more frequently sought at the beginning and toward the end of a professional career. Especially at the beginning—if you are hesitant about committing yourself to a particular location, you might want to try a salaried position with a hospital or as an ER physician, or take a *locum tenens* for a while. The best way to learn about a community is by living in it.

ASSOCIATION

The term "association" is a venerable one that in the past covered almost all situations in which the practices of two or more physicians were coordinated. It has now come to apply to a spectrum of arrangements in which some form of expense sharing is the chief characteristic. An association is almost always a step in the direction of another arrangement, because if physicians find they can get along, there are advantages to forming a group. Although an association is still sometimes based upon a loose understanding and a handshake, it is advisable that a written agreement, contract, or memorandum of understanding be prepared as its legal basis.

Most often, an association is entered into by a new physician with an established one. Both should have the same specialty. Their compatibility should be considered carefully before entering into the agreement.

The agreement itself must be specific as to the expenses that are to be shared, from major ones, such as the lease, the equipment (including the use of the depreciation allowance), and employees' salaries, down to minor ones, such as utilities and telephone. The method of apportionment of expenses must also be specified in the instrument, the fairest being according to the hours each uses the office, not the income produced. The way in which the expenses are to be paid must also be detailed. A dollar limit is usually placed on what each can spend without the approval of the other out of a joint account to which each contributes. The method of arriving at such decisions as office decoration, maintenance, furniture, procedures, purchase of equipment, supplies and, especially, all matters pertaining to personnel, must be incorporated into the agreement. If the association is formed by an older physician with a younger one, it is necessary to specify the date when the older one will retire and the younger one will inherit the practice. Most important, the manner in which the agreement is to be terminated by either party must be clearly set forth. Walkouts must specifically be prohibited.

It must be clear to all concerned—to employees, to patients, and to the community at large—that each practice is a solo practice and that the association is for the purpose of sharing the office or expenses only. If it is perceived by the public or the IRS as a partnership, there could be trouble. With all the above precautions meticulously observed, this form of association, although (or because) it is self-limiting in duration, usually works well and is an especially good way for a younger physician to become established in a community. He acquires an immediate roster of patients as the older physician introduces him to the community. The younger physician gains first-hand experience in personnel administration and business matters without bearing full responsibility for his mistakes. This arrangement also benefits the older physician who is tapering his practice and wishes to reduce expenses. However, he must be careful not to overload his younger colleague and must treat him in all respects as an equal.

It is only a small step from such an association to a true partnership of two physicians with a legal instrument as its basis. This is still called an association by physicians, despite its being a partnership legally. It may start as a partnership, or evolve from an office- or expense-sharing association. It is also self-limiting in duration, as it will almost invariably undergo change, occasionally reverting to a solo practice as the older physician retires, or, more often, expanding into a group. Three physicians practicing together is a much more satisfactory number than two, from many points of view. They provide each other with greater professional stimulation and better coverage for weekends, vacations, and illnesses. Greater economy of operation is achieved, since personnel are utilized more efficiently. There is more financial stability in times of economic hardship; in terms of prosperity, better facilities may be purchased and more efficiently utilized and maintained. Finally, more opportunity for continuing medical education is available to each member.

As stated previously, the chief disadvantage of a two-man partnership is that each partner is responsible for all the business and professional actions of the other and of the partnership as a whole.

GROUP

A group may have the legal structure of a sole proprietorship, a corporation, a partnership of individuals, or a partnership of corporations. About two-thirds of groups are corporations; less than one-third are partnerships. The other two organizational types make up only about 2 per cent. As any group can also have salaried physician employees or utilize solo practitioners as consultants or for other purposes under contract, the legal possibilities are quite complex, but unnecessary for our consideration here. So, still setting aside the legal structures, let's look at the way groups actually practice medicine.

According to the American Medical Association, "Group medical practice is the application of medical service by three or more physicians formally organized to provide medical care, consultation, diagnosis, or treatment, through the joint use of equipment and personnel, and with income from the medical practice distributed in accordance with methods previously determined by members of the group." A group may be linked to a hospital, to a medical school or other institution or may be freestanding. Also, groups may be single specialty or multispecialty, may vary as to size, and may operate on either a fee-for-service or prepayment basis.

Groups are growing in both number and size. Today, nearly 40 per cent of physicians in the United States are in group practice. The advantages start with the income distribution over an entire career. Income is satisfactory at the start, when the need is greatest, and although it may not reach as high a peak as solo private practice, it is still satisfactory in the years prior to retirement when illness occurs more frequently and stamina declines. Benefits are better than in most salaried positions once one becomes a partner or shareholder.

The space, technical services, and facilities are usually superior to those available to the solo practitioner. Supplies can be ordered in bulk for greater economy. Personnel utilization is better vis-à-vis patient-load fluctuation. There is greater professional stimulation through conferences, patient-problem sessions, journal clubs, and "curbstone" consultations. Textbooks and journals are purchased for group use, and time off for continuing medical education can be taken without loss of income. Teaching, medical society, and hospital medical staff activities usually are encouraged and remuneration provided. A group specialist can limit his practice more to his specialty than a solo practitioner can.

Coverage for nights off, weekends, and vacations is much better. Rather than being dependent on a voluntary call group that can vary from month to month, coverage is regularly scheduled far into the future so that plans can be made well ahead of time. With this coverage, better continuity of care for patients is provided than in voluntary call groups. However, if the physician joins a multispecialty group, he must be certain there are enough physicians *in his specialty* to provide proper coverage.

Physicians in group practice work fewer hours on the average than solo practitioners, and the hours are more regular. In groups of five or less, lifetime income is only moderately below that of the solo physician. In larger groups it may be substantially lower. A group physician is able to achieve a satisfactory income, even though he works fewer hours, charges comparable fees, and employs a higher ratio of personnel, because he sees about 15 per cent more patients than does his counterpart in solo practice. The greater number of ancillary services (such as laboratory and x-ray) provided in-house by paraprofessional personnel add to the gross. Start-up costs are essentially zero.

Joining a group with a good reputation tends to give a new physician "instant prestige" that might take him years to earn on his own. A subspecialist who might find referrals scarce in some areas will have more at the start from other members of the group. The transition from a training program to group practice is less traumatic than is the transition to solo practice.

One last advantage of group practice is that most business and personnel matters are taken over by managers who are educated and experienced in the field. This also provides some protection in economic downturns and from the increasing competition in areas where there is a surplus of physicians. With groups of three to five physicians this is not always true, but larger groups almost invariably employ a professional manager.

The main disadvantage of group practice is the loss of a measure of independence. Many aspects of patient management, from scheduling up to and including some medical decisions, are taken out of the hands of the individual physician. This may be difficult to live with.

Almost all business decisions are made by the organization, which may cause concern when they affect patient care. The group member may have to abide by rules and regulations of which he partially or totally disapproves. These may not constitute a serious grievance in matters relating only to expansion of facilities or equipment purchase, but when they begin to concern professional standards and methods of practice, they may become intolerable. Specialists may find that they receive few referrals from physicians outside the group. There also may be restrictions on obtaining outside consultations, tests, and procedures.

Some conflict with colleagues is almost unavoidable. Disagreements over apportionment of income are the most frequent. Depending on the degree to which personal and professional lives come together, there may be conflicts between spouses as well. Specialists have a tendency toward overspecialization that may cause difficulties when groups become large. Relationships with patients are more distant and diluted than in solo practice, with the loss of satisfaction that implies. In some groups, patients are rotated among physicians with little or no choice by either party.

These are your four principal options. Although generalizations can never cover particular situations, this chapter does give some concept of what your choice will mean to you.

5

Selecting a Location

Allow a year or so to select a location if you want to do it right. Throughout the process, try to look ahead from the conditions as they are now to five, ten, and fifteen years in the future. Changes will occur in the community, yourself, your spouse, your children, friends, and colleagues, and in all the professional aspects of the area under consideration. After all, you will be there for at least this length of time, if not for your entire career.

The first step involves a little research to gather information. It is no longer as simple as hanging out a shingle wherever you want to. Data on population, population trends, and physician numbers can be obtained from the **Bureau of the Census**, Department of Commerce, Federal Center, Suitland, MD 20233. Information on health care services and facilities is available from The **Department of Health and Human Services**, Public Affairs Officer, 200 Independence Avenue SW, Washington, DC 20201. A useful guide, **The Occupational Handbook**, which contains a section on employment opportunities for physicians, can be obtained from any regional office of the **Department of Labor.** Also write the chambers of commerce and relevant departments in local governments for the areas that interest you. Subscribe to the local newspapers. Call or write real estate agents.

There is a surprising amount of information in your medical library. Find the latest issue of **Physician Characteristics and Distribution in the United States,** published annually by the American Medical Association. This has detailed statistics on the distribution of physicians in the United States by specialty board status, sex, age, medical school and year of graduation, and it notes trends over recent years. The AMA ceased publishing **Profiles of Medical Practice** in 1980, but that last edition may still have a lot of applicable information. Consult the latest **Directory of Medical Specialists** and the four-volume **American Medical Directory.** The latter has biographical information on all United States physicians, whether members of the AMA or not, and Volumes II through IV are geographically indexed. Look at the American Hospital Association's **Guide to the Health Care Field** of the current year. Read the ads in *JAMA,* the *New England Journal of Medicine,* and your specialty journals. Other general journals and even certain "throw-aways" should be reviewed for pertinent ads. Jot down possible leads and contact them. Don't overlook the large professional placement agencies. The listings they have on file will contain a lot of information you can use.

Look through the state medical journals and write the state medical associations of your preferred areas. Many have free placement services with information packets in which positions are offered. Request the addresses of local medical societies and contact them. Your own specialty society may have helpful information, and some have placement services. Write the **Physicians' Placement Service,** American Medical Association, P.O. Box 10012, Chicago, IL 60610 and register. This service maintains complete, up-to-date information on 3000 counties in the United States. The fee is low, and for it you will be listed in the quarterly physician placement registers. Your resume will also be sent to those who request it, and you will receive these four registers, which contain a wealth of information.

As you do your research, remember that ads do not usually lead to the best opportunities. These are most often found through personal contacts. What you are doing is gathering information that will enable you to make these contacts. I do not advise placing ads, either. They are expensive, the information you can include is limited, and there is often a three- to six-month delay before they appear.

Once you have compiled your information, sift through the possible locations using a set of personal criteria first. No matter how well your practice does, if you and your family are not happy in the community, sooner or later you will want to move to one where you will be. I have assembled a list of criteria for judging how an area will suit you and your family:

- The similarity of the areas to ones in which you and your spouse grew up or have lived contentedly for several years
- Weather: especially extremes and their duration
- Social environment: clubs and other organized activities
- Recreational facilities
- Cultural amenities
- Pace of life

- Schools for your children: quality and location; busing
- Churches and religious organizations appropriate for you
- Living costs, including food, taxes, utilities
- Employment opportunities for your spouse, if desired
- Opportunities for making friends
- Shopping facilities
- Economic base: its stability and diversity
- The levels of air, ground, and water pollution
- Housing: its availability, cost, and suitability
- Crime rate
- Community services
- Community trends: deterioration as opposed to new business and housing starts
- Ethnic and cultural compatibility
- Community attitudes toward outsiders

Delete items on this list that do not apply. Add others that are of special relevance to you. Define some more clearly as they apply to you and your spouse. Then arrange them in order of your own priorities. Draw a dotted line after the top ten or so and apply these criteria to the areas you have under consideration. The areas that still interest you will next be evaluated using a list of professional criteria. With the list that follows, once again add or delete, refine more carefully, and arrange the items in your order of importance:

- Population, population trends, age profile, and other demographic indices that will affect your practice
- Socioeconomic factors such as economic base, employment, average income, and health insurance
- The number of physicians, their ratio to the population, and their average fees
- The number in your specialty, their ratio, and average income. Coverage availability.
- Community attitudes toward health matters, physicians in general, and your specialty in particular
- The number of physicians who would potentially refer patients to you, and of those you could use for consultation. The relationships between generalists and specialists in the community
- Hospitals of good quality and location, with staff membership and privileges available; check occupancy rates
- Availability of assistants and suitable office locations; cost of both
- Good laboratory and radiological facilities
- Well-stocked pharmacies and competent pharmacists
- Opportunities for continuing medical education
- Opportunities for teaching and community service
- Allied health services such as physiotherapy and visiting nurses

- Availability of qualified advisors such as accountants and attorneys
- Lending institutions suitable for your needs
- Opportunities for supplemental income, if desired
- Numbers of ambulatory care centers and of limited license practitioners

Again in order of your priorities, draw a line after the top dozen or so—you can't get them all. After screening your potential areas with this second list of criteria, you should now be down to only three or four areas. If some are still too close to call, assign numerical values to your criteria and score each area.

As a last check before you arrange to visit these areas, look over the following table of the best population-physician ratios for most specialties to be sure your areas will support you:

Specialty	Recommended Population Per Physician
Allergy	25,000
Anesthesiology	15,000
Cardiology	30,000
Dermatology	35,000
Gastroenterology	45,000
General and Family Practice	2000
General Surgery	10,000
Internal Medicine (General)	5000
Neurology	70,000
Neurosurgery	110,000
Obstetrics and Gynecology	15,000
Ophthalmology	20,000
Orthopedic Surgery	25,000
Otolaryngology	30,000
Pediatrics	15,000
Plastic Surgery	50,000
Psychiatry	10,000
Pulmonology	100,000
Urology	25,000

I would like to make a few personal comments at this point. I suggested as one criterion that you look for an area similar to one in which you or your spouse was raised. My reason is that many people experience a deep-seated psychological urge, especially as they approach their thirties and forties, to return to a childhood home, or to a place like it. Another reason is that one or two visits to a community are never enough to learn about all the facets of life there.

Cultural considerations are often given great weight when arriving at a decision on location. Cultivated friends are important, but cultural facilities are much less so. Most physicians and their families spend little leisure time at the opera, concerts, or plays. More time is spent in simpler pursuits, such as reading, hobbies, conversations with friends, and family activities. These activities can be supplemented by National Public Radio, PBS, cable TV with premium channels, a video recorder and rented tapes, records, and correspondence or extension courses at universities. More sophisticated cultural opportunities are often available in a nearby big city and can be enjoyed on a weekend away, which is a wise break for a physician and family to take from time to time.

Keeping up with new developments in your specialty and in the profession is not as easy. Reading journals, using video tapes, listening to and watching the newer FM and TV programs for physicians, and attending the occasional medical meeting never seem to be sufficient. You will need daily stimulation from colleagues in the hospitals where you practice, plus meetings and activities there, with the local chapter of your specialty society, and at a nearby medical school. Try to locate in an area where these opportunities for continuing medical education are available.

One last comment. Most of us entered medicine because of our ideals. When we finish our education and training, we often want to practice where the need is the greatest. This is a praiseworthy aim, but you should be aware that you do not have to spend your life in such an area. Contact your church or such organizations as the **Peace Corps,** Washington, DC 20526 or **Project Concern International,** P.O. Box 85323, San Diego, CA 92138. The latter is not well known, but has programs with native Americans, with migrant farm workers, in the neediest areas of Appalachia, and in developing areas all around the world. Two or three years of such service early in a career, when children are small and the spouse is also eager and more adaptable, will satisfy this need for a time. Later, it is possible to volunteer for a month or two at a time, or longer sabbaticals can be taken. And many of us can look back on years of serving the neediest of the inner cities as students and house officers in major medical institutions. The point I wish to make is that your ideals do not have to determine where to live and establish your practice.

Now let's outline the procedures for your first visits to the areas that interest you. If you plan to join a group, go on to the next chapter. What follows here are guidelines for those looking for an association with another physician and for those entering solo private practice.

You have now narrowed your choices to three or four, but don't discard your information on the other areas just yet. A visit to one of your top choices may be so disappointing that you have to think again about places you hadn't seriously considered. Before you make the trip, write to the following in each area: the local medical society, the health department, two or three physicians in your specialty, and the major hospitals. Set up appointments in advance with those who would be likely to have busy schedules. The hospital administrator can schedule appointments with the chief of staff and the chairman of your hospital division. When you arrive you will also want to contact a local real estate agent, a high school principal (who is the best source of information about the elementary schools), City Hall, the chamber of commerce, and other physicians.

One day in each area is enough if your time is well organized. Take your spouse with you if you possibly can. The most frequent reason for relocation is the spouse's dissatisfaction. While you concentrate on professional matters, she can be forming an opinion of the community by touring the area with a real estate agent, investigating the cultural and recreational opportunities, visiting religious organizations and schools, checking out the shopping, and learning the tax rates. One of you should be responsible for obtaining a map and a telephone directory to take back with you. I'll tell you why in a moment.

At City Hall, inquire about taxes and municipal services. At the Planning Commission, ask about future plans of the community. The Health Department can provide objective information of all sorts on the medical community. The local Health Systems Agency has similar information, and the executive secretary of the medical society will have more. Each hospital administrator will tell you about the hospital itself, its personnel, equipment, and facilities. Ask him about nearby office space and hospital staff membership. Request a copy of the medical staff bylaws and rules and regulations. The hospital administrators often know about the politics among physicians in the area and about practice opportunities. They are good sources for information that is usually not volunteered by local physicians. The chief of staff and the chairman of your division can tell you how the rules and regulations, and bylaws are enforced. You should ask specifically about staff membership and privileges in your specialty.

Get the names of the last two or three physicians in your specialty who have set up practice in the area. Give them a call and see if you can drop by and talk to them. You can learn from them some of the problems you will encounter and how they would handle them, given another chance. Ask about physicians who have left the area and call them. Talk to two or three physicians *outside* your specialty, especially those from whom you would expect referrals. Don't overlook pharmacists and detail men in the area—they know a lot more than you think they might.

Take notes as best you can. After you return home, review your information and have some long talks with your spouse. Then get out the map and yellow pages directory for each area. Using different colored felt pens for each, locate hospitals, possible office and house locations, physicians in your specialty, and referring physicians. Study the map and talk with your spouse again. Then decide on your first choice and write letters of appreciation to all those who have helped you in each area.

The second trip is only to the area of your first choice. Spend a couple of days looking around more carefully and getting answers to all remaining questions.

Concentrate first on selecting the principal hospital you will use. Some particulars to inquire about are:

- Current approval by the Joint Commission on Accreditation of Hospitals
- Staff organization
- The range and qualifications of specialists on staff
- Acute care facilities
- The laboratory tests available with 24-hour coverage
- Emergency room coverage
- The range of social services
- The quality of the library
- Continuing medical education programs
- Percentage occupancy and its trend
- Medical records library
- The qualifications of respiratory therapists and dietitians
- Autopsy rate
- Records of the Tissue Committee
- The presence of a full-time pathologist, pharmacist, and radiologist

Next, if you are setting up a solo practice, select your office building. Real estate agents are fond of saying that there are three things that determine property value: location, location, and location. This holds true for your office site. You will be visiting your principal hospital at least once a day—sometimes more often when a patient is critically ill or when you have a new admission. You will have various staff and medical meetings to attend, many of which are conducted at lunch time; you will also want to meet with other physicians for strengthening your ties in the medical community and for professional stimulation. Being close to the hospital makes you more available for prompt consultation and to attend patients referred to you in the emergency room. Since these visits to the hospital will usually be from your office, the principal consideration in selecting an office is its proximity to the hospital or hospitals in which you intend to have most of your hospital-based practice. The other two criteria most often considered by new physicians, closeness to home and to the patient drawing area, are considerably less important. When I say "proximity to the hospital," I do not mean actual distance so much as travel time. In other words, think in terms of minutes, not miles.

After determining your preferred locations, you have to think about the type of building in which you should have your office. Avoid a building with general businesses, even other professionals such as attorneys or accountants. The occupants should all be physicians, or at least professionals who provide traditional, ethical health care. If you locate in a building with reducing salons, chiropractors, holistic health practitioners, and "natural" food outlets, you will be associated with them by the public. There are other reasons for selecting a building with peers as occupants: professional stimulation, referrals, and informal consultations. If an emergency should occur in your office, there will be qualified physicians available to help. And the reputations of the physicians in the building will have a definite effect upon yours, especially in the first year or so.

Many hospitals own nearby medical buildings and offer favorable leases to physicians looking for office space. Their hope, of course, is that the physician-tenants will admit most of their patients to that hospital. Ask about these arrangements. Some hospitals even help finance new physicians to increase their own referral base.

Other features to consider in an office building are the proximity of support facilities such as x-ray, medical laboratories, and pharmacies. Also look for available public transportation, adequate parking, a low crime rate, the safety of access routes, elevators and wheelchair ramps for the elderly and ill, good landscaping and a pleasing facade, quality construction, adequate maintenance, an attractive entrance and lobby, and wide, well-lit corridors. But above all is *location*. It is even worth paying a higher rent than you had anticipated to get a good location.

A great deal more will be said about individual offices in Chapters 10 and 11. But while you are touring the buildings you like, keep in mind that the best shape for a physician's office is square or rectangular, not irregular. The approximate office space required for common specialties are

- Psychiatry–600 square feet
- General and specialist surgery–800 square feet
- Allergy, dermatology, OB/GYN, ophthalmology, urology–1000 square feet
- Primary care–1200 square feet

One last suggestion. If you think you have found the perfect office building, find one more. This way, when you negotiate with the landlord, you will be able to do so with confidence, knowing you have an alternative.

6

Joining a Group

In the preceding chapter, I indicated that the information-gathering phase of selecting a location was similar for all types of practice. From the first visit on, however, the process varies with the type of practice sought. Although the suggestions given for the first and second visits were mainly intended for the physician who will set up a solo practice, with some modification they are also applicable to the search for a salaried position or for an association with another physician. The same is true for the advice in the chapters that follow. This chapter, however, is addressed to those seeking a position with a group.

Information-gathering differs from that I described in Chapter 5 in only two ways. First, ignore the reference works listing physicians in the United States and refer instead to the AMA publication **Medical Groups in the United States.** This will give you the names and addresses of all groups in the areas that interest you. Second, write the **American Group Practice Association,** 1422 Duke Street, Alexandria, VA 22314. Ask for their directory and for information about their placement service. The journals mentioned in Chapter 5 also carry advertisements of group openings, and the major placement agencies do handle group opportunities.

Again, I caution against relying on ads. Some groups hire new physicians at low salaries with promises of lucrative partnership or stock ownership later. But then barriers are raised, and the physicians usually choose to go elsewhere. These groups keep filling their positions through advertisements or by using placement agencies. Some groups have high turnover rates for other reasons, while others are simply unable to fill a position through more traditional means and must resort to advertisements. As a general rule, the best opportunities are those you uncover on your own or learn about through personal contacts. Although you may discover an exception, the rule is that ads should be regarded as no more than an opportunity to make personal contacts in an area. Incidentally, if you are in your last year of training, talk to your Chief of Service. The most common source of personal leads is a phone call from one of the senior members of a group to the Chief, asking about likely candidates in his program.

While you are gathering information in preparation for your first visit, keep in mind that the ideal situation is a single specialty group with three to five members. A few of the reasons are: it is easier to evaluate all the members of such a small group, homogeneous training and interests promote compatibility, the size is small enough to be flexible, and, on average, the income is higher than it is in larger groups.

When you have obtained all the information you can, have sorted it all out, and have decided which groups you wish to investigate, it is time to set up the first visit. I would advise you to make up a list of questions you want answered, arranged in order of importance. Prepare a photocopy to use with each group. Be sure to take notes as opportunity permits. Some groups will try to avoid answering certain questions; the representatives of others may be ill-informed and rely on glad-handing to recruit new members; still others may not answer because they don't want to be bothered with details. Through it all, since you will be visiting one group after another until they begin to blur together, making notes on a prepared list of questions is the only way you can begin to cope. If you are consistent in following this approach, certain unanswered questions may stand out. They will sometimes tell you more than the ones that are answered.

Below is a fairly comprehensive list of questions. Add your own, delete those that are of no interest to you, arrange the rest in an order that suits you, then divide them up by assigning them to either the first or second visit. The wording of the questions in the list is for your reference only. You will have to be more tactful when you ask them.

1. What is the history of the group?
2. What is its philosophy?
3. How many physicians belong?
4. What specialties are represented?
5. How many physicians are there in my specialty, and how is coverage arranged among them?
6. What are future plans regarding additional physicians?
7. What are other future plans of the group?
8. What is its legal structure?
9. How is it governed and how will I participate in the process?
10. How frequently are general meetings held, and what other meetings am I required to attend?

11. Are there any power blocs or divisive politics? Are there any impairment problems among staff members? Are there any pending malpractice suits?
12. May I tour the facilities?
13. May I look at the equipment available for use in my specialty? How are new items acquired?
14. May I see the fee schedule? How is it determined?
15. What are your relationships with local physicians?
16. Are patients referred to this group from outside physicians? If so, are they returned?
17. What diagnostic and therapeutic facilities are available within the group?
18. Whom do you use for consultations or diagnostic procedures not available within the group?
19. Are there any restrictions on obtaining consultations and special procedures either within or outside of the group? How are they obtained?
20. What is the physician turnover? What are the reasons?
21. Could I have the names and telephone numbers of the last three physicians to leave the group?
22. How is day-to-day management accomplished? How are ancillary personnel hired and fired? What is the turnover? What is their level of compensation? May I see the personnel manual?
23. May I have a copy of the group policy manual or bylaws?
24. Are there any present problems in management? What recent conflicts have occurred? How were they solved?
25. What conferences or journal clubs are conducted in the group? What are the library facilities? Journal subscriptions? Computer linkage for obtaining references?
26. Are outside continuing medical education, teaching, hospital staff, and medical society activities encouraged?
27. What is the financial condition of the group? Gross income? Overhead? Outstanding debt? What does the average partner or shareholder earn?
28. How is my patient load determined? How are new patients, emergencies, and walk-ins assigned? What will my hours be? How are hospitalized patients cared for nights, weekends, and holidays?
29. Are scheduled patients rotated among physicians or will I have my own? Can undesirable patients be "dumped" on the new member?
30. What other duties will I have?
31. Will I be supervised by senior members of the group? If so, how?

32. What is the starting salary? Is this guaranteed?
33. How are productivity bonuses and other increments, such as cost-of-living adjustments, added to it? Is outside employment allowed?
34. How long before I can become a full member? What total investment is required? What are the payment terms?
35. What other requirements are there? Is board certification one of them?
36. Will I be required to purchase a share of accounts receivable? Good-will? Tangible assets? Building? Land?
37. If I leave the group, how will I be compensated for these investments?
38. How will my stock or equity value be determined both at the time of investment and if I were to leave the group at a later date?
39. What is the group's policy on providing benefits while on salary, and subsequently as a partner or shareholder? Vacations and sick leave? Life, health, disability, and malpractice insurance? Pension plan? Reimbursement for professional travel expenses, society dues, and professional journals?
40. What are the specific conditions for termination, both voluntary and involuntary?
41. Is there a restrictive covenant in the agreement? What are its specifics?
42. Is there a provision for distribution to my estate of my stock or equity in the event of my death?
43. What is the formula for income apportionment among members?
44. How are such factors as seniority and status defined in the formula?
45. How is productivity defined?
46. What are the rules on voluntary and mandatory retirement?

Notice that financial concerns are listed last. They are better left for the second visit unless brought up earlier by a group representative. They won't make their best offer until they are certain they want you.

When you are ready to make your trip, set up appointments ahead of time with those who are likely to be the most difficult to see. Schedule them so that the intervening time can be filled with other activities and appointments. Take a list of potential contacts so you can call another if one isn't available.

Plan to visit all groups in each of your selected areas on the same trip, allowing half a day for each. If possible, your spouse should accompany you. Meet the administrator or chief executive officer (CEO) of each group. He is usually the best one to ask about the history of the group and its future plans. Obtain a copy of the bylaws or policy manual from him. Then take the tour. During the tour, try to get a feeling for the working harmony of the physicians and employees. Don't be rushed—stop a few minutes to talk to several. You can pick up a lot if you are aware and alert. Examine a few office charts at random. Get a feeling for the philosophy of patient care.

If it is a small group, ask to meet all the physician members, not just one or two of the leaders. Sometimes the "black sheep" is intentionally hidden away, and this one contact may prove to be the most enlightening. Be alert for clues suggesting personality conflicts among physicians. These cause more trouble in groups than all other problems put together. If you can, meet two or three members of the group informally, preferably over lunch or dinner. During the entire process, ask the same questions of different physician members and later compare answers. Request a curriculum vitae from all physicians and reciprocate by offering yours.

Visit the hospital used by the group. Talk to the administrator and chief of staff. Find out how well the group functions and how it is regarded in that hospital. Examine a few representative charts, not ones selected for you. While you are there, obtain routine information about staff membership and privileges, and ask for application forms.

Before you leave each area, talk to a couple of physicians not in the group. Ask them their opinion of the group's methods and its reputation in the community.

Upon returning home, organize your notes and evaluate your information as soon as possible. Talk everything over with your spouse. You should be able to narrow down your selections at this time to no more than one or two areas and perhaps as few as one or two groups in each. Then, before your first impressions have faded, schedule second visits with the top two or three groups, in order of your preference. This time be prepared to make a decision on the spot. Take your spouse again if you can.

On this second visit, go with a specifically prepared list of new or still unanswered questions for each group, based upon what you learned previously. Try to get answers to all your questions. When you ask those that were unanswered on the first visit, listen to the silences as well as the answers.

This is the time to discuss financial matters. If possible, wait for them to bring up the subject. If they do not, broach it yourself. It must be brought up one way or the other, and all aspects must be clarified.

There are five basic methods of income distribution among members of groups. Usually, two or more of these are combined. Although you may become a partner or shareholder in one year, it will take a few more years before your income becomes equal to the others with any of these methods.

1. **A straight split or equal share in the net.** This is easy to administer, but it lowers incentive and invariably causes conflict, so it is almost always used *with* a productivity, percentage, or point system.
2. **Pure productivity.** This is unfair to hard-working but low income-producing physicians who are vital to the group, tends to reward those who perform procedures, and may lower quality of patient care by its emphasis on the dollar. However, when combined with a base salary or a split, this method does add incentive.
3. **A percentage formula.** This is usually worked out on the basis of data accumulated over the past year or longer. It is easy to administer, but the percentage used is always out of date, and if inequitable may be difficult to change.
4. **A point system.** A fixed number of points is assigned to each of several factors. In this system, since the factors themselves change during the year, there is a greater degree of flexibility than there is under a percentage formula. Some of the factors are shares held, seniority, board certification, professional status, workload, new patients seen, charges put on the books, referrals, and perhaps even teaching activity or papers published. Some factors may cause conflict because they are difficult to quantify or have little or no relation to income generation.
5. **Straight salary.** This is mostly used to compensate a new physician for the first year or two, but it may be used for members if combined with one or more of the above systems.

Usually, a formula incorporating a partial straight split with a partial basis in productivity works out the best. Know which factors are included in the formula, how they are defined, and how the calculation is made. Overhead is one example. Preferably, fixed overhead is divided equally, and variable overhead is apportioned by productivity. Once you understand the method used by the group, put yourself into it to see how you will alter it.

One word of advice on the initial salary. Many fine groups offer only a modest salary the first year. Evaluate it over the long term: your lifetime income will be in the millions. Don't let a few thousand dollars less the first year keep you from accepting a good position.

In addition to learning about benefits and income, on your second visit you will want to find out more about the organizational structure and decision-making process. Determine how much input you will be allowed. Ask to see minutes of both executive committee and general meetings. If any group will not show you these minutes when you are this close to joining, write that group off then and there.

On this visit, spend some of your time with those in your specialty with whom you will be working, those you will refer patients to, and those from whom you expect referrals. Schedule meetings with key members of management to get a sense of what your relationship with them will be. If your spouse can come on this trip, try to arrange meetings with the spouses of those physicians who will be closely associated with you in order to judge both personal and professional compatibility.

Determine how the patient policies are actually implemented. Will you be able to refuse certain patients? Who is responsible for treating emergencies during scheduled clinic hours? Must you accept any and all walk-ins, or are they screened? Do senior members skim most of the consultations? Will you be required to take patients who are rejected by other physicians? Ask about coverage of hospitalized patients and emergency room rotation at the hospital, two concerns that are frequently omitted in presentations.

Spend some time in the area where you will be working. If you can, practice there for a few hours. Examine and test the equipment you will be using. Talk to the personnel there at some length and observe how patients are cared for. Ask them about employee turnover.

Go back to the hospital and evaluate it more carefully this time. Talk to nurses, laboratory personnel, pharmacists, and other allied health professionals. You may pick up valuable clues at this level.

Explore some of the more sensitive areas, such as recent or pending lawsuits against the group and personnel problems. You may wish to schedule appointments with the group's accountant and attorney and get a recent financial statement.

If there are no more clues to run down, no more questions to ask, if you feel you will be satisfied with this group, and if you and your family will be happy in the community, say "yes."

A formal contract covering the first year is not absolutely necessary. It is considered to be a trial period by both sides. But a clear written agreement is essential. Sit down with the authorized representative of the group and work out all the details of the agreement. The more clearly details are understood by both parties, the fewer the conflicts later. The term of the agreement must be stated, with precise dates. Compensation during this time should be spelled out, including anticipated raises and bonuses. The same with details on all benefits, such as malpractice insurance, vacations, sick leave, and medical meetings. The retirement plan information should indicate the contributions that both you and the group make, the vesting schedule, portability provisions, tax implications, and projected income at one or more ages. A paragraph of intent must be included, setting forth details for buying in as a shareholder or partner, when this can be done, exactly what you will purchase with your investment, what the pay-out system will be, over what time, and whether or not interest will be charged on any unpaid balance.

One area often overlooked has to do with the terms for leaving the group either voluntarily or involuntarily: the appeal mechanism; the status of your vesting in the retirement plan to that date; the disposition of bonuses not yet paid, of vacation and sick leave accrued, and of continuing medical education time not used; details on the restrictive covenant; the convertibility of group benefits to private benefits; and your entitlement to a share of the accounts receivable for the termination year and to compensation for your contributions to equipment and inventory purchased.

The restrictive covenant is a clause restricting you from practicing, either solo or with another group, within a certain geographical area for a specified period of time after leaving the group. While it is true that these covenants are seldom enforced by the courts in most states and are unenforceable in a few, in general, if the terms are reasonable you should assume it is binding and act accordingly. In those states in which restrictive covenants are not enforceable, a liquidation of damages clause compensates the employer and accomplishes the same purpose. Expend your efforts early on to make the covenant a reasonable one, then abide by it. "Reasonable tests" are applied by the courts in most states. There are three such tests: (1) The covenant must protect legitimate interests of the employer, and these must be expressly stated. (2) It must be fair to the employee and imposed at the start of the relationship. (3) It must be reasonable as to time and distance. A period of two or three years for a radius of three to five miles is usually considered acceptable for most areas. The distance may be less in cities and more in rural areas.

Once all of these points have been clarified, include them in the letter of agreement. Have the group prepare the letter on its letterhead and mail it to you. When it is received, check it for accuracy and completeness. Have your attorney review it. Then sign both copies, returning the original and retaining your copy. You are in!

At the end of the first year, you will know a great deal more about the group and its workings. This is the time to use all that you have learned during that time for hard negotiations with the group, with the advice of an attorney. Then have a formal contract prepared and signed.

7

Setting Up Solo

The preceding chapter is the only one in this book devoted exclusively to the interests of those who have chosen to join a group. Although the remaining chapters offer advice for them as well as for physicians going into other types of practice, the emphasis throughout is on solo practice. It is here that the need for information is greatest. Relatively little is said specifically about a salaried position. There are reasons for this. At the end of a training program, physicians usually have held several salaried positions. The training program itself is one, and most have done some "moonlighting" or have held other jobs. Anything more a salaried physician may need to know can be readily gleaned from the advice to solo and group physicians.

On to solo practice. If you have been following the sequential suggestions so far, you have prepared a curriculum vitae, obtained a license, selected the area in which you wish to practice, and determined one or two likely sites for your office. Let's assume it is the fall of your last year of training and you plan to go into practice next July.

First, nail down that office you selected. If it is really what you want, you are better off signing a lease now to take effect next July, even though July is many months away. See Chapter 10 for specific advice on this step. If the office is ideal and alternatives are few, it may be worth offering the landlord some inducement to hold the office for you until then. As I indicated, location near the hospital is the principal criterion. If a second choice is fifteen minutes farther away and you visit the hospital four times a day, that is two extra hours consumed in travel in each day. This represents a fourth of your potential income lost. Considering it this way, it is evident that you can afford to pay something to reserve the office you want.

Next, contact the local medical society—not just for information but to join. Membership offers many advantages to a starting physician.

You can always withdraw later, if you wish. The local society is a valuable source of contacts in the medical community and of information and assistance. You can ask there about local hospitals, personalities and conflicts in the professional community, as well as part-time employment and teaching opportunities. Some societies hold practice management seminars designed especially for new physicians, and some prepare packets of information for physicians just starting out. Others operate employment agencies for medical assistants, and still others have a billing service and collection agency. You may even find that your society has a professional answering service. All societies offer ethical guidelines on matters such as announcements and office signs. The larger ones offer group insurance plans, maintain a library, and conduct continuing medical education programs. Many hospitals require medical society membership before admitting you to their staffs. If you join the state medical society, it will also have information of value. And the AMA's **Department of Practice Management** publishes literature and holds workshops periodically around the country. The documents you assembled in applying for a license (see Chapter 3) are usually those required for medical society membership as well. Allow ample time for processing your application.

Another item to take care of early is your office telephone number and its listing in both the white and yellow pages. The local medical society will provide ethical and practical guidelines for your listings. In most areas, new telephone directories are issued in January, so information for them must be submitted before November 1. In some areas the closing date is as early as August, with directories coming out in November. Most telephone companies will assign a telephone number ahead of time, list it in the directory, and forward all calls to your present home for a monthly charge before the telephone itself is installed. Or your answering service (see the paragraph to follow) can pick up calls to that number. Since your private office number and home telephone number will be unlisted, obviating the problem with directory listing, you can wait until you move into the community to arrange for them.

At this point, about six months remain before opening your office. Your spouse, with your help, is proceeding with such steps as renting or buying a home, looking over churches and schools, setting up a schedule with the movers, and attending to other personal affairs.

The selection of an answering service comes next. Don't ever use an answering machine, for obvious reasons. Once you have an office number, even though the directory is not yet out, calls may start coming in, so you will want to have settled on an answering service by January. Your medical society, the principal hospital at which you will practice, and your colleagues in the community can all make recommendations. The service you select should have a large proportion of physician customers and a good reputation with them. Before you make your final decision, find out what types of radio pagers ("beepers") are compatible with the service. These come in various sizes and with various options: tone only, tone and visual, tone and voice, memory retention, quiet vibration alert, and one- or two-way capability. Some of the newer models that transmit via satellite have a markedly extended range. It is better to buy your beeper than to lease it from the service.

Start assembling your own library of information about opening a solo practice. Contact the **Department of Practice Management of the AMA,** 535 North Dearborn Street, Chicago, IL 60610 and ask for their free **New Doctor's Kit.** This consists of a timetable for opening your practice, a list of resources and courses for you and your assistants, medical-legal forms with instructions for completion, guidelines for forming or joining a medical group, a brochure on preparing a patient information booklet, instructions on preparing a curriculum vitae, a sample patient survey questionnaire, a booklet entitled "The Business Side of Medical Practice," another called "Planning Guide for Physician's Medical Facilities," a sample universal health insurance claim form with a brief instruction pamphlet, and a list of the practice management publications obtainable through the AMA. Add a copy of the Medical Practice Act of the state where you will practice to your library.

Early in the new year, choose your advisors (Chapter 8), start planning your office design and decor (Chapter 11), and select your office furniture and equipment (Chapter 12). If you plan to buy a practice, see Chapter 9. Leasing an office is covered in Chapter 10.

This is also the time to start thinking about financing. Look into all possible sources: your own assets, family assistance, spouse's income, part-time positions you will hold, credit unions, the **National Association of Residents and Interns** if you are still in training, or the **American Professional Practice Association** if you are presently in practice. Both offer low-interest loans and can be contacted at 292 Madison Avenue, New York, NY 10017. Most physicians starting out rely on two major sources of financing: a loan from a commercial bank and the payment plans offered by the manufacturers or suppliers from whom they purchase their major medical equipment and furniture. While you are looking for sources of financing, call the local office of the **Small Business Administration.** They sometimes guarantee loans, and the advantages may be worth the red tape. Call a couple of finance companies also. Their interest rates and charges are higher than commercial banks, but their requirements are less stringent. Contact two or three savings and loan institutions. Their usual business is mortgages, but some make the kind of loan you want. Ask the local medical society for their recommendations on lending institutions in the area.

Open your practice checking account at a large commercial bank near your office and get a personal account at another near your home or the shopping center you will use. You may change banks later, but these two will be the focus of your first efforts to get a loan. Having an account at a bank improves your chances. You should have five items in hand before you go in and introduce yourself to a loan officer:

1. **A curriculum vitae.** This is not absolutely necessary, but the first factor considered by a bank is your character. A curriculum vitae is a businesslike way of giving some information about yourself.
2. **A net worth statement** (See Fig. 7–1). You can prepare your own following this guide. Type **Net Worth Statement** at the top. Date it and give your name and address. Then list your major **assets** in one column: cash, savings, checking and other accounts, any money owed to you, the fair market value of your home and car,

J. Q. JONES, M.D.
1234 Any Street
Middletown, AB 10000

NET WORTH STATEMENT

January 1, 1986

Assets		**Liabilities**	
1. Cash	______	1. Home Mortgage	______
2. Checking Accounts	______	2. Car Loan	______
3. Savings Accounts	______	3. Student Loan	______
4. Other Accounts	______	4. Other Debts	______
5. Money Owed	______		
6. Family Home	______		
7. Family Cars	______		
8. Securities	______		
9. Cash Value, Life Insurance	______		
10. IRA or Other Retirement Plans	______		
11. Family Jewels, Art Objects, Furs, Etc.	______		
12. Furniture and Household Goods	______		
13. Other	______		
TOTAL ASSETS	______	TOTAL LIABILITIES	______
		NET WORTH	______

Figure 7–1.

securities, the cash value of your life insurance, IRA and retirement plans, jewels, art objects, furs, furniture and household goods, and "other." Total these. In a second column, under **liabilities,** list mortgage, car loan, student loan, and any other debts. Total these. Subtract total liabilities from total assets to arrive at your net worth. Make photocopies—each bank will want one, and you should retain some for your personal reference and other uses.

3. Copies of your **income tax returns** for each of the last three years. If you are still a resident or fellow you may not have earned much, but reviewing tax returns is part of the bank's routine.
4. **A detailed description,** with prices, of all the major equipment and furniture you plan to purchase. They may be required as collateral. If you are going to finance them through suppliers, the bank will not be able to use them as collateral, so be prepared to offer a third-party cosigner instead. As good a credit risk as you are, the bank wants a little more than your word.
5. **A cash flow projection.** This is the most difficult item to prepare: ask your accountant to do it for you. Here are brief instructions for the rough draft you will give him. Rule off and number a column for each of the first 12 months of your practice. Use the first three lines across to give: (1) a realistic estimate of the charges you expect to post for each month; (2) the amount you expect to collect each month; (3) the difference between the first two. Allow a realistic lag in collections and use a conservative collection ratio. Don't add other income sources such as your spouse's income or part-time employment. This projection is for your practice only.

   From the fourth row down, list practice expenses for each of the 12 months. Start with capital expenditures in the first month for equipment and for leasehold improvements, such as telephones and a security system, and be sure to include deposits. For each of the 12 months, estimate rent (including deposits), utilities, maintenance, clinical and office supplies, salary and benefits for each assistant you expect to employ, insurance, payroll taxes (these will be quarterly for federal and state withholding, FICA, and unemployment), miscellaneous (such as professional dues and meetings), and interest payments on the loan you hope to get. Then total the net profit for each month, putting parentheses around "negative" profit totals. From these projections you can see when you plan to break even, and what the net result of one year of practice should be.

   Below the net profit totals, make a summary of estimated personal expenses for the 12 months. These include moving costs, rent or mortgage, utilities, car (including loan payments), food, clothing, insurance, income taxes, entertainment, payments on student or other loans, and miscellaneous.

Then subtract personal expenses from net profit for each month and add up the grand total—this is the amount you wish to borrow. To be on the safe side, try to make this a little more than you think you will actually need by overestimating practice and personal expenses and underestimating income.

With these five items ready, it is time to see about the loan. Get out your best suit, have it cleaned and pressed, and call for an appointment. Remember that banks are in this as a business. This is the way they make their money. As you apply for a loan, you are not asking a favor but offering the bank a business opportunity. Physicians are among the best credit risks, but don't be overconfident—the credit market may tighten at any time and can squeeze physicians too.

Before your appointment, become familiar with some of the terms that will be used. A *line of credit* is an approved amount that you can draw as needed, paying interest only on what you borrow. This is the best form for your loan. You have to ask for it—banks rarely offer it. A *demand note* means you receive the entire amount, pay interest on a determined schedule, and repay the entire principal at an agreed-upon date, when repayment is "demanded." This is the most common form for your type of loan. Most of the other terms you need to know relate to interest charges.

Interest can be calculated several ways, so be sure to request quotations in terms of the annual percentage rate, or APR. This must be provided to you under the Truth in Lending Law. Simple interest is that charged on the amount of the loan and paid when the principal is due. Simple interest is hard to find nowadays because banks make more with other methods. One of these is compounding, in which the interest is added to the amount borrowed so that you wind up paying interest *on the interest.* Another is add-on, in which you make equal monthly payments of principal and interest during the term of the loan, paying it off by the end of the term. You are actually paying interest throughout the year on the amount you have already repaid, so this comes out to about twice the simple interest rate. Perhaps the most common is the discount installment loan. Here the interest is deducted right at the start. You receive the stated amount of the loan less the interest, but it is the stated amount that you repay in installments. The bank makes money on the interest you prepaid throughout the year, so the effective cost to you is 1 or 2 per cent greater than add-on! It will help if you not only understand each of these methods of charging interest, but calculate the cost of each, figured for the amount that you want to borrow, before you go into the bank. Use for your estimate of simple interest one or two per cent over the present prime rate.

During your discussion with the bank officer, be ready to elaborate on any details. Be businesslike and confident in manner. Discuss but don't decide—you want to shop around a little more. Take any forms he offers and leave any material he requests. Ask about life insurance charges on the loan and whether you can avoid these by signing over one of your present policies. Inquire about early repayment without penalty. Refuse to accept "points," if at all possible. Request interest-only payments for the first year, then a repayment schedule over two or three years. If variable interest tied to the prime is offered you, insist upon a one and one-half or two-point cap. This first visit is the best time for your toughest negotiations. He knows you will look elsewhere. When you are finished, make no commitments—just stand up, thank him, and leave.

The loan officer will discuss your loan with a loan committee or the Board of Directors. They rely on five "C's" to decide upon a loan. *Character* is appraised by your appearance, dress, grooming, and professional and credit references. Be sure to bring addresses and phone numbers for these with you. Have a list of your credit card numbers, and a TRW or other credit report may also prove useful. *Capacity* to repay is the second criterion, judged by your cash flow projection. *Collateral* or cosigner is the third. *Conditions* refer to those prevailing in the community. Have in hand the homework you did when you selected your location, with such data as the number of physicians in the same specialty in your drawing area. *Capital* is the last "C," which is taken directly from your net worth statement.

Talk to at least one other commercial bank, preferably two or three, and make notes for later comparison. You can borrow from more than one bank, but there is no advantage in doing so, since you must disclose all loans to each. However, it may be advantageous to finance the furniture and equipment through one or more major manufacturers or suppliers. Since manufacturers can manipulate their profit margins, they frequently offer lower interest rates than commercial lenders. Obtain bids and information on payment plans. Demand a guaranteed delivery date and in-transit insurance. Then calculate once again the amount you will need to borrow and call the loan officer of the bank that made the best offer. Go in to see him with all forms completed, negotiate any final items, and sign on the dotted line.

I would advise against leasing any equipment. Leasing no longer offers a significant tax advantage. It is more costly, and you are not building equity. It is done today only if, for some reason, you have to limit your immediate cash outlay. But, even then, it might be preferable to reduce your purchases instead, or to compromise with used furniture and reconditioned equipment.

With your financial arrangements out of the way, other items of business to take care of approximately three or four months before opening your office are:

1. Apply for staff membership and privileges at the hospitals you wish to use. The Membership or Credentials Committee will want to check your documents and interview you, so some delay of your approval should be anticipated. Temporary privileges during this delay are usually granted. Apply to two or three hospitals in case the staff of one hospital is closed. Sometimes the closure is not evident at first glance.

   There are good reasons to concentrate your activities in one hospital if you can: locating your office near this hospital reduces travel time; you will be more likely to develop a good working relationship with the administrator and nursing supervisor and thus have more influence over the quality of patient care; your activity on staff committees will be more in-depth; and you can devote the time necessary to acquire an authoritative staff position.
2. Consult your advisory team (refer to Chapter 8). If you have decided to have a professional management consultant, see him first. The other advisors will then fill in the gaps. Request that your attorney prepare a summary of the various laws and regulations affecting personnel hiring and firing, collection, and other areas of business management in which you might stumble over some obscure statute. Discuss with your accountant the bookkeeping systems for your office and have him outline applicable state and federal tax regulations. Ask your insurance agents for their recommendations and rates on your professional insurance: office overhead, office liability, all-risk and floaters, fidelity bond, umbrella liability, workers' compensation, employee health insurance, disability, and nonowner automobile. These are discussed later in this chapter. Inquire into the group policies offered by your medical society and professional organizations, comparing them with your agents' policies and rates. Research the professional liability coverage available in your area. Review your personal insurance requirements as outlined in Chapter 26. You don't need to make any decisions yet, but this is the time to look into all insurance.
3. Write (or call 202-254-8255) the **Drug Enforcement Agency,** 1405 Eye Street, NW, Washington, DC 20537. Request Form DEA-224, the application for a DEA registration number and narcotics license. Triplicates can be obtained from the agency by checking Block 4 on DEA-224. Also ask for the "Physician's Manual" and put it in your library. It outlines what you should know about

storing, dispensing, administering and prescribing controlled substances. If you have a DEA number now and will practice in the same state, notify them of your new address. If you will practice in another state, a new DEA number is required. Some states have independent systems; the State Board of Medical Examiners will tell you if yours is one of them.

4. Ask your local medical society for the name and address of the Medicare fiscal intermediary that administers Part B in your area. This intermediary will issue your Medicare provider number upon application, provide information on Medicare itself, and inform you of the prevailing fees in the area.
5. Contact the State Department of Health and Human Services (or its equivalent) for information about Medicaid, if you are going to accept Medicaid patients. Obtain guidelines and a provider number.
6. There is usually one Blue Shield and one Blue Cross office in each state. Ask your local medical society for the addresses and obtain appropriate information from each. You will have little to do with Blue Cross because it works directly with hospitals, but you want to learn what you can, since patients often ask questions about it.
7. Most communities require a business license. Contact the county/city clerk to inquire about this. You may want to have your accountant take care of this and the next two items.
8. All employers must have an identification number from the IRS. Call the local IRS office and obtain an application form (SS-4). Once this form is completed and submitted they will issue your employer identification number and provide you with employee withholding tables, instructions, and forms.
9. Most states require a state employer identification number, which may or may not be the same as the IRS number. Inquire at the state employment office to find out.
10. Write to at least three major cataloguers:

Bibbero Systems Inc.
1300 North McDowell Boulevard
Petaluma, CA 94953

Colwell Systems, Inc.
201 Kenyon Road
Champaign, IL 61820

Control-o-Fax Creative Systems Inc.
3070 West Airline Highway
P.O. Box 778
Waterloo, IA 50704

Health Management Systems
1455 Broad Street
Bloomfield, NJ 07033

Histacount Corporation
Walt Whitman Road
Melville, NY 11747

Medical Arts Press
3440 Winnetka Avenue North
Minneapolis, MN 55408

Physicians Record Co.
300 South Ridgeland Avenue
Berwyn, IL 60402

Safeguard Business Systems
470 Maryland Drive
Fort Washington, PA 19034

Request catalogs, samples of their medical records systems, accounts receivable/accounts payable systems, payroll systems, appointment books, and other office forms. Inquire about the preparation and printing of customized forms. Some have useful instruction books for your medical assistants and toll-free numbers for them to call if they have problems. Compare materials and prices, but read the appropriate chapters in this book, especially Chapter 13, before you order.

11. Order outside signs for your office. This is one "perk" your landlord may provide if you ask him. The local medical society can give you professional guidelines, but these are not legally binding—the city sign code is.

When you have taken care of these items of business, you will be within two or three months of your opening date. It is time to make decisions on professional insurance. See Chapter 26 for guidelines on your personal insurance. As suggested there, most personal policies should be placed through professional societies and organizations at group rates. One or two personal policies can be obtained through an independent agent who specializes in life, health, and disability insurance. These policies are high-commission items, and the agents handling them are often more interested in making sales than in providing the quality of service you want for your professional policies. The latter should be obtained through a second agent who specializes in casualty insurance, also in conjunction with your medical and professional societies.

The first step in planning your professional insurance program is to identify the risks involved and the coverage you wish to have on each.

The major item is professional liability. I hesitate to call it "malpractice insurance" in view of the type of suits prevalent now, only a few of which actually involve malpractice. Any liability policy you have covering cars, boats, property you own and your office (except for certain malpractice policies which include office liability) are separate and distinct from your professional liability insurance. These liability policies offer no protection for your professional actions. Look into medical society plans, doctor-owned companies, and insurance trusts created by groups of physicians. "Going bare," or practicing without professional liability insurance, is extremely risky and is not advised. Most hospitals now require proof of adequate coverage for staff membership.

Since the malpractice crisis of the middle 1970s, there has been a change in the type of professional liability offered by most insurers. "Occurrence coverage" is the traditional form. This protects you against any claims arising out of your professional practice in the year covered, no matter when the claim may be made. The shift has been to "claims-made" coverage, which protects you only against the claims that *arise* while the policy is in effect. When you consider that statutes of limitations in various states run from three to six years following the date of discovery (in the case of minors that long after their age of majority), the pitfalls of this latter type of policy are easily seen. On the average, malpractice actions are filed three to seven years after a given incident occurs. Claims-made coverage initially is less expensive, but you must buy an additional endorsement at some time to cover you for the "tail," so the total cost comes out about the same. Be sure that the cost of the "tail" is stated in your policy as equal to the premium for occurrence coverage the year the tail is purchased. Do not rely on verbal assurances of the future cost. The "modified claims-made coverage" works much like a claims-made policy, but has a buy-out provision to cover the tail when you discontinue practice.

The amount of professional liability insurance you should carry depends mostly on your specialty and the area in which you practice. Although a deductible may be offered, the expense of a legal defense against a fraudulent claim, plus the time and stress involved, make it wise not to have a deductible even if one is available. The standard basic coverage is $100,000/$300,000, and at least this much is recommended for all specialties, with an umbrella. Some physicians may feel comfortable only with an umbrella of additional coverage of from $2 to $4 million over the basic policy. Check the provisions of your umbrella carefully—some *do* provide protection against personal liabilities if your personal liability policies reach the lower limits of the umbrella.

Most of the rest of your professional protection is grouped under the term *casualty insurance*. This type of insurance is low-commission compared to life, health, and disability, so you would be wise to use only one agent for all your casualty coverage. This way, the total commissions offer sufficient incentive for the agent to provide good service and fair claims adjustments.

Public liability insurance for your office is the most important part of casualty coverage. This protects you against damages from any accident that may occur on your premises, and should be coordinated with your landlord's policy to protect you against accidents in public areas and parking lots. Although such accidents are infrequent, a physician is a prime target for suits. Coverage should be written to at least $100,000 per incident. An "umbrella" raising it to at least $1 million is recommended and may be obtained for a small increase in cost.

A basic fire and theft policy covering your office contents, extended by a physician and surgeon's equipment floater, is essential. Be sure the policy covers outside signs and awnings, leasehold improvements, and the contents of your bag. Replacement cost coverage is advisable to avoid the large additional outlay often needed to make up the difference between your coverage and the actual costs of replacement. Fire and theft policies are often integrated into an "all-risk" package protecting the office and its contents against most hazards, including coverage for loss of earnings when the office cannot be used. This is even better protection and is recommended if available. Your accounts receivable records must be insured either way. Although you may plan to safeguard your A/R records by keeping them in a fireproof cabinet or by having an aide make copies to take home, it seems that when a fire or other catastrophe occurs, it is just the one time that someone has neglected to take these precautions. This type of insurance does not automatically pay you the balance of your accounts receivable. It does compensate you for the cost of recreating your records and of additional collection efforts. It will also pay the amount you are unable to collect, provided that you can present acceptable evidence. If you will have valuable works of art in your office, you should have a fine arts floater to cover them. One useful precaution is to take photographs of your office and equipment and keep them in a safe deposit box.

Although your automobile may be used primarily for professional purposes, or be owned by your professional corporation, in this book it is considered a personal possession, so your car insurance needs are discussed in the section on personal insurance in Chapter 26. One type of automobile coverage that is not on your own vehicle and is considered professional is nonowner liability. It protects you if an employee has an accident and claims that at the time a service was being performed for you. Sometimes an assistant may volunteer to run an errand for your office and you are totally unaware of it. You are still vulnerable. Ask your agent about this coverage and be sure to have it.

Business interruption or office overhead insurance compensates you only for the actual expenses incurred if your practice is interrupted due to disability or specified catastrophes. It does not provide very good insurance for the premium. Much of your risk is protected by the continuing income from your accounts receivable and by your personal disability policy. Not only is this coverage limited to the expenses incurred, but some companies quibble indefinitely over payment and demand excessive documentation. I do not think it is worthwhile, but you should evaluate your own need for this type of coverage.

A fidelity bond, usually one providing blanket coverage on all employees, is advisable. It not only deters embezzlement, but provides you with assistance in tracking down cases of suspected embezzlement. You should know ahead of time that the insurance company will not reimburse you for your loss unless you are willing to pursue legal action against the embezzling employee.

Workers' compensation coverage is required by every state for your employees. If you are incorporated, you can elect to be covered yourself. You may be insured through a central fund in some states, but in most you can select a private carrier. The cost is determined by the number of employees, their classification, and the size of your payroll.

There is still a lot more to do during the last month or two before opening your office, but the hardest part is now behind you. The next six chapters give you guidance on the most important tasks that remain.

When these are done, hang up your shingle, send out invitations for your office open house, and order the champagne!

8

Choosing Advisors

As I suggested in the preceding chapter, your advisory team should be selected about six months before you open your practice.

The first member to consider for your team is a professional practice management consultant. It seems that almost all books on practice management are written by these consultants, who invariably put forward one of their number as the most essential on the advisory team. Two "throw-away" journals on medical economics and physician's management give the same opinion, as do occasional articles appearing in more prestigious journals. But again, these are written by management consultants. The authors support their case in two ways, by citing horror stories of mismanagement they have encountered and by asserting that physicians who use management consultants have higher net incomes and better organized practices.

Let's look at their two reasons. Although the horror stories are testimonials which we were taught to disregard, they are usually true, albeit overstated. They are like the mismanaged cases we received from the "local medical doctor" when we were house officers. We learned later that these disasters occurred only every year or two at most in his practice, and were not representative. We didn't know about the 40, 50, or 60 patients a day he treated satisfactorily. As for the second contention, those physicians who pay attention to managing their practice are the ones who turn most often to consultants. In most cases their practices were running better than average before they called in a management consultant. A higher income and a smoothly operating practice do not usually result from a one-shot consultation.

There is one circumstance in which a professional management consultant can really help. The disasters that occur almost always happen to those physicians who do not apply simple management principles. You are reading a book that contains all you need to know about managing a medical practice. There is no mystery to it. With about half the brain power you needed to get through medical school you can absorb these principles and put them into effect. But if you have a strong aversion to business affairs, then by all means select a competent management consultant. Do so early on, and stay with him. The physicians who need them the most call upon them too late.

There are two major organizations that can supply names of Certified Professional Business Consultants in your area:

The Society of Professional Business Consultants
221 North LaSalle Street
Chicago, IL 60601
(312) 346-1600

The Society of Medical and Dental Management Consultants
4959 Olson Memorial Highway
Minneapolis, MN 55422
(612) 544-9621

There is also a large firm with franchises in most major cities:

The PM Group
1109 Comerica Building
Battle Creek, MI 49016
(616) 962-2684

Note that I recommend only a Certified Professional Business Consultant. Those who are will have **"CPBC"** after their names. Check into this credential: your consultant must have it. If none of these organizations can provide the name of a CPBC close to you, choose one at a distance rather than a consultant without this credential in your area.

If you do decide to have a management consultant, call him in *before* you have a problem. You will benefit most when you know the least. Their fees may be a bit lower when you are just starting out because they hope for larger fees later on as your practice begins to prosper. Ask for fee quotations up front.

Their backgrounds and the services they offer vary. The best have a formal education in business management and accounting, with years of experience in the business side of medical practice. They can assist you in the very first steps, such as selecting an office, negotiating a lease, and hiring employees. They can advise you on sources and methods of financing, train your staff, guide you in organizational matters, and help in setting your fees and collecting. Some can also do your accounting. Best of all, perhaps, they can help you select your other advisors and coordinate them. Later they may uncover problems you didn't know you had and prevent others from arising. You do have to keep in mind that their ethics are those of the business world, which are quite different from those in medicine; accordingly, you should take some of their advice with a grain of salt.

If you do not choose to have a practice management consultant, the most crucial member of your team is the accountant. Select him carefully, since he will set up procedures that will remain in place for years and be difficult to change. And there is no substitute for the continuity that one good accountant can provide over the years. When you select one, be sure to ask him his fees and hours first, or his bill may come as a shock. You can get all the accounting service you need in about four hours a month. Tax returns are extra.

Don't try to pick him out of the yellow pages. Ask your colleagues who their accountants are, and how satisfied they are with them. Other medical professionals and even your banker may have good suggestions. Above all, the accountant must be experienced in working with medical practices. At least half his clients should be physicians. And it is best if the accounting firm is matched in size to the individual physician, association, or medical group. Avoid the "big eight" accounting firms, even if one of their accountants does work with physicians. They have more expertise than you need, and their fees are substantially higher.

Screen the names you have been given using four criteria. Professional qualifications come first. Accounting is a licensed profession in almost all states. The accountant must be a college graduate in accounting and must pass an examination before he can be a **Certified Public Accountant** and use the designation **"CPA"** after his name. This is an indicator of a certain level of competence and is the simplest one to look for. It is not absolutely necessary that your accountant be a CPA, but if he is not, evaluating his competence is much more difficult.

After his professional credentials, his interest and experience in working with physicians is the most important consideration. The third criterion is his personality: he has to be receptive to your ideas and able to communicate clearly to you and to your aides. As a fourth qualification, he should be skilled in tax matters. Less crucial is his expertise in investments, retirement plans, and estate planning.

Initially you will be utilizing him in setting up the financial systems for your office. He will establish efficient methods for billing and collecting, and for handling staff payroll and benefits. He will also provide a system of suitable accounting procedures with internal controls and quarterly reports—monthly reports are an unnecessary expense. He will also handle all tax matters, both office and personal.

For the long haul, his tax philosophy has to be compatible with yours or a falling out will eventually occur. One caution in this area. Physicians tend to regard their accountants as absolute arbiters in all tax matters. The truth is that they vary widely in their skill in this arena. All tax matters are based on law, and the real expert is a tax attorney. Whenever you have a complicated problem, it is your prerogative to call in a tax attorney for consultation.

An insurance agent is the next most important member of your team. But the selection can be tricky. There is more variation in knowledge and ethics among insurance agents than with any other profession represented on your team. And you can't select just one agent. All agents fall into two categories and you need one in each—those that specialize in life, health, and disability, and those who sell property and casualty insurance. The knowledge and standards of the former are usually lower than those of the latter. Find out first what your medical and professional societies offer. The policies recommended by these organizations are selected and monitored by committees of your peers and are obtainable at group rates. On average, group policies have premiums 25 per cent lower than individual policies.

However, you need to have at least one disability policy that is noncancellable and guaranteed renewable, and these are not available on a group basis. So you have to find one good agent for this and another one for your casualty insurance. Several large companies are "direct-writing." That is, their agents are employed by them and represent them exclusively. In general, the premiums are somewhat lower and the service is satisfactory. The problem is that the savings on premiums may not be worth the bias their agents tend to have toward their companies rather than their clients when it comes to settlements. For this reason, I recommend selecting an independent agent in each of the two fields. Again, ask your colleagues. Find out about the companies each represents by consulting **Best's Insurance Reports,** which provides independent ratings of all insurance companies.

As you narrow your choices down in the life/health/disability field, you will find that you need to evaluate designations of competence put forth by the insurance industry itself, such as "million dollar round table" and similar bits of braggadocio. The use of this phrase often indicates that an agent has been putting most of his efforts into sales. In many cases, he is not giving his clients the best rates and coverages (often obtainable through other companies), and he is not taking the time to ensure that the settlements for his clients are just and equitable. Avoid any agent with this description. Another such designation is **"CLU"** (Chartered Life Underwriter) for agents who specialize in life insurance. In order to derive sufficient income from this one source, an agent has to hard-sell expensive whole life, minimum-deposit, universal, or variable life insurance, rather than the low-cost term that you should have. Avoid these agents as well.

In the property and casualty field, however, there is one designation that does mean something. **"CPCU"** (Chartered Property Casualty Underwriter) after the name of an agent signifies a certain amount of expertise in his field. Contact the **Society of Chartered Property and Casualty Underwriters,** Kahler Hall, Providence Road, Malvern, PA 19355 for names of agents in your area. The one you select must be familiar with the special problems of physicians and their practices. Be sure to check on his performance in handling claims.

One caution: try to have no more than one agent in each field. Resist the temptation to do favors for patients who happen to sell insurance, or to throw a policy to a third and then a fourth agent who offer you what appear to be better deals. There are two very valid reasons for limiting the number of agents you use. First, you need to coordinate your coverage. If an agent has placed several policies for you, he is more amenable to looking over policies you obtained through your medical or professional societies to avoid gaps and overlaps. Second, when it comes to a settlement, an agent who has a lot of income at risk from the other policies he has placed for you is more likely to stand up to any one company on your behalf.

Selecting a competent attorney is even trickier. First, go to a major public library or a law library, and ask to see **Martindale-Hubbel's *Directory of Attorneys.*** Jot down the names of several qualified attorneys in your area. After each name in the Directory you will find such information as pre-law school, law school, specialty, types of clients, and rating by other attorneys. Legal ability is rated *A, B,* or *C.* After five years in practice, an attorney can be rated *B*, after ten, *A*. Only about 10 per cent of attorneys ever attain an A rating. The letters *u, v* and x refer to such characteristics as reliability and morality—*u* is unsatisfactory, *v* is satisfactory and x is unrated.

Call the State Bar Association to ask if any on your list has been disciplined, then check with your colleagues about those left on the list. The best recommendation you can have is from a satisfied client. A business lawyer in a medium-sized firm is the legal profession's closest equivalent to a general practitioner. Try the top one on your list with a simple legal matter, such as reviewing your lease, to see if he communicates clearly and if his personality is compatible with yours. If he comes up short in these areas, consult the next one on your list about another legal problem, such as the purchase of your home. Ask about those to whom he refers for special problems and check *their* rating in the Directory.

The legal field is as specialized as medicine, although not as formalized. It is best if the same general attorney handles both your personal and professional legal matters. Before settling on your final choice, make sure that your spouse is satisfied with him. Your lawyer must be trusted by you both as an advisor and counselor. He will not necessarily be a friend, but he should be a friendly person.

A bank officer is sometimes included as a member of the advisory team though not as often today as he was in the past. Unless you are in a rural area, you should be able to consult a more qualified financial planner. Write the **International Association for Financial Planning,** 5775 Peachtree-Dunwoody Road, Suite 120-C, Atlanta, GA 30342 for the names of *certified* financial planners or *chartered* financial consultants in your area. Be sure they have one of these designations. Then screen the names given you by asking your colleagues and interviewing each one personally.

In my opinion, a stock broker does not belong on your team. I recommend in Chapter 26 that your only venture in stocks and bonds be through no-load mutual funds, a strategy that bypasses brokers altogether. See that chapter for the rare occasions a broker should be called upon for advice. There are many reasons for avoiding stock brokers, not the least of which is the fact that their sins are mostly sins of commission.

9

Purchasing a Practice

Because of the increasing competition now among physicians, especially in desirable areas, more established practices are being put on the market and sold than ever before. Purchasing a practice is an excellent way for a new physician to acquire a furnished office in an advantageous location, with good equipment, trained personnel, and established patients. He can also learn about the business side of private practice from the selling physician. There are advantages for the latter, too, who may want to relocate or retire. But both the buyer and seller must know how to evaluate a practice properly. Even a physician who has no intention of selling should know how to evaluate his practice. He may be making a divorce settlement, getting a loan at the bank, bringing in an associate, doing some estate planning, or may just be curious.

There is no simple formula for determining the value of a practice. In a sale, the tax consequences are especially complicated. The buyer and seller should always consult with their respective accountants, practice management consultants, and attorneys. Some firms specialize in evaluating practices and handling their sale or purchase:

Durham Medical Search, Inc.
268 Main Street, Suite 600
Buffalo, NY 14202

The Health Care Group
Suite 400 GSB Building
One Belmont Avenue
Bala Cynwyd, PA 19004

Health Resources, Ltd.
River Road Professional Building
P.O. Box 14188
Kansas City, MO 64152

Professional Practice Sales, Inc.
540 Frontage Road
Northfield, IL 60093

VR Professional Practice Brokers
P.O. Box 154
Captiva, FL 33924

The following discussion is aimed at enabling the purchasing physician to understand the essential elements in the transaction. It is *not* a do-it-yourself guide, but it is sufficient to help you prepare the necessary information for your advisors.

The elements that must be considered in assessing the value of a practice are these:

1. **Gross Earnings.** This is a more fragile item in a medical practice than in the average business. Here the income potential depends upon the public perception of the individual practitioner, and other intangible factors. One cannot just project prior gross earnings. Keeping this one caveat in mind, determine the gross earnings of the previous year, adjust this figure for any trend evident over the past few years (being sure to deduct income from other sources that may be coming through the office), then multiply it by an estimate of the percentage of patients who will remain after the practice is sold. The result is the first part of the overall value of the medical practice.
2. **Tangible Assets.** No pun intended, but there are some intangibles to consider here. The selling physician sometimes has a strong attachment to his furniture and equipment, or they may not be to your taste. First, therefore, decide what you will want to use. Second, determine the original purchase price, then adjust it for inflation. Calculate the present book value (the original purchase price less depreciation). A point midway between these two is the best estimate of their present value. This sum is the second part of the practice value, and is added to the adjusted one-year gross income.

   Supplies and medications are not usually included in the sale of a practice. The selling physician has no further use for them, and the buyer may not want most of them. However, in those cases in which a substantial inventory is on hand that you *can* use, their value may be estimated in the following way. Most practices maintain about two months' worth of supplies in the office. Take the total purchases for the past year and divide by six. This gives a rough estimate of the value of supplies on hand, which is added to the value of the tangible assets. There is no need for an inventory unless unusual circumstances prevail. Bear in mind that the selling physician will tend to use up the supplies and medications during his last month or two. Just expect this depletion and accept it.

3. **Clinical Records.** These present a problem. The selling physician may want to sell them, and it *is* possible to calculate a value. If patients are properly notified of the transfer, and if the selling physician remains for a reasonable period—say two or three months—to introduce you, perhaps 60 to 70 per cent of the active patients will make at least one more visit to the office. Each extra month of introduction will add 5 to 10 per cent. So an estimate of value can be made. The problem is that it is unethical to assign a value to clinical records and include this value in the sale. It would also alter tax consequences of the sale for one or both parties.

   The more ethical course of action is to ask the selling physician to remain at least two or three months. Have him introduce you, and offer patients the opportunity to transfer their records either to you or to another physician of their choice. This introduction is then one component of goodwill. However, it *is* acceptable to make an adjustment in the price of the practice for the actual cost of transferring the records to other physicians.

   An agreement should be included in the sale document requiring the buyer to preserve the medical records for a specified period and to make them available to the seller in the event of a legal action involving the latter.

4. **The Lease.** The value of the unexpired term of the lease rarely enters into a purchase unless all of the following conditions prevail: more than a year remains; the lease is transferable; the rent is favorable and will continue to be so as other rents in the area change. Under these circumstances, the advantage of the lease can be calculated easily and added to the other assets.

5. **Leasehold Improvements.** These are usually the property of the seller and consist of built-in cabinets and the like. The value to the seller at this point is probably zero; their value to you depends entirely upon the use you can make of them. First, check the seller's lease to see if these improvements become the landlord's property automatically, or if the premises must be restored to their original condition when the term of the lease expires. In the first case, the improvements would have no value to you; in the second they would represent a considerable liability. If neither of these situations pertains, and if the leasehold improvements are substantial, in satisfactory condition, and of use to you, then 50 per cent of their original cost is a fair estimate of their value. This is added to the total assets.

6. **Accounts Receivable.** These represent, in theory at least, an advantage for two reasons. They would provide a cash flow to you

during the first few months, and there is a tendency for patients to return for care to the office where they are already making payments. But one physician's accounts receivable can be difficult for another physician to collect—so difficult, in fact, that in most circumstances they should not be included in the sale. It is better for the selling physician to take the accounts receivable with him and continue his own collection. If he cannot, or if you want them for a good reason, they can be included by using the following formula: (1) adjust the total by calculating and applying the actual collection ratio over the last year. This usually involves taking about 10 per cent off. (2) Estimate your ability to collect them and make a second adjustment. (3) Deduct the expense of the collection process itself, which is usually another 15 per cent. (4) Then remove all accounts older than 90 days, which usually results in a reduction of another 5 per cent or so. (5) Age those that remain and make further adjustments on this basis. The remaining amount, usually about 60 to 70 per cent of the total accounts receivable, is added to the assets.

7. **Goodwill.** Think of this as the purchaser's potential for generating future income from his predecessor's reputation and success. Goodwill is very difficult to assess, but it is a highly significant factor in determining the value of a practice and the issue must be addressed. The doctor-patient relationship is a delicate one, and in certain circumstances a surprisingly low proportion of the patients will continue with a purchasing physician. Some of the factors that affect the value of a practice are community characteristics, including population trends and economic base; the location of the office in relation to the drawing area, to hospitals, and to other medical services; the availability of parking and public transportation; the number of physicians in the community, especially in the same specialty, and their patient loads; other competitors, including ambulatory care centers and allied health personnel; the reputation of the selling physician; the number of new patients seen over the preceding several months; the length of time he remains to introduce you, and his manner in doing so; the quality of the employees and the likelihood of their remaining; the compatibility of the purchaser's and seller's personalities, practice patterns and objectives, and social or religious affiliations if strongly held; the amount of the office overhead; the efficiency of established collection procedures; and whether or not the office telephone number will be retained.

The value of goodwill is something that must be negotiated between the selling and purchasing physician after considering all these factors. It usually averages about 25 per cent of the previous year's gross. Add the amount agreed upon to the other assets.

You may hear the term "going concern value" used by accountants in reference to equipment, furnishings, and other attributes of a practice that function as an effective unit. Ignore this term, since this value is already included in goodwill.

8. **Covenant Not to Compete.** This has no value *per se* but is mentioned as a separate item for two reasons. Failure to include an effective covenant in the agreement of sale can entirely negate the value of the goodwill that was so carefully calculated and negotiated. And the value assigned to the covenant has important tax consequences.
9. **Miscellaneous.** Cash equivalents (such as the practice accounts, petty cash, stamps, and unexpired magazine subscriptions) are included at their actual value. Determine any outstanding liabilities and deduct them. Specify the items that are to be excluded in the sale. The land and building are *not* included—if they are to be purchased, they are handled under a separate agreement.

When all of these values are added up, the grand total is the value of the practice. A pay-out plan is then agreed upon, suitable interest on the unpaid balance is determined, and the negotiations are concluded. The agreement is then typed up and reviewed by the advisors of both parties. You and the seller sign it, and each retains a copy.

There are tax implications for both sides that will need to be considered as the value of the practice is being determined.

The selling physician must determine his basis in furnishings and equipment. This basis is arrived at by deducting the accumulated depreciation from the original purchase price. If the furnishings and equipment are sold for more than this basis, he realizes a gain that is taxed at capital gain rates. At the same time, you as the purchaser can depreciate the items at your purchase price. If the accelerated rates of the Economic Recovery Tax Act of 1981 still prevail, this is a substantial advantage to you. A tension is thus set up between the parties. The seller wants to reduce the amount assigned to this asset, while you will press for some of the value of other items to be shifted to this one. Leasehold improvements come under a similar consideration. Disagreements may also occur in deciding the price paid for supplies and medications, since it is taxable income for the seller, whereas it is a deduction for you.

Goodwill is subject to especially complicated tax considerations. In general, it is considered to be nondepreciable; therefore, the selling physician's basis will be the price he originally paid for it, which, if he began the practice, was zero. The difference between the basis and the selling price of the goodwill is taxed at capital gain rates on the selling physician's return. The purchase of the goodwill is not a deduction for you, and the only tax advantage you can derive is obtained on a subsequent sale.

That portion of the purchase price allocated to the restrictive covenant is considered by the IRS to be compensation for what the selling physician would have earned if the sale had not taken place. He is taxed for it at ordinary rates rather than capital gain rates. However, the covenant is depreciable by you over the covenant period and constitutes another possible point of disagreement.

One more factor complicating tax considerations is the fact that the seller is probably in a higher tax bracket than you are. And the sale itself has tax implications, depending upon whether it is on a cash or installment basis. Each principal in the transaction will seek to obtain the most advantageous tax position possible. The best approach to take on the tax aspects is to agree first on a price for the practice, then settle the tax questions so that the seller receives the same net from the sale. You can see why it is important to have your team of advisors involved and to follow their recommendations.

10

Leases and Landlords

Even if you are among the fortunate few who have the financial resources to buy an office condominium or a medical building, it is still best to lease office space for the first year or so that you practice. No amount of research can uncover every last wrinkle in the local social, economic, and medical environment, but a year of living and practicing in a place usually will.

If you have followed the advice in Chapter 5 on selecting a location, you have found office space in a suitable professional building in the best location available. As that chapter suggests, you ought to find at lease one other satisfactory office as a precaution, in case of problems in negotiating an acceptable lease.

Get the keys to your preferred office from the landlord or his agent, ask for a blueprint, and insist on inspecting the premises without him. Take your practice management consultant or contractor, or both, if possible. Walk again through the grounds and building, look around, and talk to two or three physician-tenants in the building to get an idea of how the landlord operates. It is a good sign if the building is nearly filled. Be sure the public areas are safe, accessible, and attractive. Measure the usable square footage of the office space to make sure you aren't being charged for the width of the walls or outside corridors. Note the dimensions of each space to enable you to plan the location of your furniture and equipment. Look for any evidence of water damage. Check the location of electrical outlets; be sure that they are "hot" and provide the voltage you require. Try the faucets to see if they turn easily and do not leak when turned off. Note any repairs required for the floor or walls. Test the soundproofing in areas where noise will be produced or confidential conversations will be held. Open and close all doors and windows to be sure they operate smoothly. Check to be sure the outside doors are solid in construction and equipped with deadbolts. Check the heating and air conditioning.

Be sure the hot water is truly hot. Turn on all lights to see if the ambient lighting is adequate. Note which walls are weight-bearing or contain plumbing and therefore cannot be altered. Test toilets for excessive noise, leaks, and inadequate flushing. It is advisable to have an inspection by a pest control firm for rodents, roaches, termites, and other pests.

All of these suggestions are made on the assumption that you will be looking at finished office space. Raw office space that you must complete yourself requires a longer lease of five years or more, so it is not a wise choice if you are moving into a new community.

When you are satisfied with your inspection, return the keys to the landlord or his agent. If you express an interest, he may fill in the blanks on a printed lease form and present it to you for signature with the assurance that it is the standard lease form all tenants sign. *There is no such thing as a "standard lease."* All leases are designed by attorneys to protect the landlord, not the tenant. This is the time to remind yourself that landlords are much more experienced in negotiating with tenants than tenants are in negotiating with them. But don't let this deter you. Most leases are negotiated, and "standard" lease forms can be amended before being signed. So you will not be an exception by any means. Do not sign the lease at this time, just take it with you.

Call your attorney to set up an appointment during the next day or two. While your inspection of the office is still fresh in your mind, make a list of the damages you wish to have repaired. If you aren't able to get some items on the list taken care of by the landlord, a list of these preexisting damages should be attached to the lease when you sign it. Retain a copy of this list to avoid problems recovering your security deposit after the lease expires. Prepare sketches and specifications of the leasehold improvements you will have done. Be sure that major items of furniture and equipment will fit or that the space can be modified to suit them. There is no point pursuing negotiations if space limitations will prevent your occupying the office.

Now study the lease itself. The language can only be decribed as dull and the plot as thin. Yet this document can oblige you to put up with undesirable conditions for a long time. It is a fact that 50 per cent of physicians want out of their leases for one reason or another within two years. So you have to study it even though it lacks literary merit.

The easiest way to start is by reading over the entries the landlord has made: the description of the property, your name, the rent that he is asking, the due date of the rent, and so forth. Five to 7 per cent of your anticipated gross is about right for rent; pay no more than 10 per cent for utilities and rent together. Other details that should be checked at this time are the landlord's name, the square footage, grace period, and late charges if the rent is not paid on time. Make sure all of these items are correct and acceptable.

Now to the finer print. Note the duration of the lease, requirements for termination, options to renew, and escalator clauses. Be especially alert for double escalators. Try to obtain a one-year lease with annual options to renew for at least two or three years. Landlords prefer a longer lease, usually three years, with renewal options. Notification of renewal time should be the landlord's responsibility, not yours. Escalator clauses increasing the rent on renewal ought to be based upon indices that are directly applicable to the cost of office space, such as an increase in property taxes, not upon such unrelated factors as your income or the nationwide Consumer Price Index. Note the deposits required and the conditions under which they will be returned to you. Usually there are two deposits: a cleaning deposit that is rarely refunded in full, even if you have the place cleaned on your departure, and a separate damage or security deposit, for which the list of prior damages is your best protection against unfair claims.

Make sure there are escape clauses that allow you to terminate the lease in the event of your death, disability or military service, and that release you from rent if the premises are rendered untenable by disasters such as fire or flood. The landlord should be restricted to renting space in the building only to suitable professionals, and you should have the right to share or sublet the space to such a professional without obtaining the landlord's permission. The landlord usually bears the expense of supplying your street sign and of adding your name to the building directory.

Negotiate for the right to make the leasehold improvements you want without the landlord's prior approval. Assume the responsibility of having them done yourself. Don't let the landlord do them unless you are unable to borrow the money. Otherwise, you may be stuck with low-grade materials, sloppy workmanship, and delays over which you have no control. And your higher rent will form the basis for future increases that will remain in effect long after you have paid for the improvements. Make sure you do not have to return the premises to their original condition at the end of the lease. If you accept this provision, at the expiration of the lease the landlord may make you pay his estimate for this work, which could be substantial. He may then rent the premises just as they are, letting the new tenant make his own alterations under the same terms. Insist that the improvements remain your property on expiration of the lease, so you can either sell them to the new tenant or take them with you.

In studying the lease, notice how ordinary maintenance is accomplished, what is considered "ordinary maintenance," whom you contact for this service, and who bears the expense. Look for clauses stipulating periodic redecoration and replacement of worn carpeting or defective fixtures at the landlord's expense. Be sure you do not bear any obligation for maintenance outside the office. This is the landlord's responsibility, and his acceptance of it should be in the lease. The maintenance of outside lighting, security, parking facilities, grounds, and building exterior should all be specified. Look for wording in the surrender-of-possession provision that allows you to return the premises in the same condition "except for reasonable wear and tear." Make sure there are no unreasonable restrictions on the hours you can practice. The utilities should be listed individually in the lease with the responsibility for the payment of each specified. Those you pay should be metered for your office only. The parking spaces you require must be guaranteed. Don't depend upon an empty lot next door or on street parking.

Then meet with your attorney and discuss the lease with him. His function is to explain any item that may not be clear to you, detect illegal clauses, point out omissions, suggest changes beneficial to you, and counsel you in regard to the negotiations with the landlord. He may wish to represent you in these, but this is not usually helpful. Trained in the adversarial mode and not bearing responsibility for the outcome, an attorney often alienates the landlord without winning you the concessions you are seeking. Review the lease also with your practice management consultant if you have one, and call your accountant to discuss the financial terms.

Now you can return to the landlord with the unsigned lease and the list of changes you wish to make in it. Have in mind a rough order of their importance to you, but leave the rent for last. Only when you have won as many concessions as possible, and the lease has been altered accordingly, is it time to discuss the rent. First try to reduce the monthly amount. If this fails, request the first few months free. Many landlords will offer this sort of inducement if you are the type of tenant he wants and other office space is available in the same building or nearby. If this tactic also fails, try for a lower rent at the start, raised in stepwise increments, to average out to the same total over the life of the lease. Then press for an allowance off the top to cover the leasehold improvements you will make.

When you have the best deal you can obtain, sign it, and you have the office in which you will set up your practice!

11

Office Design and Decoration

There are so many different sizes and styles of medical offices that some assumptions have to be made before we can begin to discuss office layout. One is that you will not be converting a fine old house somewhere in New England into a home-office. Those went out with buggy whips. Another is that you will not be saddled with the responsibility of designing a large multiphysician suite. Groups this size wisely utilize experts to plan such arrangements. However, most of the burden of designing a one- or two-physician office falls squarely on the shoulders of the private practitioner who is solo or taking on an associate. This chapter is intended to help that practitioner. Further assumptions are that your lease allows you to remodel and that you are not located in an older building with fixed walls that would prevent any alteration in the layout. Most modern office buildings provide space as a "shell" within which non–weight-bearing walls may be moved or altered easily. Other assumptions are that the shape is rectangular, and that the total area is approximately that suggested in Chapter 5 for your specialty.

Before you begin to design your ideal suite, gather together all the information you can. Your medical library will have several good books on the subject. Medical Economics publishes **Designing and Building Your Own Professional Office** by Murray Schwartz, D.D.S. An excellent booklet, **"A Planning Guide for Physician's Medical Facilities,"** is obtainable from the AMA. If you prefer to contract with a consulting firm, a good one is Zirkle, Lee and Associates, Inc., 4747 Table Mesa Drive, Suite 200, Boulder, CO 80303. Beyond these sources, the best information comes from other physicians who have faced this problem before you. Visit their offices and ask each what he likes about his, and what he would do differently, given the chance to do it again.

It helps if you approach the project by dividing it into three somewhat overlapping parts. The first, the layout, is up to you, although you will want to use ideas and suggestions from many sources. The second is selecting the furniture and fixtures. You will pick all the professional and business equipment, but the choice of furniture will depend more upon the advice of an interior designer. The third part is the decor, which is almost entirely the responsibility of the interior designer, guided by you and your spouse. The major spaces that concern the designer are the waiting room, the consultation room and the hallways, but he will also have suggestions for the business office and employee lounge.

Select an interior designer before you go any further. There are three categories. The most qualified ones belong to the **American Society of Interior Designers** and use the initials **ASID** after their names. Contact the Society at 730 Fifth Avenue, New York, NY 10019 for names in your area. These individuals are independent contractors who work either by the hour or for a fixed sum negotiated in advance. If you order your furniture, carpet, and drapes through this type of designer, you can take advantage of the considerable discounts they receive. The savings may actually pay for his services. In the second category is a designer who works for a furniture store or supplier and receives his compensation from commissions on what you buy. His advice may be incomplete and slanted toward sales of goods carried by his employer.

In the third category are the amateurs who design mostly for the fun of it. They cannot obtain discounts and lack formal training, although they may have natural flair. You undoubtedly have friends in this category, but because disputes may arise, I'd advise keeping them as friends and not hiring them as designers. As a professional yourself, you will probably be best satisfied working with a professional designer, one who is a member of the ASID Once again, ask your colleagues for their recommendations.

Now to the layout. The best advice I can give you is that old dictum of architects: form follows function. List all the tasks that will be performed in your office. Decide where they will be done and who will be doing them. Project a year or two down the line when you will have your full complement of personnel. Once the tasks have been delineated, prepare a flow chart consisting of blocks representing the tasks, connected by arrows showing their usual sequence. This will be the usual patient traffic flow. From it, an outline of the best layout for your office will emerge. Before you draw your actual design, find out about local zoning ordinances, building codes, OSHA regulations, and state laws regarding the handicapped. Even if your state has no special laws regarding the handicapped, you still may want to make your doors, halls, and restroom accessible to them.

On quarter-inch graph paper, draw the outer walls of the office to scale. Show the fixed elements—doors, windows, toilets, sinks, and weight-bearing walls. Sketch in non–weight-bearing walls lightly with dotted lines. Now determine the dimensions of major items, such as waiting room chairs and other large furniture, examining room tables and cabinets, and business office equipment. Prepare scale cutouts from stiff paper for these items. Then, using a pencil with a good eraser and the scale cutouts, you can let your imagination loose. Draw various arrangements and designate them as Plan 1, Plan 2, and so forth. When you have selected the best two or three plans, set them aside for a few days before you make your final decision. It's surprising how many good ideas occur to you during that time.

Among these thoughts will be some about the purpose of your medical suite and the ways in which the design and decor can reflect this purpose. It is a place for you to provide care and comfort to those who are ill and anxious, so the colors you select should have the desired effect on your patients. Most people find light blue and green soothing and cooling. Yellow is bright and a bit startling. Browns and beiges with touches of orange are warm and welcoming. Red and black are usually avoided for obvious reasons. Textures, rounded edges, comfortable furniture, and attractive art also project your purpose. On the other hand, clutter and crowding arouse anxiety. Surfaces are important. Stainless steel, plastic, shiny finishes, and abstract art increase patient discomfort and anxiety. Rich, plush fabrics, gold or silver finishes, and fine antiques inevitably raise concern about the cost of your care. Your office is a place to express your personality and taste *if* that expression is appropriate and dignified. It is not the place to assert your vanity or that of your decorator without concern for the responses of your patients.

Other design factors that enhance patient comfort are separate thermostats for different rooms so that those clothed and unclothed will be comfortable; soothing ambient light but with good lighting provided where needed for reading; and fresh air without smoke or odors.

Sound is an important factor in patient comfort that is often overlooked. There are four aspects of sound control. Its *production* can be limited and controlled through intelligent selection, placement, and maintenance of necessary noise-producing equipment. Confidential conversations should be conducted quietly in areas where they cannot be overheard. Sound *absorption* is maximized with the use of carpets, drapes, upholstered furniture, and acoustic tile ceiling. Sound *transmission* is reduced by walls with offset studs, solid-core doors with jambs and weather stripping, and baffles in the heating and air conditioning ducts. And, finally, noise can be *masked* by background music.

You will find that if your design puts concern for your patients foremost, you and your staff also benefit. You will work more efficiently with less fatigue and stress, and have more energy and higher spirits at the end of the day.

Think of safety, too, in designing your suite. Avoid hard corners and sharp edges, loose throw rugs, passageway obstructions, slippery floors, unstable furniture, and the like. Install either smoke detectors, heat detectors, rate-of-rise detectors, or combinations thereof. Ask your local fire chief which sensor is best for you and what type of alarm you should have.

Remember, as you are reflecting on your design, that the three areas most likely to become cramped as your practice grows are the business office, hallways, and storage. Allow them adequate space now.

Plan to take some simple security precautions. The outer doors should be solid-core with strong frames and deadbolt locks. The door between the waiting room and the rest of the office should also be strong, with a secure lock for use during lunchtime to protect your staff. Provide a safe place for their purses and other valuables during the day. Security is a concern of patients too. It is a good idea to install a hook in the examining room on which a woman can place her purse or a man his jacket and keep either within sight. If you have coat, boot, or umbrella racks in the reception room, they must be located where your receptionist can keep them under observation. Good locks are necessary on the windows so that a burglar would have to break a window to enter. If window guards are installed, be sure that quick escape is possible in the event of a fire. Plan to use an inexpensive engraving tool to put identifying numbers on typewriters, copiers, and similar equipment. In addition, large equipment can be bolted to countertops. Talk to the local police department and alarm companies about burglar alarms.

Think about materials for the floor, walls, and ceiling. If you plan to use a computer, you may want to install antistatic floor covering. Recommended carpeting materials are nylon and polypropylene, known by brand names such as Antron and Herculon. Small patterns—tweeds are the best—are recommended to camouflage dirt and stains. A level loop is the most durable, yet still pleasing in appearance. In your private office you may want a deeper pile. Areas most commonly carpeted are the waiting room, hallway, and your consultation room. Surprisingly, carpet holds up well in the business office and examining rooms. Common areas should have a commercial-grade carpet glued to the floor without padding. Good padding increases sound absorption and makes the carpet itself feel deeper, so you will probably want to use it in your consultation room. Consider having all carpet treated to resist stains initially and then renewed periodically as required. Areas not carpeted are the restrooms, laboratory, and procedure rooms. The uncarpeted floor areas are covered with either vinyl-asbestos tiles or sheet vinyl. The latter is preferred because it has fewer seams to open and trap dirt. A process called seam-sealing is recommended for closing the cracks between the widths of sheet vinyl. A cove base is also advisable. This is a rounded base cemented to both the wall and the floor that reduces the accumulation of dirt and makes cleaning easier.

Painting walls is less expensive than papering. Although paint becomes marked easily and cannot stand much scrubbing, it is easily touched up. A completely new paint job will be required every year or two. Wallpaper is more attractive but is easily torn and cannot take cleaning. It should be used only in your consultation room, or perhaps in your reception area if you are prepared to replace it every two or three years. Vinyl wall covering is the most practical choice because its tough surface can be washed repeatedly, and it comes in attractive textures and colors. It may last ten or twelve years with proper care, which more than offsets its higher price. If you can afford it, I would recommend this for all your walls.

A dropped ceiling with acoustic panels works best in most circumstances. The ceiling should be attractive. You won't notice it, but your patients on the examining table will.

While you are considering all these options, you will be making minor adjustments to your plans and appending notes. The final alterations can be made and the best layout determined if you then walk through the rooms in your imagination, considering each area and its function as your patients will experience them. Let's do this together.

The first area encountered is the waiting room, more euphemistically referred to as the reception room. It will open off the entry, and the entire area should be under the observation of your receptionist at all times. The best shape is rectangular, usually about 12 × 15 feet in size for one practitioner. It will be smaller for certain specialties and larger for busy primary-care physicians. The size required is also affected by the shape and the number of doors and windows. The reception area size can also be calculated by allowing 15 to 20 square feet per person waiting. This number, and the number of seats to be provided, is twice the peak number of patients you expect to see in one hour, including emergencies and "work-ins." This space has to be increased in ethnic areas where family members tend to accompany patients, and doubled for pediatric and geriatric practices for the same reason. Incidentally, this is the same number to use in figuring the parking spaces required for your patients, provided you and your employees park elsewhere.

Individual seating is preferred. Patients tend to sit at either end of couches, leaving the center unoccupied, so this space would be wasted. The chairs should have firm seats, about 16 inches from the floor. Arms are advisable so that ill, elderly, or pregnant patients can rise from them easily. Theoretically, not *all* need to be firm and have arms, but it seems that all too often handicapped patients tend to choose the most comfortable chairs without thinking how they are going to get out of them until the time comes to do so. Most of the chairs should be back to back in the center, not facing each other unless it is unavoidable. Patients would rather look at plants or art objects than each other. The best covering for chairs is a sturdy fabric. Avoid plastic in this area if you can.

Once you have determined the number, size, and location of the chairs, the other furnishings for the waiting room are easily arranged. Subdued overhead or indirect fixtures provide adequate ambient light, but some floor or table lamps should also be provided for reading. You may wish to add your own special touch with potted plants, an aquarium, or a table offering coffee or tea. In some areas, plants can be rented, and in most a service will take care of aquariums. Even if you do not treat children, an alcove for them with toys, books, and small chairs will be appreciated by mothers who have to bring their small ones. It is not advisable to have a TV or a clock in the reception room.

The magazines in medical offices have always been the subject of stale jokes. Subscription services can advise you about the most popular and appropriate titles for your area. It is a good idea to obtain all of your magazines through a subscription service so that the renewal dates coincide. As a general rule, approximately ten magazines are recommended, none older than one to two months, kept in plastic covers to protect them and to prevent their easy removal from your office. The older issues can be taken home after two months. Travel or picture books on tables provide a nice touch. Be sure that no medical journals are left in your waiting area. A bulletin board, a holder for your patient information booklet, and a rack for other general health information pamphlets are options. Depending upon the weather where you practice, a boot and coat rack or an umbrella stand just inside the door may be required.

The reception area gives the arriving patient his first impression of your office, so overall dignity and good taste are important. Your interior designer is the one who can advise you best on colors and their coordination, the texture and quality of materials to be used on floors and walls, and the durability of these materials.

Background music here and throughout the office is an excellent touch. It diminishes the effect of business office noise and helps ensure privacy both for telephone conversations and for private discussions in the examining rooms. The least expensive way to provide music is to have an FM receiver tuned to a suitable station, with unobstrusive speakers in various parts of the office. Four or five speakers with individual volume controls operate well with a standard hi-fi receiver. If there is no suitable FM station in your region, a cassette deck with a loader that handles several tapes will do as well. The best location for speakers is in the acoustic ceiling, covered by a grill that matches the acoustic tile.

A restroom for the patients measuring about 4 × 5 feet and equipped with a paper cup dispenser should be close by the waiting room. Be sure to follow ordinances on accessibility for the handicapped. It is wise to have this restroom under the visual control of your receptionist. Don't worry about decor here—this room is functional. I suggest a wall-mounted toilet, a plastic laminate wall covering, and a sheet vinyl floor. If it is possible to arrange its location next to your laboratory, a small two-way compartment for urine specimens preserves privacy.

Patients are next taken to an examining room, so let's look at these. Most physicians need three examining rooms. Of course, there are exceptions to this rule: a family practitioner might fully utilize four or more, a specialized internist only two, and a psychiatrist rarely even has one. If the doors are close together, you will save steps. All should be as soundproof as possible. Have a chart rack on each door. A signal system to indicate whether a room is occupied is not necessary for a solo practitioner, but is useful in a suite with two or more physicians.

Standard sizes for an examining or treatment room are 8 × 10 to 10 × 12 feet, but certain specialists, such as ophthalmologists, might want one larger room for particular equipment or procedures. Doors must allow wheelchair access.

This size allows enough space in each room for a sink and wall-mounted cabinets, low and high. Counters are covered with plastic laminate—in a color of your choice—with a matte finish to reduce glare. Drawers should be sturdy and riding on ball-bearing rollers; shelves should be shallow and adjustable. Any protruding corners ought to be rounded to prevent injury. Waste receptacles are located in a lower cabinet with a hinged door. Remember that cabinets and other wall-mounted furnishings are depreciable if they can be detached from the wall.

All examining rooms should be identical in size and shape, if possible (Fig. 11–1). Avoid mirror-image reversals: doors, cabinets, light

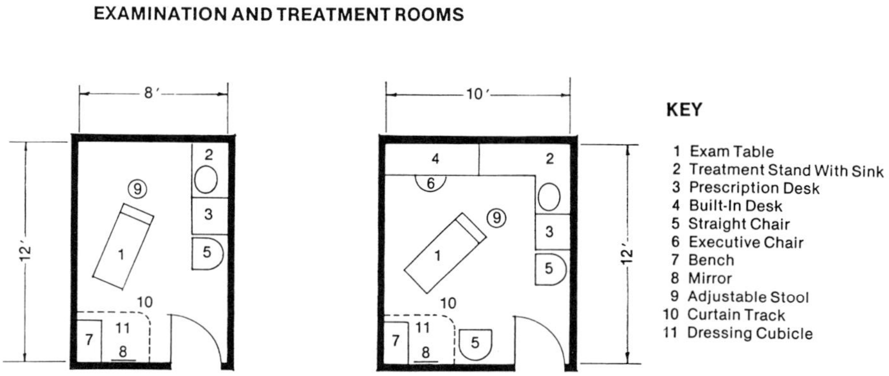

Figure 11–1.

switches, sinks, wall-mounted instruments, and electrical outlets should be in the same location in each. Place the examination table diagonally so it faces away from the door, with your stool and floor lamp at the far end. This arrangement protects the privacy of the patient in the event the door is inadvertently opened—which happens occasionally despite the best precautions. Put a mobile over the table for the patient to look at. Plan the storage of equipment and supplies to be the same in all rooms—within reach whether you are seated on the stool or standing beside the examining table. Post your storage plan inside cabinet doors. Although fluorescent lighting is too harsh to use elsewhere, here it allows a better physical examination. Watt-for-watt, fluorescent bulbs are four times more energy efficient than incandescent bulbs, and they last much longer. All sinks are wall-mounted and stainless steel, fitted with levers or foot controls for the faucets. The examination rooms, not your consultation room, are where your diplomas, certificates, and civic awards should be displayed.

An area set aside in each examination room for patients to have some privacy while changing is much appreciated by them. The simplest solution is a curtained-off corner with a chair, hook-and-hanger combination, and a small mirror. Provide cloth gowns, not disposable paper ones.

Most of the furniture in the examining rooms comes under the category of professional equipment and will not be discussed here. Patients should never have to wait in examining rooms for any appreciable length of time. But if you anticipate an occasional short wait, a comfortable chair, magazines, and a good reading light should be provided. Physicians sometimes put a set of scales in each examining room, but since the standard reference charts are for patients wearing shoes and indoor clothing, there is no advantage in doing so. Patients weigh the same in the corridor outside, and one set of scales located there is adequate.

Your otoscope and ophthalmoscope should be rechargeable types, not those on long cords. The hose of a wall-mounted sphygmomanometer will entangle you and your patient enough during physical examinations. Last, give some thought to softening the cold, sterile feeling that all examining rooms have with the use of soft colors and perhaps some art on the walls.

You will have to pause now to decide how you will make entries in your medical records. Some physicians sit at a desk in the examining room. This puts patients at ease, but sit-down-stand-up cycles are fatiguing. They also tend to be time-consuming, and the desk takes up space. Others prefer to stand at 40-inch-high fold-out desks mounted on the wall. This is more efficient and still acceptable to patients. Either of these two ways, patients are made aware of this time that is spent on their behalf, and any doubtful points that occur to you while you are writing can be cleared up before you leave the room. Other physicians use a hand-held dictating machine which can be used in two ways: at a stand-up dictation desk outside in the corridor or some dictation done in the examining room, with confidential items added outside. Either way gives all of the advantages of dictated records (more complete, legible, and less time-consuming) but all of the problems as well (lost tapes, errors in transcription, and delays in typing the chart entries). Some physicians try to write all notes in their consultation rooms between patients, but when the office gets busy, there is a tendency to stack the charts on the desk with a promise to get to them later. At the end of the day it is surprising how many charts have been given this promise, and by then details are difficult to recall. Probably the best method all around uses either style of dictation, while making every effort to minimize the inherent problems mentioned.

You may want to plan a central station for your clinical assistant. This can be as simple as a stand-up desk in the corridor central to the examination rooms.

Most suites also have a procedure room, which is slightly smaller than the examining rooms. If you will not be doing surgical procedures, this room can be used by your assistants for such activities as completing histories, patient education, autoclaving, giving injections, performing electrocardiograms and physical therapy, changing dressings, drawing blood for laboratory tests, and obtaining vital signs.

Nothing will be said here about radiological facilities. Office x-rays are taken today only by certain specialists such as orthopedists and pulmonologists, with state-of-the-art equipment operated by licensed technicians. Consultants are available to advise these specialists on space, wiring, shielding, and other requirements.

Most laboratory tests, too, have left physicians' offices because of quality-control problems. Although two or three sources provide materials and methods for quality control, in the rush of private practice this is one of the first things to go. Most assistants are not professionally trained and may be distracted at the wrong time by their other duties. It is better to have all laboratory tests done at a reliable laboratory except for a few simple "stat" tests for the convenience of patients. This situation may change in the future if the price of the newer automated dry analyzers comes within reach. You may wish to anticipate this development by setting aside space in your procedure room and installing a sink, counter, and electrical outlets.

Specimens are best obtained in your office, however. Patients are already there and prepared to have specimens taken. They do not have to drive to a laboratory, which may be at some distance or difficult to find. Specimens are obtained by your personnel, in whom your patients have confidence, and at the proper times and under conditions that you control. In most commercial laboratories, the areas in which specimens are taken are unattractive and sometimes unclean. Their personnel are more concerned with performing the laboratory test than in pleasing your patients. Space and equipment for preparing specimens should be provided in your procedure room.

Your consultation room is the least "efficient" space in your entire office, but as time goes on it will be the most valued. It should not be shared, even with another physician. You will need a place for rest, refuge, telephone calls, and reading. There are times, too, when you will need to talk with distraught patients or relatives. If you ever have a twinge of guilt because this room is reserved mostly for you, just arrange to see some patients there who need follow-up without examination.

The size of the consultation room depends on your personal preferences and available space. The decor can suit your own taste. Indulge yourself a little with quality wall covering, deep carpeting, and drapes in quiet good taste. Put your finest art objects here. Shelves will be needed for textbooks and journals. Furniture for your consultation room will consist of a fine wood desk (not metal or plastic—patients tend to judge you by the quality of your personal desk) with adequate drawer space. A swivel-type executive or adjustable chair for you, and two or three comfortable chairs for patients will be needed. Perhaps a table with a lamp between the chairs and a credenza for storage, which will give you that "clean desk" look, could be added. Most offices are laid out so your private entrance is to this room (see Fig. 11–2).

An adequate storage area is sometimes forgotten during initial office planning, but it will be acutely needed in the future. First, try to obtain

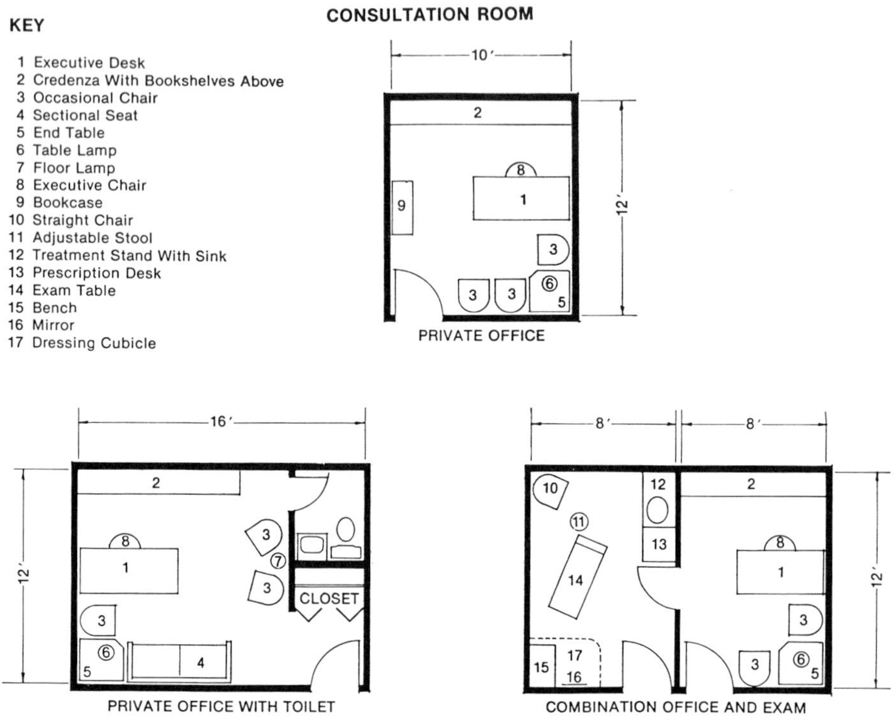

Figure 11–2.

dry, temperature-controlled storage elsewhere in the building at less than your per-square-foot rent. If it is not available, plan for one 4 × 6 or 6 × 6 foot closet in your suite, furnished with shallow adjustable shelves. In most solo practices it is not economically worthwhile to bulk-order supplies, so storage for that purpose is minimal. But, over the years, it is surprising how many other items will need to go into your storage closet.

In addition to the restroom for patient use, you should have another for you and your staff. It is not necessary to have your own private restroom off your consultation room, but some physicians like this convenience.

Hallways have to be about 4 feet wide in order to permit the passing of two persons comfortably. Allow 5 feet if you can. As I suggested previously, check your state laws and local building ordinances on halls and doorways with regard to accessibility for the handicapped.

A combination lounge and staff conference room about the same size as an examining room will have many uses. It is an informal place where employees can relax when there is an opportunity, enjoy coffee breaks and conversation, and in which you can hold periodic staff conferences. It should be clean, light in color, with the same wall and floor coverings as your examining rooms. A table with the appropriate number of chairs, a refrigerator, and a sink are the essentials. You can also have a microwave, coffeemaker, posters, bulletin board, or whatever other conveniences the staff chooses. You may want to put in cabinets for additional storage. This is a good place to locate locked cabinets for controlled substances, injectables, and drug samples. The size of the lounge area is determined by the space that is left over when all of the more essential areas have been provided for.

Now we come to the business area. This has been kept for last, but is actually first in terms of usage, in expansion requirements for the future, and in the number of people who will be working there. It also is the first place that patients stop to look at after they come in the door and walk through the waiting room. So, careful planning needs to be given to this area. Minimal space for one assistant is 125 square feet, with approximately 75 square feet for each additional person. If you can, add 100 square feet or so for various future requirements. If possible, separate the business office into two sections. As displayed in Figure 11–3, the business office itself is not divided, but a full partition could be constructed by extending the one separating the two parts of the reception desk.

One section of a divided business office is for receiving patients. In it, the receptionist sits behind the counter, with the telephone and the appointment book, and welcomes each arriving patient. A sliding glass window between this area and the reception room is *not* advised, since it tends to seem too impersonal and exclusive to your patients, and this is not how you want them to view you or your staff. However,

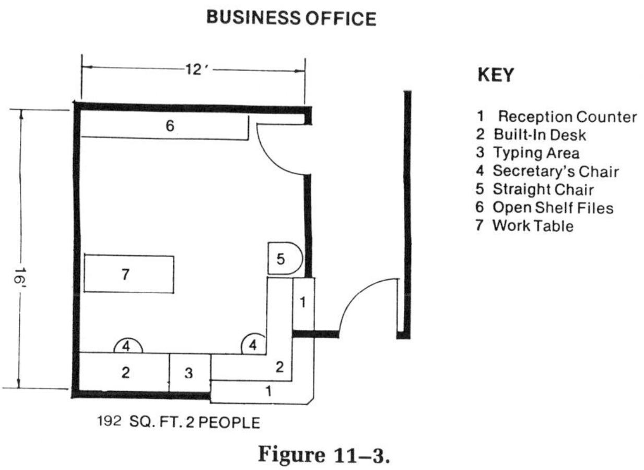

Figure 11–3.

having this section always open to the waiting room requires that your assistants be discreet in their conversations, both in person and on the telephone. The ledger card tray and photocopier are usually located in this section, as well as a desktop transcriber, with earphones and a foot pedal for transcription. Patient charts may be stored either in this section or in the adjacent one described in the next paragraph.

The other section of a divided business office, separated if possible by a soundproof wall from the first, is for collections. It is used for calls and work that is best done out of earshot of the patients who are sitting in the reception area. In this section there is another window at which patients report to pay their charges for the day before departing. Discussions about charges and payments are thus kept confidential. A doorway in the corridor separates patients standing at this window from those in the waiting area or at the reception desk.

In both sections, there are no desks as such—just built-in counters without drawers if possible, because all sorts of things seem to find their way into drawers and get forgotten. The usual counter height is 29 to 30 inches. A portion three or four inches lower is needed for the typewriter. Front-to-back counter depth of at least 20 inches is necessary to provide adequate working space. Counter space beyond 26 inches is out of convenient reach and not well utilized. A built-in business carrel is a good idea and will find many uses.

Give some attention to the quality of the chairs in the business office. Your assistants may spend five or six hours a day in them so they should be comfortable. A good chair is about 18 inches wide and deep, with screws or levers allowing adjustment of the height of the seat, and the position, angle, and tension of the backrest. Often these chairs are adjusted at the time they are received, and the instructions thrown away. Then two or three years later, when you have a new assistant, you may have forgotten how to adjust them. Tape the instructions underneath. Wheels or castors are convenient on business office chairs. In your own office, which will have a thick carpet and pad, you will need either oversized castors or a large acrylic mat under your chair.

Let's take a long look at chart storage options, because whatever method you choose will come to dominate your business area. The oldest method, once physicians stopped using small cards for their notes, is the ordinary office filing cabinet. These are readily available, protect the charts against dust and dirt, can be insulated to offer some degree of fire resistance, and can be locked to provide protection against theft, vandalism, and curiosity. However, the weight of the charts requires ball-bearing roller suspension, increasing the expense of the cabinets. The time and effort required to open and close the drawers many times a day is excessive. The drawers, when open, require nearly twice the floor space of the cabinets themselves, and frequently interfere with personnel movements. The three-drawer cabinet is too limited in capacity, but the taller ones become unstable when the top drawer is open. The charts in the top drawer are nearly inaccessible, while all the space from the top of the filing cabinets to the ceiling is wasted.

Then lateral filing cabinets with drawers that open only a little over a foot were developed. These hold the charts sideways, and some come with covered shelves. The covers provide protection for the charts, but they are often not closed by personnel, even at the end of the day, negating this theoretical advantage. Lateral cabinets do conserve office floor space, since they are bolted to the wall for stability, and thus can go higher than standard filing cabinets. More charts can be seen at a glance when the sliding covers are open, so filing and retrieval are easier. In fact, this type of chart storage has only two disadvantages. One is the failure of any combination of cabinets to utilize *all* the length and height of the wall space available in any particular office. The other is the expense, which is prohibitively high.

These disadvantages have led many physicians to choose built-in open-shelf storage, which is what I would suggest. You first have to decide whether your charts should lie on their fold with the tab containing patient identification at the bottom projecting toward you, or whether they should rest on their bottom edge with the tab on the side projecting toward you. The depth and spacing of the shelves are determined by this decision. The way to figure the length of shelf space required is to estimate the thickness of your average chart as one inch, and multiply it by the number of active charts you expect to have. Although the shelves will go from floor to ceiling, the top shelf will be for inactive charts, while the bottom will be used for storage of heavy supplies.

This completes the tour a patient would take through your office. You now have all the information you need to return to your graph paper and create the office that will best meet your requirements.

12

Business Equipment

The selection of professional equipment has been left entirely to you, because it depends so much on your specialty. But some items of business equipment are necessary for all physicians.

Buy or lease? The tax advantages of leasing office equipment have been eliminated by the 1982 Tax Equity and Fiscal Responsibility Act (TEFRA). This leaves only three reasons for leasing: an item with a high rate of obsolescence, one that is needed for only a brief time, or one that is beyond your budget. The latter is not valid—if you are caught in a cash-flow crunch, it is better to borrow money, settle for less equipment, or purchase second-hand items.

If you *do* lease, watch out for the pitfalls. The major one is the method of valuation of the equipment at the end of the lease period. Be sure the lease contract states that the "fair market value" at the end of the lease period will be determined by a reliable method and will not be artificially inflated by the leasing company. Alternatively, a purchase option at a stated price can be made a part of the contract. Another potential trap is that the lease period may be so long that certain items will become obsolete during the term of the lease. Get a clause in the agreement allowing you to cancel or upgrade during the lease period. A third trap has to do with cumulative hidden costs—such as repairs, maintenance, casualty losses, personal property tax, and loss of the investment tax credit. A fourth is the penalty for early termination of the lease. By following the advice of your accountant and attorney, and by watching out for these particular traps, you may avoid getting caught in them—and others.

Now to the equipment itself. The most heavily used item is the typewriter. Your assistant will insist upon an electric typewriter with a good correction feature as a minimum. Look at reconditioned machines if you are pinched for funds. Either a good standard type bar electric (Royal or Olivetti) or one with a stationary carriage and a movable typing element, such as the IBM Selectric, is satisfactory. If you will turn out a lot of correspondence, much of which is standard format, consider one of the less expensive electronic typewriters. Most established physicians can afford and prefer a mid-range electronic. A microcomputer with a word processing program is also a possibility, discussed in Chapter 31. A maintenance contract is advisable in any case.

Some years ago, an office copier was optional equipment, but now it is essential. There are many types available. The best for a medical office is a desktop model with an automatic feed that uses ordinary paper. Don't bother with the other bells and whistles that will be offered you. Just test it before you purchase it. Notice the quality of reproduction and the ability of the machine to handle the types of originals you will be using most frequently. Make sure the copier will fit in the space you have and can be operated conveniently there. Choose a major manufacturer such as Ricoh, Canon, IBM, 3-M, or Xerox whose local representative has a good maintenance service with a loaner provision. A maintenance contract is advisable.

You can't get by without a printing calculator. Many excellent ones are on the market at reasonable prices. Perhaps the best are produced by Canon with Texas Instruments and Casio not far behind. Pick a quiet one with large keys to reduce entry errors. A printed tape is not only valuable as a permanent record, but makes it easier to correct errors when entering figures. The most convenient size uses 2¼ inch tape. You will probably want such features as a light-emiting diode (LED) or other display, at least one memory, a multiplication and division constant, fixed and floating decimal, a % key, an add mode, two clearing keys—one for the entry and another for the register—and an item counter. Other features are convenient, but optional. A service contract is not necessary.

Dictation equipment is not essential for some starting practices. If it is in your case, the simplest setup is one desktop combination dictation-transcription unit. When you wish to dictate you can take the unit to your desk, and when you are through return it to where the dictation is to be transcribed. Later on, you can add a matching second unit that will stay in your consultation room. The desktop units are more rugged, with better voice quality and more versatility than the portable ones. Your typist will appreciate other features they have that the portables do not, such as speed-up and slow-down, tone control, and rapid scanning with cues. However, a small portable unit in addition to the larger machine really comes in handy. You can dictate anywhere you wish with one of these—in the hospital, in your car, or at home—and then drop off the tape. If you are on an extremely tight budget and this is your only dictation equipment, just drop off the whole unit for transcription. If you select one that can use standard household current with an adapter, your assistant can plug in earphones and a foot pedal and transcribe directly from the portable unit. Make sure all your units use the same standard cassettes. The newer microcassette units are approaching their larger portable brothers in quality and features, but they are not there yet. The micros are only slightly smaller, the tape is more likely to break or tangle, voice quality is poorer, and on occasion the proper cassettes may be difficult to obtain. A service contract is advisable for desktop units, but not for the portable ones.

A postage meter is neither necessary nor economical, except in large practices. If you are concerned about the theft of stamps, order your return address envelopes *prestamped,* and monitor your stamp usage. A postage scale, however, will save you effort, time, and money by eliminating delayed and returned mail, extra trips to the post office, and wasted excess postage placed on mail "just to be sure." An electric letter opener is not expensive, is a lot of fun, and does save time. The same is true for a postage stamp affixer.

A check protector is not a necessity, but if it makes you feel more secure, get one. This device embosses your checks with the correct amount, making the check almost impossible to alter.

Office telephones are now a major item. Since the restructuring of AT&T and its Bell System, the installation cost is substantial, and ongoing costs have increased to about three or four per cent of the gross in most medical offices. The general rule now is to buy your phones. The break-even point is between two and three years. You then have equity, certain tax advantages, and the equipment is yours to take with you if you move. I would advise this approach:

1. Decide on the ideal number and location of telephones in your office, so that you can plan for the future and, if you wish, install the wiring and modular jacks now in the four or five best spots. In any case, get switching equipment that will allow later expansion. The ideal is usually one or two wall-mounted phones—to conserve desk space—in the business office (one in the reception and one in the collection section), one desk telephone in your consultation room, perhaps one wall-mounted telephone in the corridor near the examining rooms (out of earshot of patients), one in the lounge, and one in the patient waiting area adjusted to prevent outgoing long distance calls. But you will probably start

with only two instruments: one wall-mounted to the left of your receptionist who presumably is right-handed, and one desk telephone in your consultation room. Both should be push button, which is three times as fast as dial for a 7-digit number, in colors coordinated with the rooms in which they are located, and the standard six-button style. These have two buttons for your trunk lines, two blank buttons for reserved numbers in sequence, and rotary capacity. The fifth button is for hold and the sixth for intercom. Only one number is listed, and if this line is busy, the call is automatically transferred to the next line.

2. Contact your telephone company and at least two interconnect companies. Investigate the latter carefully in terms of their reputation, the length of time they have been in business, the reliability of their equipment, their service, and their prices. Discuss with all three the features you want for your office among all those available: intercom, volume control, automatic rollover, privacy safeguards on extensions, call alert notifying you of another caller on the line, conference call capability, automatic redial, computerized speed dialing, power failure transfer, monitor on hold, automatic dialing of frequently called numbers, and call forwarding. A chime is much more pleasant than a bell. One of the new small headsets that weigh less than an ounce and fit behind the ear will allow your receptionist the use of both hands. A cordless telephone may work well in your office. These now have double the frequencies previously available. The new frequencies are no longer subject to eavesdropping over AM radios, and the crackling and static caused by home appliances and transformers has been greatly reduced. Consider a cellular phone for your car. The cost—even to lease—at the present time is high, but should decline rapidly over the next few years.
3. Next decide on the telephone equipment you want. Obtain bids from the two interconnect companies you have selected, and compare them with what your phone company offers. If you select interconnect companies carefully, you can obtain equal quality equipment at about half the price of the phone company. The interconnect company will install wiring and equipment, and will be responsible for maintenance and servicing. Service is usually free for a year, after which a service contract can be purchased.

   It might be worthwhile to purchase one telephone company phone and put it on the shelf. At a later date when you have any difficulty, you can plug this phone into a modular jack. If it works, the problem is with the equipment and the interconnect company should be called. If it does not, the problem is on the line and the telephone company should be called. This will avoid putting you in the middle of a dispute between them. If the phone company telephone does work, you can use it while the equipment in your office is being checked.

A hospital extension is inexpensive and invaluable. You can reach the floor or lab quickly, and the nurse can reach you without delay. If you wish, you can use the hospital operator to place long distance calls and save your aide's time.

If you plan to make many long distance calls, you should request a guide to the many companies competing with AT&T from the **Better Business Bureau,** 257 Park Avenue South, New York, NY 10010. Several firms will analyze your pattern of calls by computer and determine the least expensive long distance company for you for a fee.

Some items having to do with fire safety were discussed in the previous chapter: detectors, alarms, sufficient outlets to minimize the use of extension cords, and a master shutoff switch. Some other suggested fire safety items are an urn near the entry for people to put out their cigarettes on coming into your office, signs prohibiting smoking, and at least two fire extinguishers. Ask your fire department about these. Fire extinguishers are most often located in the business office, the laboratory (if you have one), and the employee lounge. The newer models rated "A, B and C" are best. This rating means that they can put out any type of fire. The telephone number of the fire department should be prominently displayed near each telephone.

At least one three-drawer filing cabinet will be needed for copies of correspondence and other miscellaneous items. "Fireproof" models can withstand a temperature of 1300° Fahrenheit for one hour, but they are much more expensive. The filing cabinet, whether fire resistant or not, is the place to put your ledger card tray, appointment book, checkbooks, cancelled checks, tax returns, and other vital business records at the end of each day. A regular cabinet offers some fire protection, and compressing the ledger cards in their tray offers more for them. An extra copy of the ledger cards should be run off monthly or whenever statements are prepared, and a designated assistant should take these home. If you take your photocopy of each day's appointments home also, reconstruction of most of your accounts receivable is possible if the ledger cards are destroyed in a fire. The filing cabinet should have a lock, and both you and your assistant should have keys.

You will need a number of small items such as a rotary file, desk calendar, cancelled check box, petty cash box, cardholder, and nameplate, but these pose no difficult decisions.

One last item that is not strictly business equipment is the reference library for your front office. A dozen well-selected books for your assistants will make your practice run much more smoothly, will save you time in constant reminders, will enable your assistants to look up various information that you may not even know, and will provide a better quality of patient care and better continuity in the event of personnel turnover.

Those suggested are:

1. One easy-to-read book on general medical matters. Choose from the following: Jane Brody's *Guide to Personal Health*, *The Family Medical Guide* put out by the AMA, or the latest *Merck Manual of Diagnosis and Therapy*.
2. A standard English dictionary of good quality, such as *Webster's New Collegiate Dictionary*.
3. A medical dictionary. Perhaps the best is *Dorland's Illustrated Medical Dictionary*.
4. A recent edition of the *ICD*, often referred to erroneously as the *ICDA*. Don't order the latter. It is the *International Classification of Diseases and Accidents* and is a work used for mortality classification that has no place in a medical office. The *International Classification of Diseases*, or *ICD*, which you do need, is a three-volume set. To further distinguish this publication from the *ICDA*, the words "Clinical Modification" are appended in the title and the standard abbreviation accordingly is *ICD-CM*. the current edition, at this writing, is the ninth, so a more correct abbreviation is *ICD-9-CM*, but "ICD" will do for everyday conversation in your office. This is obtained from the Superintendent of Documents, U.S. Government Printing Office, Washington, DC 20402. If you wish to save money at the start, the second volume is the one most often used.
5. The latest edition of *Physician's Current Procedural Terminology*, or *CPT*. This is an annual publication giving uniform nomenclature with code numbers for medical, surgical and diagnostic procedures. The current one at this writing is *CPT-1985*, and it can be obtained from Order Department, American Medical Association, P.O. Box 10946, Chicago, IL 60610.
6. You will receive *Physicians' Desk Reference* and *Physicians' Desk Reference for Nonprescription Drugs* every year from Medical Economics. A good location for the previous year's editions is at the front desk.
7. A secretarial handbook, if you will be doing much correspondence. *The Elements of Style* by W. Strunk, Jr., and E. B. White is a classic. *Webster's Medical Office Handbook*, published by G. & C. Merriam Company, is another good one.

8. The latest edition of *Instructions for Patients* by H. Winter Griffith, M.D.
9. The AMA produces drug instruction sheets that at the present time cover 81 frequently prescribed medications. Also available is USPDI Volume II, entitled *Advice for the Patient* and Griffith's *Drug Information for Patients*. This AMA series is being expanded and is perhaps the best. Choose one of these three and use it for each medication prescribed. Photocopy the pertinent sheet and hand the copy to the patient. Package inserts are inappropriate, yet it is your obligation to provide patients reasonable and comprehensible information on each medication: the result expected, possible side effects, and precautions to observe.
10. A *Zip Code Directory*, obtainable from the Superintendent of Documents, is a convenient publication to have, but it is bulky. By law, first class mail without a zip code has to be delivered, so if you wish you can get by without a directory, or use the one at your local post office.
11. The *Postal Manual*, obtainable from the same source, is also bulky, but your local post office has a series of smaller brochures summarizing essential information on various aspects of the U.S. Postal Service.
12. And to tie it all together, get the wonderful guide that has remained in use through 25 years and five editions, The *Medical Office Assistant* by P. M. Frederick and M. E. Kinn published by W. B. Saunders Company. It is half administrative and half clinical. A workbook has been prepared to go with it, and the combination can be used by your assistants to prepare for certifying examinations. The authors have put an amazing amount of information between the covers of this book, and no medical office should be without it.

13

Forms and Printing

Depending upon your specialty and style of practice, there is an optimum number of printed items and standardized forms that will enhance office efficiency. Beyond this point, however, having more will only confuse personnel and clutter the office. Most physicians fall well short of that point. The following are suggested as a reasonable minimum, to which you can add as you see fit for your own practice.

ANNOUNCEMENT CARDS

My opinion may be a minority one, but I think announcement cards no longer serve any valid purpose, although they may have in the past. Try to imagine a typical situation 50 years or so ago. In almost every region across the country there was a physician shortage. The only requirement for a new physician then was that he have an M.D. degree and a license. Then, printed announcement cards mailed or appearing in the local paper would attract a number of patients directly, and indirectly by referrals from fellow physicians. Currently, most physicians entering practice are specialized or subspecialized. There is now a surplus of physicians, and patients are much more sophisticated. A card in the mail or an announcement in the paper will not induce a patient to visit that physician, nor will it give enough information for another physician to use it as a basis for referring patients. Announcements now are only informative, and there are better ways to let the community know you are there. But if you do wish to send them out, you can at least keep the cost down. Contact a pharmaceutical firm that prints announcements at no charge to you. Eli Lilly Company is one, and its address is in the *Physicians' Desk Reference*. Your local medical society may run the envelopes through its addressing machine at no cost or for a nominal charge. Then your major outlay will be for postage.

LEONARD S. TAYLOR, M.D.

ANNOUNCES THE OPENING OF HIS OFFICE FOR THE

PRACTICE OF GENERAL MEDICINE

2100 West Park Avenue

Champaign, Illinois 61820

Office Hours	Telephone
By Appointment	367-6671

Figure 13–1. (Courtesy of Colwell Systems, Inc., Champaign, Illinois.)

The usual format is on a $3\frac{3}{8} \times 5\frac{3}{8}$ inch panelled card of good quality white or ivory vellum stock (see Fig. 13–1). Your name and degree are at top center, under which is the message: "Announces the Opening of his Office for the Practice of ____________________." This is followed by the office address. In the lower left corner is "Hours by Appointment" and in the right corner, your telephone number. Matching envelopes have your return address printed on the flap. Type style is simple and dignified, and black ink (raised or flat impression) is used. The medical society and the local pharmaceutical representative will have several examples.

PROFESSIONAL CARDS

The standard size for a professional card is $2 \times 3\frac{1}{2}$ inches (see Fig. 13–2.) Good quality white medium-weight vellum should be used, with black raised-impression printing (or the more expensive steel-plate engraving) in a conservative type style. Your cards are a reflection of your professional standards, so you want to avoid colored or "see-through" parchment stock, odd sizes, and ornate or colored print. These are used by some physicians to attract attention, but they are not in keeping with the dignity of the profession. The card should give the following information. In the center is your name, followed by your degree. Under this is your specialty, expressed in a way that is easily understood by patients yet professionally correct. In the lower right corner is your address with zip code, and in the lower left a statement about your availability, such as "Hours by Appointment," with your telephone number. Include the area code if appropriate. You will probably need a thousand or so to start. The reverse side of your card can be used for a map if your office is difficult to find, or printed to serve as an appointment card. Check the specifications and

Donald L. Donohugh, M.D.
Internal Medicine

BY APPOINTMENT
(714) 544-5680

13420 NEWPORT AVE.
TUSTIN, CA 92680

Figure 13–2.

prices of the major cataloguers listed in Chapter 7. Compare them with what your local printer offers. In most cases, it is better to go with a cataloguer for these and all other items in this chapter.

LETTERHEAD STATIONERY

Standard letterhead stationery is 8½ × 11 inches. You will have little need for the smaller executive or half-sheet sizes. Select high-quality paper, at least 25 per cent cotton-fiber bond, and 20 to 24 pound weight (the number signifies the weight of a ream). Both tradition and the dignity of the profession dictate that the stationery be white and the printing black in capital letters. It may be raised-letter or steel-engraved as you wish. The information on the letterhead is, from top downward: name and degree in the top line, specialty in the second, and the address below these (see Fig. 13–3). If your practice is incorporated, "A Medical Corporation" must appear on all your forms and stationery. (Do not, however, add "P.C." after your name at the bottom of a letter—a corporation cannot sign anything.) Usually the telephone number, with area code, is the bottom line.

There are only two or three "no-no's" here. The worst is printing your name "Dr. J. P. Jones." The title "doctor" is a form of address or

DONALD L. DONOHUGH, M.D., F.A.C.P.
A MEDICAL CORPORATION
INTERNAL MEDICINE AND CARDIOLOGY
13422 NEWPORT AVENUE, SUITE B
TUSTIN, CALIFORNIA 92680

(714) 544-5680

Figure 13–3.

salutation and does not belong on a letterhead. Another is the use of a logo. And some women physicians feel they should declare their femininity with colored print and stationery or with ornate type styles. I feel that the profession should be indifferent to gender and that nothing in the traditional format described declares the physician to be male or female. A good rule to follow is that all declarations of individuality are better reserved for personal stationery.

The number of matching blank sheets to order will depend upon the length of the letters you customarily write. The cost per sheet is about half that of the letterhead. If you are uncertain of your requirements, start with two sheets for every letterhead sheet. Instruct your typist that typing is always done on the "felt" side, the one from which you can read the watermark when the sheet is held against the light.

Matching envelopes, of course, are of the same quality and color paper, using the same type style. Gummed flaps are satisfactory unless you plan on a voluminous correspondence, in which case self-sealing flaps will save time. The return address is at the upper left of the front of the envelope, *not* across the end or on the flap. It consists of your name and degree, omitting your specialty, and your return address with zip code (see Fig. 13–4).

PRESCRIPTION BLANKS

The standard size for prescription blanks is 4 × 5½ inches, on 20 pound white bond in pads of 100, set in black capital letters (see Fig. 13–5).

There are a few variations on this format. If a carbon sheet is placed behind each blank, or if NCR (no carbon required) treatment is used, a copy is automatically made. Either way, the insertion of a firm surface behind the copy is necessary to prevent the impression from carrying through to the next sheet in the pad. Making a copy may be an advantage in states that require filing one for Schedule II and III narcotics, but a copy added to the medical records has no legal validity. You still must write the medications you have prescribed in the record itself. However, a blank placed over the appropriate place in the record with a carbon so as to make a copy *in the record*, which is then signed, is valid. I do not feel this latter system is worth the trouble. Another variation is a multiform prescription blank on which up to five drugs can be written. This makes it temptingly easy to prescribe an extra drug or two when good practice of medicine indicates you should not. Also, the patient may add one of his own. Another objection is that some medications cannot be written on the same prescription blank by law. So I do not recommend the use of this form, either. One

DONALD L. DONOHUGH, M.D., F.A.C.P.
A MEDICAL CORPORATION
13422 NEWPORT AVENUE, SUITE B
TUSTIN, CALIFORNIA 92680

Figure 13–4.

variation that may be worthwhile in high risk areas is the use of "alter-proof" blanks, printed much like checks, so that erasures are easily detectable.

Prescription blanks should be printed with sequential numbers in one corner to help detect theft. Your DEA number should *not* appear on the form. Knowledge of your DEA number makes forgery of a prescription for narcotics simpler and unlawful telephone prescriptions a snap. Prescriptions requiring a DEA number are few in the average practice, and it takes little effort to write it on those few. If you treat children, adding the age of the patients after their names aids the pharmacist in checking your prescribed dosage against body weight.

Have the notation printed at the bottom left, "Label All Medications," so that your patients will know the name of the medication they are taking. Or have the word "label" next to a box that you can tick, if

LEONARD S. TAYLOR, M.D.
2100 WEST PARK AVENUE
CHAMPAIGN, ILLINOIS 61820

101

TELEPHONE 352-7656

NAME____________________ AGE______

ADDRESS____________________ DATE______

℞

☐ LABEL

REFILL______TIMES

☐ MAY SUBSTITUTE

☐ MAY NOT SUBSTITUTE ____________________, M.D.

Figure 13–5. (Courtesy of Colwell Systems, Inc., Champaign, Illinois.)

you wish to maintain discretion. Another space should indicate whether you wish to have refills or not, and if so how many. Add one more space to indicate if you wish to permit generic substitution by the pharmacist. Follow your state law in this regard. Giving the pharmacist permission does not mean he will use it. Surveys have shown that such substitutions save patients only about 15 per cent on the average, and run the risk of impurities, variations in bioactivity, and absorption differences, so exercise your discretion unless state law requires you to permit substitution.

One or two additional precautions should be mentioned. Use only one pad at a time and keep it out of sight when not in use. Lock the others up. Never use your prescription blanks for doodling, for diagrams to show patients, or for memos. Don't even write on the back and discard them—some of those in the narcotics trade rummage through the trash behind medical offices. They can use crumpled prescription forms with diagrams or notes on the back to obtain controlled substances. If you are careless in any way, you will have problems with the Drug Enforcement Administration and your State Board.

PATIENT REGISTRATION FORM

The patient registration form is the basic document from which information is taken for making up ledger cards, for insurance billing, and for skip tracing, which will be described in Chapter 22. The registration form is also the source of numbers and addresses for contacting a patient or the patient's relatives in emergencies, whether at home or at work. A good form to start with is illustrated in Figure 13–6. You will develop your own after some months in practice. The standard registration forms provided by cataloguers are rarely satisfactory for any individual practice, but they will print your own design.

The first item is the patient's *legal* name. Your assistant checks that it is correct and legible when the form is filled out. This name is then used consistently throughout the office. Items on the form must be updated when changed and all other records corrected.

Scattered throughout the form are several questions to assist in skip tracing, and the use of these will be explained in Chapter 22. The social security number is required on insurance forms. Information about the person or physician who referred the patient to you is valuable in practice analysis. The name of a financially responsible person is required for minors and eliminates billing confusion after a divorce or separation. The name of the nearest relative not living with the patient or of a close friend may be important in emergencies and is also useful in skip tracing. You may want to change this item to,

REGISTRATION FORM
(Please Print)

Patient's Full Name ____
(Last) (First) (Middle Initial)

Address ____
(Street) (City/State) (Zip)

Telephone (____) __________ How long at this address? ________ Own/Rent ____

Previous Address ____

Date of Birth __________ Status: ___ Single ___ Married ___ Widowed ___ Divorced

Sex ___ M ___ F Social Sec. No. ______________ Driver's Lic. No. __________

Referred By ____

Patient's Occupation ____

Employer Name/Address ____

Business Telephone (____) __________ Ext. _____ How long employed? ________

Spouse's Name ______________________________ Business Tel. __________

Home Address (if different) ____

Spouse's Business Address ____

Name/address of financially responsible person:

____

Name/Address/Telephone Number of nearest relative not living with you:

____

INSURANCE INFORMATION

Do you have medical insurance? __________ If yes, please fill in the following:

Name of Carrier ______________________________ Policy No. ________

Name of Carrier ______________________________ Policy No. ________

NOTE: If above patient is a minor, please sign below.

I hereby authorize ____________________, M.D. to examine, treat and/or hospitalize my son or daughter.

____
Parent or Legal Guardian

Reviewed by ______________ Date ______________

Figure 13–6. (Courtesy of Colwell Systems, Inc., Champaign, Illinois.)

"In case of emergency, contact:". An entry for allergies is frequently added.

The insurance information section may be expanded. A typical expansion is:

INSURANCE INFORMATION

Do You Have Health Insurance? If yes, please fill in the following:

Person Responsible For Payment		Address	
City/State		Telephone	
Blue Shield (Give Name of Policyholder)		Certificate No.	
Group No.		Coverage Code	
Champus Sponsor's Name	Service No.	I.D. Card No.	Expiration Date
Branch of Service		Duty Station	
Other, Write In The Name Of Insurance Co.		Policy No.	
Medicare	Medicare No.	Medicaid	Program No.
County No.		Account No.	

An assignment block may also be added for the signature-on-file provision on insurance claim forms:

I hereby authorize ____________________, M.D. to furnish to the above insurance company(ies) all information which said insurance company(ies) may request. I hereby assign to Dr. __________________ all money to which I am entitled for medical and/or surgical expenses relative to the services rendered, but not to exceed my indebtedness to said physician and/or surgeon. It is understood that any money received from the above named insurance company(ies) over and above my indebtedness will be refunded when my bill is paid in full. I understand I am financially responsible to said doctor for charges not covered by this assignment. I further agree, in the event of nonpayment, to bear the cost of collection and/or court cost and reasonable fees should this be required.

________________________________ ________________________________

Insured or Guardian Signature Patient's Signature

The release-of-information authorization of this block is optional. Courts have held that the submission of insurance information by the patient to the physician constitutes implied consent to release the required information to the insurer.

If you treat children, include space for authorization of treatment by a parent or guardian (see Fig. 13–6).

At the bottom of the form is a space for your receptionist to initial and date after having checked the form for completeness and accuracy.

A LIFETIME ASSIGNMENT FOR MEDICARE PATIENTS

The Health Care Financing Administration permits use of a lifetime assignment form whether you are a participating physician who accepts assignment on all Medicare patients or one who accepts assignment on a case-by-case basis. With this form in your records, you do not have to obtain a signature each time a claim is filed. The patient signature space (block 12 on the claim form) should be filled in with the words, "patient request for payment on file." You can buy a rubber stamp for that entry, or if you're using a computer the legend can be automatically keyed in. The signed lifetime assignment form should be kept with the medical records and a notation of its existence made on the patient's ledger card.

Lifetime Assignment for Medicare Patients

________________________ ________________________

Name of Beneficiary Medicare HIC Number

I request payment of authorized Medicare benefits be made either to me or on my behalf to (name of physician, i.e., corporation or solo name) for any services furnished me by that physician. I authorize any holder of medical information about me to release to the Health Care Financing Administration and its agents any information needed to determine these benefits or the benefits payable to related services.

________________________ ________________________

Date Beneficiary

PATIENT QUESTIONNAIRE

See Chapter 17 for suggestions.

CLINICAL RECORDS

The folder, medical history form, physical evaluation form, continuation or progress sheets, and other optional forms in the clinical record, such as flow sheets, are discussed in detail in Chapter 20. A medical history form designed to be completed by the patient is extremely useful in private practice. Rarely does a physician have the time to sit down and ask the many questions that he learned to ask when he was a medical student. Instead, most perform a hurried and abbreviated history. If you use a self-administered form, do not hand a patient the form 10 or 15 minutes before you see him and expect anything like a complete or accurate history. However, if the form is given to a patient to fill out at home where he can take the proper time, consult records, and question relatives, it constitutes a valuable portion of the clinical record. Such a form is also handy for new hospital admissions or consultations. If the hospitalized patient feels well enough to complete the form, it assists a great deal in the initial evaluation. In any case, go over the completed form with the patient as soon as possible, taking all the time you need. Question the patient on all omitted, positive, and dubious answers, and follow through all clues. When your notes are added to the patient's entries and it bears your signature, the form constitutes a valid history.

You can start your practice using one of the standard history forms for your specialty obtainable from any major cataloguer. But after a few months of practice, it is better to develop your own and have it printed.

OTHER PRINTED FORMS

The *telephone log* is described in Chapter 18.

The *appointment book* is covered in Chapter 19.

The preparation of a *patient information booklet* is outlined in Chapter 14.

Five forms are required for employees. Four of these, the *employee application form*, the *employment agreement*, the *attendance record*, and the *periodic evaluation form*, are discussed and illustrated in Chapter 16. The fifth, the *compensation record* for use with the "one-write" disbursing system, is explained with a sample form in Chapter 24.

The *pegboard, day sheet, receipt-charge slips, "superbills," ledger cards, statement envelopes*, and *collection letters* are all discussed in Chapter 22.

The *universal claim form, insurance carrier record,* and *summary log* are illustrated in Chapter 23.

The forms and double-window envelopes required for the "one-write" disbursing system and the components of the inventory system are listed and explained in Chapter 24.

Allow ample time—a month or more—for delivery of your printed items.

MISCELLANEOUS

Among the many miscellaneous items to be ordered at about the same time as your forms and stationery are rubber stamps. They will find many uses. Obtain the self-inking variety to avoid the mess and clutter of using and storing different colored inkpads. The most frequently used stamp will be the one applied to the reverse of incoming checks to endorse them for deposit. This reads "Deposit to the Account of ______________" with your name and bank account number. Another stamp frequently used is a large one, "Allergic To ____________" with red ink on the front of the chart to reinforce whatever other method you have for calling attention to patient allergies. A date stamp will be used a lot. Do *not* order a signature stamp. The problems that such a stamp can create, even if kept under lock and key, far outweigh any possible advantage.

And before you place your order with a cataloguer, browse through the catalog. You will find a surprising number of ideas and gadgets to make your office run more smoothly.

14

Patient Education

As patients become better informed and more inquisitive, physicians accordingly are improving their efforts in patient education. This is another topic that is neglected in medical school and residency that the physician in private practice must learn on his own. Despite the general improvement most physicians are showing in this area, there are still too many who make only a minimum effort. Some offer a cliché to explain a test or other procedure, or report only one diagnosis to the patient even if several are made, or tell him the intended effect of a medication without mentioning major side effects. Even "informed consents" are sometimes less than informed.

We all know that the days of the autocratic physician are long past. There was a time, perhaps, when a physician assumed absolute authority in the physician-patient relationship, mumbled an esoteric term to the patient about his diagnosis, and scribbled a prescription in Latin–which the pharmacist (alchemist?) filled without labeling the container. The patient's role was totally passive. Not so today. This scenario began to disappear around the turn of the century, although some vestiges still linger today.

Consider with me some of the reasons for offering an effective patient education program:

1. At the time of a serious acute illness or surgical procedure, the emotional state of a patient will improve if he thoroughly understands what is going on and is reassured. In the educational process, you will learn more about his anxieties and fears. When a patient has a more positive attitude, there is usually a better outcome. The same is true if his network of family and friends is well informed.
2. In chronic illnesses, a comprehending patient will be able to assume a greater degree of independence and self-care. The long-term

management of his health care will thereby be improved, he will have a more positive attitude, and the outcome will be better.

3. With minor intercurrent illnesses, a well-informed patient will tend to report all of the significant symptoms and will not distract you with those that are not. He will be calmer and more cooperative in undergoing the tests you recommend, and more compliant in taking medications. The patient will also be more inclined to report any complications or adverse effects of medications or treatment promptly and accurately.
4. If you make the effort to educate your patients, they will be more likely to detect early signs of disease and to seek your care in time.
5. Even more important, the *prevention of disease* is much more effective with the patient as an informed partner. He is motivated to take better care of himself and to alter lifestyles that adversely affect his health.
6. Finally, an educated patient will do more to enhance his *wellness*. This is our highest purpose in medicine—not just to treat disease, but to enhance the happiness and well-being of our patients.

There are other benefits that are less tangible. The physician-patient relationship is strengthened. An informed patient might favorably influence a friend toward better health, or he might take action to raise the standards of health in the community. I am sure you can add to this list. One final thought: a physician who obviously cares and is willing to take the time to explain usually has no trouble maintaining a busy practice.

You are the key to the whole program. You are the one with the greatest knowledge of a test, disease, or procedure—and of the patient. You also have his respect and attention or he wouldn't be in your office. So you have to start the process in every case. But you may not be able to follow through because of greater need for your skills elsewhere. So you should also outline a program, assemble materials, and train your assistants to carry on where you leave off. Your medical assistants will become health educators and extend your efforts. At their level, they have a unique role. A patient may be more likely to confide certain information to them; they can increase the interest of the patient in his condition and treatment; they sometimes give a less technical, more understandable explanation; they will enhance motivation; and they can tailor the standard educational material to fit the individual patient. Then it is up to the patient to continue the process with the educational material he takes home. These are the three most important phases of patient education—your efforts, those of your assistants, and those the patient makes on his own.

There is still another phase, one which is all too frequently omitted. That is the follow-up. You initiate it with your inquiry, but your medical assistant continues it. She should ask about details, reinforce the patient's efforts, resolve any additional questions or problems, and continue to motivate and to provide emotional support.

That is an outline of the method. Now for the materials. These fall into three categories: those produced entirely by you or your assistants, those produced commercially but modified in your office, and published materials that are used without alteration.

The most important of the educational materials produced by you is the **Patient Information Booklet**. An outline of an effective patient information booklet will be given at the end of this chapter. The second most important are the handwritten instructions and diagrams drawn during explanatory talks with individual patients. The third are your "Letters to Patients" covering the health issues on which you are an authority or which frequently arise in your practice.

The materials that you modify are only slightly less effective. The mainstay should be a book of the type of **H. Winter Griffith's Instructions for Patients.** This contains information on more than 250 medical problems, their treatment, and complications that may occur. It also includes diagrams and diet plans. The instruction sheets are kept in a three-ring binder, so that they can be easily removed and photocopied. The copies can be altered by you to suit the individual case, and then handed to the patient. You will want to add the AMA drug information sheets and other items to the binder. Your medical assistant will reinforce these materials with additional explanation, with demonstrations when appropriate, and by tailoring the sheet to the patient by adding his name and by altering certain instructions.

There are an unbelievable quantity and variety of educational materials available that are not readily modified or adapted in your office. These are less effective educational tools for this reason, but you can select the best, handing out only those that are appropriate in each case and reinforcing them orally. This method of use lends them additional authority. Set up a small lending library located in your reception room. Books can be checked out from your receptionist. It will surprise you how few you lose—a phone call will usually serve to recover the occasional overdue book.

I would advise against handing out any materials provided by pharmaceutical firms. These inevitably favor the products of these firms, and your patients are sufficiently sophisticated to detect this bias. They look to you for balanced, reliable information and will think less of you if you utilize such materials. All too often, if you take the time to read them, you will see that they do not contain exactly what you want your patients to know.

Sources of educational material that *are* recommended include:

American Cancer Society, Inc.
777 Third Avenue
New York, NY 10017

American Diabetes Association
2 Park Avenue
New York, NY 10016

American Heart Association
7320 Greenville Avenue
Dallas, TX 75231
Information
Clearinghouse
Public Health Service
P. O. Box 1133
Washington, DC 20013–1133

American Lung Association
1740 Broadway
New York, NY 10019

Arthritis Foundation
3400 Peachtree Road, NE
Atlanta, GA 30326

Center for Health Promotion
American Hospital Association
840 North Lake Shore Drive
Chicago, IL 60611

Center for Health Promotion
and Education
Centers for Disease Control
1600 Clifton Road NE
Atlanta, GA 30333

Consumer Information Center
Public Documents Distribution Center
Department 20
Pueblo, CO 81009

Food and Drug Administration
Consumer Communications
5600 Fishers Lane (HFE-88)
Rockville, MD 20857

March of Dimes
1275 Mamaroneck Avenue
White Plains, NY 10605

National Clearinghouse for
Alcohol Information
P. O. Box 2345
Rockville, MD 20852

National Health Information
Clearinghouse
Public Health Service
P. O. Box 1133
Washington, DC 20013–1133

Planned Parenthood Federation
of America
810 Seventh Avenue
New York, NY 10019

President's Council on Physical
Fitness and Sports
450 Fifth Street NW, Suite 7103
Washington, DC 20001

Public Affairs Pamphlets
381 Park Avenue South
New York, NY 10016

Sex Information and Education
Council of the United States
(SIECUS)
80 Fifth Avenue
New York, NY 10011

Superintendent of Documents
U.S. Government Printing Office
Washington, DC 20402

The Nutrition Foundation
888 17th Street, NW
Washington, DC 20006

For skeletons, models, charts, and similar materials:

Armstrong Industries
3660 Commercial Avenue
P. O. Box 7
Northbrook, IL 60062

Clay Adams, Inc.
Webro Road
Parsippany, NJ 07054

Denoyer-Geppert Co.
5235 Ravenswood Avenue
Chicago, IL 60640

General Biological Supply House, Inc.
Div. of MacMillan Science Co., Inc.
8200 South Hoyne Avenue
Chicago, IL 60640

Medical Plastics Laboratory
P. O. Box 38
Gatersville, TX 76528

NASCO
901 Jonesville Avenue
Fort Atkinson, WI 53538

A. J. Nystrom Biological Model Co.
3333 North Elstron Avenue
Chicago, IL 60618

Ward's Natural Science
Establishment, Inc.
P. O. Box 1712
Rochester, NY 14603
or
P. O. Box 1749
Monterey, CA 93940

If you wish to use audiovisual presentations, write:

Audiovisual Resources Section
National Library of Medicine
8600 Rockville Pike
Bethesda, MD 20209

Bell and Howell
Audiovisual Products Division
7100 North McCormack Road
Chicago, IL 60645

Dukane Corporation
Audiovisual Division
2900 Dukane Drive
St. Charles, IL 60174

Eastman Kodak Co.
343 State Street
Rochester, NY 14560

National Archives Trust Fund Board
National Archives Building
Washington, DC 20408

National Audio-Visual Center
General Services Administration
Washington, DC 20409

Public Health Service
Audio-Visual Facility
Centers for Disease Control
1600 Clifton Road NE
Atlanta, GA 30333

With video cameras, blank tapes, and VCRs so reasonable now, don't overlook the possibility of preparing your own video tapes.

Now for the preparation of an effective **Patient Information Booklet.** Its primary purpose is to help your patients utilize your services more effectively. But there is another reason to have one. In an average practice, about one-tenth of your time and one-fourth of your staff's is spent in repeated explanations. A well-prepared booklet will let all of you devote more time and attention to patient care.

You really can't order one from a cataloguer. You have to do it yourself. The way to begin is to jot down all the routine information that you think your patients need to know, then arrange it in a presentable format. Rework the wording to eliminate medical jargon and to ensure that your thoughts are expressed as clearly and as helpfully as possible. Then have your assistant type it up and run off a few dozen photocopies. This is your first patient information booklet! It will function fairly well while you add to your own copy answers to common patient questions, staff suggestions, and new ideas and knowledge you gain from experience. Scrounge samples from the offices of other physicians in your specialty to add more ideas.

When you are ready, prepare your "second edition." When you do, guard against a few common failings. In the hands of some physicians, a patient information booklet becomes a litany of things *they* want done and is no longer what the patient wants or needs to know. Medical jargon tends to creep back in. Long and convoluted sentences do, too. And, as it lengthens, it may become somewhat dull.

Here is a suggested outline. The first items are your name, address, and telephone number. If you wish, provide directions to your office from the nearest arterials and instructions on where to park.

Next, a clear explanation in lay terms of what your specialty is and the training you have had. Don't be modest about your credentials. Then state the type of patients you treat and those you do not accept. If there is anything unusual in the way your practice is organized (as a partnership or corporation, for example), add a sentence or two of explanation. Describe your staff, the function of each member, and the ancillary services your practice provides. The hospitals in which you practice come next, with their addresses. Conclude this section with a statement of your policy on house calls.

Next describe your system for scheduling appointments. Start with the hours you see patients, then the hours your assistant is there to make appointments. Describe briefly how they are made, both in person and on the telephone. State your policy on "work-ins." Request that cancellations of appointments be at least 24 hours in advance. Describe your reminder and recall systems. If you charge for unkept appointments, or have any other unusually stringent policy, it should be set forth clearly in your booklet. A request that all patients be on time for appointments should be followed with the assurance that you respect the value of their time and will make every effort to adhere to your schedule.

Your policy on patient telephone calls during office hours, their triage, and your "call-back" times should be explained briefly. You might want to add that all telephone advice is given without charge.

This is a good place to say something about emergencies, either during or after office hours. Briefly sketch the categories of emergencies as they are laid out in your office manual (see Chapter 15), and explain how they are handled when you are in the office or on call. Outline how your answering service functions and how you arrange coverage for your practice when you are not on call. List numbers for paramedics, the local poison center, the emergency department at the major hospital where you practice, and appropriate crisis centers.

Next, give your policy on prescription refills: how many you normally indicate on the prescription, whether you allow more on request, and if so, how the request may be made. State that the pharmacist is instructed to label the containers for all prescriptions. Outline under what circumstances generic substitution is authorized by you. If you do not give new or refill prescriptions over the telephone, say so and give your reason.

Special studies performed outside of the office (such as x-rays and laboratory tests) should be explained: where they are done, by whom, how the billing is handled, and how the results are given to patients. Add that if the patient must have special preparation or observe certain precautions, instructions will be provided by your office in writing.

One paragraph should cover your fees and collection routine. Start with how your fees are determined, and set out your policy on time-of-service payment. Give the dates of the month that statements are sent. State at what point accounts are considered to be past due and the collection procedures that are then used. Add that your policies conform to the Federal Truth in Lending Act. If you reserve the right to charge interest on any unpaid balance, say so. If you charge for preparing insurance forms, this should be clear. You may wish to mention that a copy of the charge slip and the patient's cancelled check are adequate evidence of receipt of payment for both medical insurance and personal income tax purposes. This is a question often asked of your aides. Conclude this part with an invitation to discuss any problems with you or your assistants.

It is extremely important to state your policy on health insurance in this booklet and to restate it orally as often as necessary. If you take the firm stance that an insurance policy is a contract between the patient and his insurance company, and that a separate contract exists between the patient and the physician in which the patient has complete responsibility for payment, then say so. You can soften the impact of this somewhat by adding that exceptions are made on occasion, and that your staff is willing to provide information, answer questions, and assist patients in preparing their insurance claim forms. If you will use a multipurpose claim form (superbill), instruct the patient on how to use it in filing his own claim. If you are a participating physician in Blue Shield and accept the Blue Shield determination as payment in full, tell your patients this. If you are not, make this clear. Describe the Medicare physician participation program. If you do not participate, give a reasonable explanation of why you chose not to. Clarify what your position means to your patients. Explain that Medicare does not cover some 40 per cent of the average bill because of their method of calculating allowable fees, their many exclusions, and their deductible. If you do not say something about these limitations, patients may think you are overcharging them. If you accept Medicaid patients, explain the restrictions and regulations briefly. If you do not, make this fact clear, along with your reasons. Cover Workers' Compensation the same way.

Assure your patients of the confidentiality of their medical records and information. Describe how information is given to relatives, friends, and employers. Explain the use of your release form. This is an appropriate place to add that summaries and opinions for attorneys will be charged for in advance, as will the preparation of disability and other reports.

Add anything else you wish, such as a personal resume of members of your staff, and, as the last item in the booklet, invite suggestions so that you and your staff may render more effective and efficient service.

When your **Patient Information Booklet** assumes a final form, you will want to have it printed. Either the printer or a graphic designer can suggest the best paper, type style, and general format. Thereafter, minor alterations can be made with pen and ink. Reprinting will not be necessary for at least a year or two, unless there is a major change in your practice.

The most effective way to use the booklet is to have your receptionist hand two copies to all new patients at the time they fill out the patient registration form, with instructions to keep one handy and to give the other to anyone who might be interested in becoming your patient. A supply is also made available in your reception area.

15

The Personnel and Procedures Manual

There are still some physicians in private practice who do not have an office manual or who get by with only parts and pieces of one. Their number is being steadily reduced by several factors in the current medical milieu. One is the proliferation of federal and state legislation concerning the legal rights of employees. Many physicians, especially those in solo private practice, have found themselves in conflict with some of these regulations and have been penalized. Employees have become increasingly conscious of their legal rights in regard to regular hours and benefits, so that a clear-cut policy on overtime, vacation, sick leave, and holidays is necessary. Moreover, the knowledge and training required of a medical assistant have increased over the last two decades, while the turnover rate has slowly risen. These two factors combine to make a manual a greater necessity than ever. Still another factor that has arisen since the middle 1970s is the increasing vulnerability to malpractice actions of those physicians who do not have clear and consistent standards for clinical procedures performed in the office.

These are some of the negative reasons—most of the other reasons for having a personnel and procedures manual are positive, as you will see throughout this chapter. You really should have a manual before you hire your first employee or see your first patient, but this presents a problem. You are busy setting up your practice and you do not yet have the experience required to prepare a truly top-drawer manual. The best way out of this dilemma is to send for **The Medical Office Procedures Manual** produced by the Colwell Company. This consists of a three-ring, loose-leaf binder containing the outline of a fairly comprehensive office manual, with blank lines on each page for you to fill in. It is accompanied by a workbook that suggests entries for each blank. You can even pull out entire pages that are not applicable to your practice and insert your own. So in a few hours with a ballpoint pen, you can have a manual that will serve in a satisfactory manner for the first few months of your practice. When you get around to making up your own manual at a later date, this one will be its basis. If you make changes in it as you go along, its preparation will be merely a matter of handing it to a typist.

So much for the shortcut. The rest of this chapter will be a guide for preparing your permanent manual. The loose-leaf binder format should be retained, so that any page can be changed without retyping the whole.

The first page of the manual should have a statement such as, "I have read and understand the contents of this manual," with spaces below for the signatures of your employees and the date signed. If you wish to give each aide her own copy, include a phrase acknowledging receipt. The next page or two comprise the table of contents. Without one, it is surprising how difficult it can be to find an item quickly when it is needed.

Now to the text. Begin by stating its objectives in a paragraph to this effect: "The purpose of this manual is to provide guidelines to enable all personnel to understand the conditions of their employment, to ensure fair and consistent treatment, to clarify the tasks of each, to outline the office organization, and to set down standards for clinical procedures." You might conclude the paragraph with a brief description of the contents of the manual and the manner in which you wish it to be used in your office.

The second paragraph is the best place to set forth the goals and philosophy of your practice, its history, and one or two other characteristics that you want to emphasize. Conclude with the hope that this manual will help your employees maintain the high standards that your patients deserve and that all personnel wish to provide.

The third paragraph describes the physical facilities, starting with parking (emphasizing that employees should park away from the prime areas your patients use), the building (if noteworthy), and the office, with some of the principles of its design. It concludes with a brief description of the major items of equipment and their purpose.

In the fourth paragraph, cover the various positions in the office, with a title and abbreviated description for each, followed by an organizational chart showing their interrelationships. The job descriptions may be put in the appendix to the manual. Mention the necessity of "cross-training," so that one employee can help with the duties of another in an emergency, or perform them herself if another employee is absent due to illness, vacation, or other reasons. Either here or elsewhere mention staff conferences—their purpose, frequency, and agenda. Emphasize that they are mandatory.

This leads into the next paragraph: your code of conduct for employees. Items you might wish to touch upon include appearance and grooming, courtesy to patients and fellow workers, pleasant voice and manner, uniform and name tag requirements, with perhaps specific comments on such matters as smoking, the importance of washing hands frequently, applying makeup only in the restroom, hair style, using perfume, chewing gum, wearing flashy jewelry, and having long nails or colored fingernail polish. Use this paragraph to discourage political or religious activities and the solicitation of donations in the office. Conclude with guidelines on how you and the staff should address each other, and how all should address patients.

The subject of office hours follows and comprises the next paragraph or two. Distinguish among the working hours of employees, the hours the office is actually open, and the hours that you see patients. If you plan to have part-time employees, address this topic with a general phrase to the effect that their working hours will be decided individually, and compensation will be adjusted to allow for the lack of fringe benefits provided them. Such a general phrase is all that is required, and inclusion here is simpler than greater detail later in the manual when you come to describe salary and benefits. One other topic to handle here is your afternoon or day off. Emphasize that this is the time for employees to attend to such business as billing, insurance claim preparation, collection and stocking supplies. It is *not* an afternoon off for them.

A mention of punctuality is pertinent, and more than a mention is necessary concerning overtime (see Chapter 16). Introduce the topic with a sentence to this effect: "The primary purpose of every person in the office is to help patients who are ill, and all must accept the fact that practice hours will be irregular." Go on to cover the following points in your own words. No more than 40 hours total per week will be worked, and extra hours will be only on your specific authority. Your choice then will be either to compensate them with time-and-a-half pay or to allow compensatory time off during that same week. No work is to be taken home in the evenings or on weekends; no employee with a key to the office is to come in late in the evenings or on weekends to work extra hours without your authorization; no employee having lunch in the office is to perform any duties whatsoever unless authorized by you. However you word this section, *be firm*, because many physicians suffer legal consequences due to vagueness on these points. End the paragraph on a positive note by adding that office hours may be adjusted to suit individual preferences, or whatever you wish. A copy of your lawyer's summary of the federal wage and hour law might be put in the appendix of the manual.

The subject of holidays follows. You have to select which you want to observe. Six are standard: New Year's Day, Memorial Day, Independence Day, Labor Day, Thanksgiving, and Christmas. These should be specified so that there will be no misunderstanding. Employees must work the full business day before and after these holidays to receive pay for them. You can add that if the needs of the patients permit, the office may be closed the afternoons preceding Thanksgiving, Christmas, and New Year's Day. As your practice develops and more employees are added, you will be able to make individual exceptions, but initially the same clear standard should be set for all. Some holidays will fall on a weekend, so you have to decide ahead of time how you will handle this situation. It is best to close on the subsequent day you take your afternoon or day off, *not* on the Monday after the weekend.

Your vacation policy is the next subject. Mention that it applies to full-time employees only, and, again, that part-time employees are subject to individual arrangements. Usually two weeks (ten working days) is provided *after* one full year of employment, and three weeks per year after three years of employment. To promote employee retention, work out vacation increments for up to ten years on the job. Decide if you wish to have vacation time accrue monthly or only at the end of each year, and what you would like to do about unused vacation time. As a general rule, unused vacation time is neither compensated for nor carried over to subsequent years. Employees must take their time off during the year earned or forfeit it.

Other items of vacation policy should follow. Vacations may be taken at any time during the calendar year, but requests that coincide with your own vacation will be given first priority, with second consideration given for periods of low practice demand. You may require that one week be taken during your vacation, if you wish. Emphasize that patient needs are paramount, and that vacation scheduling is subject to these needs. Requests are made at least two months in advance, and vacations must be taken in periods of one week or more. The request is always in writing to avoid misunderstandings. If two employees happen to request the same vacation period you should state how you will handle this situation: either grant vacations according to seniority, the date the requests were received, or some other system.

Clarify your policy concerning employees who request a vacation before any has been accrued. This is usually for urgent reasons having to do with family matters. The usual solution is to allow those who request unaccrued vacation time to take it without pay. If you give it with pay, state that the vacation time taken will be deducted from the employee's pay if she is terminated or resigns before the vacation time used has been earned. Giving two hours off is customary on Election Day, and five paid days are usually allowed for jury duty.

Emergency leave must also be dealt with. I prefer to use that term, although some personnel administrators like to use "personal days," because the time off is not always given for true emergencies. They often classify sick leave as "personal days," which just confuses everyone. You will need to include a sentence to the effect that each request will be considered on its own merits, with a total allowance of perhaps two paid days a year. More than that will be considered leave of absence without pay. You might want to add that any holidays other than those listed, whether taken for religious or other reasons, will be treated as emergency leave.

Your policy on sick leave is next. This is an area in which there is a lot of abuse and often a great deal of misunderstanding on both sides. You may want to emphasize first that it is to be used only when the illness truly prevents performance of duty, but that on occasion it may be taken to avoid possible adverse effects upon the patients. Verification is important. If you wish to be rather rigid, insist upon a statement by a physician if more than 24 hours is taken. Also, proper notification should be given. The method of accrual should be stated clearly. This ranges from one-half day per month after three months of employment to the same as the allowance for vacation time. The former policy is more common than the latter. Any absence greater than the time that has been accrued is treated as leave of absence without pay. Although you can set your own policy, sick leave is not normally subject to the two exceptions sometimes made for vacations: it is never given before it has been earned, nor is it ever cumulative from one year to the next. It is not wise to pay employees at the end of the year for sick leave not taken. If you decide to do so, at the most, pay a maximum of 10 days at half-salary for unused sick leave. If you wish to encourage attendance, you might instead offer dinner for two to those who have not taken any.

Attendance records ought to be mentioned next. Put a copy of the form you use in the appendix of the manual. This is a good place to slip in additional emphasis on punctuality. If an employee is unable to report to work on time, it should be her responsibility to telephone you or your office manager no later than one hour before the beginning of working hours. State how you will handle occasions when an employee is late. If anyone fails to show up for work without calling in, you may wish to say that she will be terminated unless extenuating circumstances are presented. Conclude with something on how you will handle brief absences for important reasons, such as visits to physicians. This is best done informally, with the approximate time being made up by working longer one day during the week.

Maternity leave must be covered. Ask your attorney about applicable federal (and sometimes state) law, and conform to it. Six weeks without pay is the norm, but some negotiation for each case is advisable. You should point out that the employee is entitled to receive all sick leave and vacation time accrued to that date, and only the remainder of the maternity leave will be absence without pay. Your guarantee of employment after maternity leave is the main point that should be in conformity with federal law. You may want your attorney to review this paragraph and to put a summary of the applicable statutes in the appendix to the manual.

Salary should be the next topic. Describe your method of arriving at starting salaries, the dates at which you give cost-of-living adjustments and how they are arrived at, the basis for raises and the dates they are effective, your method of determining bonuses and when they are given, and the approximate salary range for each position. See Chapter 16 for details. The payment periods should be specified: weekly, biweekly, semimonthly, or monthly. They are usually semimonthly. If this is your policy, specify the days of the month. The difference between semimonthly and biweekly is substantial, amounting to two weeks per year.

Three or four paragraphs will be required to summarize the various benefits offered to your employees. Perhaps three or four benefits can be made available in a solo practice—more in larger practices—but the number any one employee can choose is limited to two or three. This is sometimes called a "cafeteria plan." Mention those benefits required by law: workers' compensation, federal and state unemployment insurance, and the employer's contribution to FICA. Employees usually need to be reminded that these are continuing costs to you.

Among the available benefits are health insurance, life insurance, disability insurance, uniform allowance, time off with pay and expenses for continuing medical education, free parking, one or more retirement plans, and a profit-sharing plan. Stress those benefits that have retention potential, and, when appropriate, give the estimated incremental increases over a ten-year period of employment. The number of employees in a solo practice is not large enough to obtain favorable rates in the life, health, and disability field, so emphasis should be put upon retirement, profit-sharing, and short-term perquisites.

The details of the plans that you offer, the names of the insurance companies, the agents' names and telephone numbers, and the numbers of the policies should be given in the appendix of your manual. You might want to give the estimated dollar values and the approximate tax benefits.

Follow this portion on benefits with your policy on the provision of medical care for employees and their families. Each employee should be encouraged to have her own personal and family physician, but you might want to treat minor acute illnesses, dispense samples, or perform certain laboratory tests free of charge. Remind them of their coverage under workers' compensation for any accident or illness that is work related.

Next, explain the guidelines you observe in the selection, evaluation, and termination of employees. Chapter 16 will help you formulate these. The wording of your manual must be in conformity with state and federal laws.

On the topic of employee selection, include the sources of applicants, the method for advertising vacancies, the application procedure (with a sample application form in the appendix), the criteria used in the screening process, in reference checking, and in making the final decision, the purpose of the employment agreement form (with a sample of it in the appendix), and the length of the probationary period. You should coordinate the probationary period with your state law on unemployment compensation, because the amount of your contribution to this fund is based upon the size of your payroll *and* upon the claims made by past employees. If your probationary period is properly selected and stated, there will be no increase in your contributions to the fund when an employee is discharged during that time.

On the subject of staff evaluation, cover your indoctrination system, the periodic performance evaluation (with a sample form in the appendix), and the use of individual personnel records.

Termination is a subject that must be treated in detail. Start with a brief statement on your grievance procedure. This is usually informal in a small office, so a sentence stating that any employee having a problem should contact the office manager and/or you is all you need. The statement on your termination policy must be in accordance with state and federal laws, so I suggest you have your attorney review it. List those offenses for which an employee may be dismissed without notice, severance pay, or any other benefits. These include dishonesty, insubordination, gross negligence, misuse of controlled substances, working under the influence of drugs or alcohol, violation of confidential information, and a somewhat general, "gross unprofessional conduct."

In most states, two weeks' notice by the physician or the same by an employee is required for termination. However, the latter requirement is not enforceable, and two weeks' salary can be substituted for the former. Many states alow you to withhold accumulated vacation time if your employee does not give proper notice. Ask your attorney and cover this point in your manual.

Some states require a written letter of warning to an employee. If yours does, it is best given during the last performance review and signed by both of you, with a copy kept in the individual's personnel record. A face-to-face interview upon termination is also required by many states. If this is true in yours, make it clear that this will be provided. Confidentiality concerning the reason for termination is required to varying degrees by many states, and if applicable in yours, assurances should be given in your manual. Conclude with a statement that termination will not be for reasons of sex, race, religion, or age, but will be strictly related to demonstrated inability or unwillingness to perform the duties required by the position.

It is advisable to have at least two or three sentences covering the duty of your employees to respect the confidentiality of information about patients. Point out that it is improper to reveal information about a patient to *anyone*, even to another member of that patient's family, without the patient's consent. Casual conversations in the office or on the telephone should be avoided, and even those required during the care of a patient must be conducted in a professional manner out of earshot of other patients. This is a good place to add that unofficial conversations at any time on any subject are discouraged, except in the employees' lounge. End this paragraph by pointing out that the confidentiality code embraces *all* information about the patient—medical records, letters, and even entries in the appointment book.

Telephone procedure could be the next topic. Take whatever you like from Chapter 18 and summarize it. Add any thoughts of your own. State your policy on personal telephone calls during office hours. Usually the placing of personal calls by your employees is prohibited except on breaks or lunch hour, and more than an occasional incoming call is discouraged. Be sure to cover the handling of emergency telephone calls. Provide standard questions to ask to determine the nature and extent of the emergency, then set out the courses of action you wish your employees to take when you are in the office and when you are not. Some of this can be taken from your procedures for handling medical emergencies in the office, which will be described later.

Two or three paragraphs on handling mail will be necessary. Go into some detail, using the following outline:

1. Outgoing mail. Your letters are a reflection of the standards of your office, so typing should be neat and free of error. Signature stamps are never used. One copy is placed in the subject file and another in the chronological file. The latter is not often used, but when the subject copy is misplaced, it can be a godsend. Copies of all correspondence are confidential and kept in the file cabinet under lock and key when the office is closed. All outgoing mail, once placed in envelopes and addressed, is kept out of the view of patients.
2. Incoming mail. This should first be sorted into categories that you establish, with the appropriate action for each category spelled out in the manual. Some suggestions are:
   A. Category 1—all advertising material or "junk mail," including samples from pharmaceutical companies. All advertising is to be discarded upon receipt except for certain "throw-away" journals you want to look at. These are placed on your desk for you to go through and rip out what interests you. All samples are to be removed from their mailing containers and placed on your desk for your decision. Set up a storage system for the samples you wish to keep based upon the categories in the *Physicians' Desk Reference.* Inspect them every two or three months and discard those that are approaching their expiration date or that you no longer wish to retain. Samples to be discarded should be disposed of by flushing them down the toilet or using the garbage disposal. One caution: keeping samples provides a great temptation for your assistants to use them, or give them to their family, friends, or the patients. You are legally liable for any such action. The storage area should therefore be locked and the key retained by you. Some states have regulations concerning such inventories—ask your attorney.
   B. Category 2—personal mail. Although a lot of mail is marked "Personal" to get your attention, most of it is just advertising material. Therefore your assistant can be permitted some discretion. She might open envelopes on which the word "Personal" is printed, but leave unopened on your desk those on which "Personal" is either handwritten or typed.
   C. Category 3—statements and invoices. The assistant in charge of supplies and disbursement should review these first for correctness, insuring that the supplies have actually been received, the services provided, or the equipment delivered. Then they should be filed in an alphabetically indexed accordion file according to supplier, with your standard procedure followed thereafter.

D. Category 4—general mail, or all that remains. This is almost all first-class mail. Your assistant should open it and take the appropriate action. If it is from a patient, her first step is to verify that the address on the patient registration form conforms to that address. If your decision or action is required, the envelope is clipped to the letter along with relevant documents, so that when you dictate a reply you can refer to the correspondence and use the correct address. If the letter is in reference to a clinical rather than a business matter, it should be attached to the patient's chart after she has verified that the information referred to in the letter is in the chart.

It is a good idea to scoop up all mail as it comes into the office about once a month and go over every piece with your assistants. This not only ensures that your system is working well but allows you to make adjustments to it. It is also an excellent way to pick up comments from patients on the quality of your practice, to learn about account complaints that might have been kept from you, and to find out that a journal you subscribed to or notices of medical meetings were being discarded as "advertising."

The next topic in your manual describes your procedure for making appointments and scheduling patients. Take whatever you need from Chapter 19. Put in a sentence of two about your patient registration form, describing its use and importance, and stressing the necessity for accuracy, completeness, and periodic updating. Put a copy of the form in the appendix.

Follow this with a description of the way in which patients should be received by the front office, how your patient information booklet is to be distributed, some ways in which waiting might be minimized, and the way in which the patients should be conducted to the examination rooms and prepared. Some physicians have a sign-in book at the reception desk with space for changes in address or other items. A sign-in book is just as depressing and impersonal to the patient as the closed glass partition usually found in the same offices. A cheerful question at some point during the patient's reception is a much better way of getting this information.

Next, describe your medical record system, using Chapter 20 as your guide. Reiterate that no chart is to be removed from the office for any reason.

The next section is on fees. Start with how these are determined and periodically adjusted. Cover the use of charge slips, ledger cards, day sheet, time-of-service collection, routine billing, and collection procedures on delinquent accounts by summarizing the discussions in Chapters 21 and 22. At the conclusion, two or three sentences explaining permanent financial records and the role of your accountant would be appropriate.

A separate paragraph on insurance claim forms and their preparation will be necessary, and this can be adapted from Chapter 23. Motivation is everything (well, almost), so stress the importance of preparing these forms completely and correctly.

The most common clinical procedures performed in the office might be the next topic. Give a brief description of each, including patient preparation, the instruments and arrangements required, and the type of assistance that is needed. Your specialty will have its unique procedures, but some are common to most practices: taking vital signs, physical examinations, determination of visual acuity, audiometry, pelvic examinations and Pap smears, proctosigmoidoscopy, injections, instrument care and sterilization, sterile precautions, casts or dressings, electrocardiograms and physical therapy modalities. At least two or three sentences should make it clear that an assistant must be within earshot any time you are examining a patient of the opposite sex, and *in the room* whenever a pelvic examination is being done. End with your policy on consent forms.

Next, include a short section on procedures to be followed in the event of a fire, earthquake, tornado, or other emergency situations requiring a plan for evacuation or for seeking special shelter.

Medical emergencies that occur in the office or nearby must be anticipated, and a full treatment of this subject will comprise one of the most important parts of your manual. Put considerable thought into this section. The instructions to your staff should allow for three situations: (1) you are in the office; (2) you are readily available within a few minutes; (3) you are unavailable, and your assistants must act alone.

First, list half-a-dozen or so of the most commonly encountered emergency situations. These could include syncope, choking, shock, anaphylaxis, acute asthma attack, acute abdomen, chest pain, cardiac arrhythmia, cerebrovascular accident, seizure, poisoning, bleeding, burns, and other major injuries. Describe each sufficiently so that your aides can recognize actual cases. Then outline the proper action for them to take in each of the three situations in the paragraph above.

You can assemble your own emergency kit, but commercially prepared ones are available. The best are those prepared by **Banyan International,** 2118 East Interstate 20, P.O. Box 1779, Abilene, TX 79604. These come in a durable aluminum case with handle and security seal. They are easily opened so that the contents are displayed and readily available;

these contents range from simple first aid kits to sophisticated resuscitation and surgical equipment. Banyan also has a good system for updating cardiopulmonary and other drugs by regular mailed reminders that contain check-off lists to use for ordering.

Community resources for medical emergencies should also be listed in your manual. You do not need to list the current numbers, just refer your employees to the lists you keep at the telephones. The numbers there will include police, fire, paramedical service, hospital emergency rooms, nearby consultants, the poison control center, crisis centers, and ambulance services.

Describing the medical emergencies and what to do about them in your manual is not enough. Springing for a good kit still does not take care of it. You must hold regular training drills. Schedule these once a month on what would otherwise be your day or afternoon off. Ask one assistant to volunteer as the victim, give her a note on the symptoms to display and call upon her acting ability. Supervise the response of your other assistants, then sit down with them and critique the whole performance afterward. Document each of these drills. If a patient has one of the emergencies that you have prepared and drilled for, this record might be your best defense in the event of a lawsuit.

All personnel should be certified in cardiopulmonary resuscitation. Courses are conducted regularly at local hospitals, by the **American Heart Association,** and the **American Red Cross.** Keep records of staff certifications and make sure they are up to date.

The next topic concerns hospitalized patients. Start with the hospitals used, explaining how admissions are handled, reports filed, hospital-based charges processed, and hospital surgery and procedures scheduled. Outline a standard system for making appointments to see patients after discharge.

Nonemergency community resources applicable to your practice would be worth including here, as would the names and numbers of the physicians that you most often use as consultants. If these change frequently, list them in the appendix and refer to that list.

Something should be said about laboratory tests. Describe how specimens are obtained, labeled, and processed. State which tests are done in your office and which sent out, naming the outside laboratories used. Explain how telephone reports and lab slips are handled, and how results are relayed to the patient. Another paragraph should cover special tests and procedures done outside the office: where they are done, special preparation or instructions required, and how the charges are handled.

You may want to include a paragraph or two on miscellaneous subjects: checking inventory, ordering supplies, stocking clinical areas, housecleaning, replenishing your bag, precautions to be observed with prescription pads, narcotics control, duties of personnel during your vacations, and maintenance procedures for major items of equipment.

The last paragraph of your manual reiterates the purpose stated in its opening paragraph, but in different words. The last sentence welcomes any suggestions or questions the assistants might have.

The preparation of a good office manual sounds like a lot of work, and it is. That's why it was so often put off by many physicians in the past. But it will save you and your employees much *more* work through the months and years ahead. It will also help avoid misunderstandings and conflicts, raise morale, increase efficiency, and promote better patient care. It is more than worth the time and trouble taken to prepare it.

16

Office Staff

Once you have your "shortcut" manual prepared, you are ready to hire your first employee. Do this at least two months before opening your door. You are about to take the most important step of all in setting up practice. Three-fourths of all medical office problems concern employees! Personnel management is the area most physicians do least well, so this chapter will be an extensive one.

Throughout the book I try to present the most information where the need is greatest. The assumption of the first part of this chapter is that you are just starting out and will be handling the hiring process yourself. This is the time that you are the least experienced and need the most advice. The rest of the chapter is more for the established physician.

One comment before we proceed any further. You already suspect that my suggestions for managing personnel are going to be detailed, and you are right. Some new physicians may be tempted to skip over much of this chapter with the rationale that there is no need to get into this the way businesses do. Let me put it this way: you *are* in a business and have to set up *some* sort of system. Why not start with one that is complete and proven successful for physicians, and that is modeled upon those used in the business world by experts in personnel management? It *is* more trouble at the start, but in the long run a well-structured system will save you a great deal of time and trouble. If you are still skeptical, then promise yourself you will simplify this system when you have enough experience to do so knowledgeably.

The first employee in your office is crucial in many respects. She will be the one with the longest experience, the one who has received the fullest training by you, and the one whose personality and ways of operating will influence all subsequent employees. So choose wisely and choose well.

Because ours is a litigious age, before you do anything else, obtain a summary from your attorney of the federal and state legislation relating to employees and employment that is applicable to your practice. Every step in the hiring process must comply with these laws—from your first inquiries, through advertisements, telephone screening, and the personal interview, to the final decision. The same is true of periodic performance reviews and termination.

The most significant federal legislation affecting employee hiring and firing is summarized below. Most states have, to a greater or lesser degree, followed this in preparing their own laws.

1. The 1964 **Civil Rights Act,** as amended in 1972 by the **Equal Employment Opportunities Act,** outlaws job discrimination on the basis of race, color, sex, religion, and national origin. This act applies to any business or activity that receives federal aid, which of course includes Medicaid and Medicare funds. Some state laws are even more restrictive, prohibiting discrimination on the basis of weight, number of dependents, and other factors. In general, courts apply whichever is the more restrictive law, state or federal.
2. The 1967 **Age Discrimination in Employment Act**, as amended in 1978, makes it illegal to discriminate against the 40-to-70-year age group. Although this act applies only to employers with 25 or more employees, many states have similar legislation that smaller operations are subject to.
3. The **Fair Labor Standards Act** of 1938, as amended several times, applies to all businesses engaging in interstate commerce. If you order any supplies or equipment from out of state, or see a patient who is a resident of another state, this Act applies to your practice. It sets guidelines for minimum wages, the work week, and overtime.

It is not necessary to obtain the legislation itself and attempt to wade through the legal language.. This is what you pay your attorney for. He can give you a simplified breakdown of all applicable federal and state laws in two or three typewritten pages.

After obtaining this summary from your attorney, the next step is to look over the list of tasks that will be performed in your office and assign each one to the person who will be responsible for it. You already prepared this list when you designed your office. The division is easy with the first employee. There will be two groups—nonclinical for her and clinical for you, for the most part, with some overlap. Give thought now as to how your second employee will fit in, and tentatively divide the tasks three ways.

The third step is to prepare a job description for the first employee. There are five elements in any job description:

1. The job title
2. A brief description of the duties
3. Prerequisites in terms of education, skills, and experience
4. The actual tasks the employee is expected to perform, divided as to primary and secondary
5. The limitations of the position. Specify the tasks that the employee will *not* perform, the person she is directly responsible to, and her authority boundaries in relation to others in the office

Here is how a job description might go for the first employee. The job title would be "Medical Receptionist," with the description of her duties as follows: "Greeting patients and other visitors, answering the telephone, making appointments, accepting payments and issuing receipts, and keeping financial records." You may wish to end with a general phrase such as, "Miscellaneous office duties as assigned." The prerequisites might be: "A high school graduate, with ability to type and file and experience in public contact, preferably in a medical office." Most of the fourth and fifth parts of the job description can be adapted from your divided list of tasks. These are only suggestions to get you started. The final form is your own.

With the job description completed, the next step is determining a salary. Ask your colleagues what they pay, and inquire at the personnel offices of your hospitals about salaries for similar positions. Remember, hospital employees must work nights, weekends, and holidays, so their pay scale is a little higher. You can also request the latest wage survey from **The Information Office,** Room 1539, **U.S. Bureau of Labor Statistics,** 441 G Street NW, Washington, D.C. 20212. Look up your geographical area and find comparable positions. When you have settled on a range, pick a salary toward the top of the scale. Low salaries tend to result in low everything else—quality of employees, morale, energy, efficiency, and attitude—with the one exception of high turnover. Cheap help is *not* cheap.

Next decide on the benefits you will offer. Most office employees are more interested in take-home pay than in benefits. Some already have health insurance through their husband's employment. Still others might prefer flexible hours more than any benefits in order to care for small children at home. As I have said before, it is best to offer an array of benefits from which each employee can choose two or three, and adjust the dollar differences to be comparable for all.

Then you have to select the source from which you will obtain your first employee. The most qualified candidates are graduates of an accredited medical assistant school. If you are in an urban area, you will find several schools listed in the yellow pages, but most of them will not be accredited. Call the **Committee on Allied Health Education**

and Accreditation of the AMA, which accredits such schools, and ask for the names of approved institutions near you. Each school has a placement service, which will provide names of members of the latest class to graduate as well as of past graduates wanting to change positions. If there is no such school near you, the same caliber of employee may be found in one of the 500 local chapters of the **American Association of Medical Assistants.** Their headquarters is located at 20 North Wacker Drive, Suite 1575, Chicago, IL 60606. Ask them about chapters in your area. Those medical assistants who are not graduates of accredited schools but individually pursue equivalent courses of study with on-the-job training also receive certification by the AAMA, boosting total membership to over 12,000 nationwide. Certified medical assistants are entitled to use the initials **CMA** after their names. Those who go on to acquire additional qualifications in administration use the designation **CMA-A,** while others attain similar expertise in clinical areas and use **CMA-C** after their names.

The second best source of quality applicants is a community or junior college with a two-year program in the health sciences. A business program is almost as good. Although the candidates will not be as suitably trained as a certified medical assistant, there are other advantages to using this source. Some screening was done when the applicant was admitted, and further screening took place throughout her education. Some of her education will be applicable to your office. You can get a transcript of her grades and obtain reliable references from faculty members who know her well. These colleges also have placement services you may wish to use.

As you pursue sources that are less likely to yield well-trained candidates, you may have to remind yourself that you are primarily interested in aptitude, a trait composed of intelligence and willingness to learn, and secondarily in a friendly and engaging personality. The skills that your first employee needs to have are really rather basic. If she has aptitude, she can learn all she needs to know while your practice is developing—through your instruction, from the reference sources in the front office, by taking courses, and by using audio or video tapes. On the other hand, if an assistant is highly trained and experienced but a bit rigid, she will run your office exactly as she did those of her previous employers. This may not suit you at all. So although it is certainly desirable, experience is *not* necessarily the first quality to look for. I place it after aptitude and personality.

The third best source is the personnel department of the hospital you use. These departments keep a file of recent applications, and many applicants have already been interviewed and evaluated. Inquire, too, at any large medical groups in your area—they maintain similar files. Do not hire current hospital or group employees unless the contact is initiated by the employee and the person is just too good to pass up. When you do, be sure you smooth ruffled feathers as best you can.

An employment agency is usually a poor source, but you may find an exception. State agencies are particularly poor, but private ones are often little better. Many seem to operate on the theory that if they inundate you with a large number of unscreened applicants, you might in desperation hire one—and the agency can then collect its fee. But you may find an agency that specializes in medical office assistants, screens applicants carefully, and gives an impression of each before you interview. If you have such an agency in your area, use it. Most physicians who do offer to reimburse the employee for all or part of the fee and distribute this repayment over a year's time in order to encourage retention.

If there is a placement service at your local medical society, it may be a superb source. One more you can use when you are ready to hire your second employee is your first—she will let the word out, make inquiries, and may discover a jewel. You can also tell your colleagues you are looking if you want to, but doing so rarely turns up applicants.

I have listed the most commonly used method—the placement of a newspaper ad—last because I have tried to rank sources by the quality of the candidates that result. I don't know how to rate this source, because it produces a large number of applicants with all sorts of backgrounds, and quality may be there or it may not be. So I would suggest using a classified ad *along with* one or two of the other methods.

The overwhelming response from newspaper ads is both a blessing and a curse. The best way to cope with it is to place a "blind ad" asking that a resume with a handwritten cover letter be mailed to a rented post office box or to a box number at the newspaper. The only drawback to using a blind ad is that it inhibits an applicant who is currently employed and is worried about contacting her own employer. But since such applicants are few, this is a minor objection. I do not recommend putting your telephone number in the ad with the intent of screening the applicants this way. In a rural area where you expect only a few applicants you might, but not otherwise.

There are seven ingredients in a good newspaper ad:

1. The title of the position you want to fill, preferably in large capital letters to attract attention
2. The type of practice (with two or three words that describe it in an appealing way) and its general location, not the actual address
3. The duties that are to be performed, described broadly but briefly
4. The experience required

5. A statement on salary. This is almost a necessity, but a precise dollar value should not be given. Even stating a salary range has certain disadvantages. A phrase such as "Salary according to experience" is best
6. The date the position will be available
7. The means of contact

Think of some dignified way to attract attention to your ad, such as putting a border around it. Select the newspapers that are most widely read in your area by the type of applicant you seek. If there is a large city nearby, run an ad in a paper of that city also. Many assistants will commute or be willing to move. Place ads in at least two and possibly three papers. Just before you send the ad in, review it to see if it is correct and to make sure there is no discriminatory wording in it.

While you are waiting for the replies, prepare a form letter to send the applicants who are rejected. Each should be individually typed and addressed, but the body of the letter can be the same for all. A good letter of rejection contains four elements, worded as you wish:

1. Appreciation for the application
2. Assurance that the application has been given careful consideration
3. A statement that another applicant more closely meets the requirements of the position
4. A closing sentence advising that the application will be kept on file in the event of a future opening

Before the first reply to your ad comes in, obtain the application form you want to use from a cataloguer and make photocopies. Modify it as you wish, but be certain the modifications are legal. I have found the Colwell form satisfactory with the addition of a question on smoking habits, a request for the telephone numbers of previous employers and references, and deletion of the questions on birth date, children, and illnesses. (See Fig. 16–1.) Questions most likely to be in violation of the law are those concerned with religion, race, gender, marital status, age, criminal record, maiden name (father's surname may indicate national origin), number of children, and employment of the spouse.

When you receive a resume with a handwritten cover letter, notice how much you can tell about an applicant by the completeness and neatness of the resume and from the letter itself. When you find illegible handwriting and serious problems with grammar, spelling, or punctuation, you should reject these candidates outright. This is largely what the job consists of.

If you receive a large number of acceptable applications, telephone screening will be necessary to select the top three or four. There are two principles to follow in making these calls. Use a guide to keep your questions legal, and write all your notes on a sheet of paper that is later destroyed. I have found it convenient to clip a piece of paper bearing only the applicant's name to a blank application form, and then tick off the questions on the form that I wish to ask. If you use the application form for your *notes,* it may be inadvertently filed. The sheet you have written on is then clipped to the resume and letter, and the same application form is used again as a guide for the next telephone screening. Stick to the questions on the form and ask the same questions of each candidate. Even telephone screening must follow federal and state laws. In addition to the answers to your questions, you can tell a lot about an applicant from her voice, her use of correct English, her pronunciation, her manner in responding to questions, and her telephone personality. These are also important parts of the job.

When most of the replies to the ads are in, set up personal interviews with the top three or four candidates. Interview all of them before making your decision. Schedule half an hour for each at a time when you will not be rushed, distracted, or interrupted. Try to have all the interviews on the same day to be better able to compare applicants.

When each applicant arrives, greet her in your reception area, introduce yourself, and give her a copy of the job description and an application form to fill out before the interview. If the interview will be delayed for any reason, leave her your Personnel and Procedures Manual to read.

The interview itself usually begins with a tour of the suite, which is a good ice breaker and also allows you to observe her when she is not posing. It also gives her a good opportunity to ask questions about the practice. When you have completed the tour and are seated in your consultation room, start by asking a bland question, such as "How was the traffic?" Then review her resume, cover letter, the notes you made during the telephone screening, and her application. Note any gaps in education or employment history. It helps put her at ease if you look up from time to time and tell her a little more about yourself, your practice, and your office. Be honest or you will have difficulties down the line. But don't describe the job at this point or she may tailor her later answers. Ask her if she has any questions, then try to answer them truthfully. Continue the interview with questions that arise naturally from the completed application form. Don't ask questions that are already answered on the application—just have her amplify and clarify. Phrase questions so that they are open-ended and cannot be answered with a simple yes or no. Get her to volunteer

Classification ______________________________
(Not to be Filled in by Applicant)

Date ______________________________

APPLICATION FOR EMPLOYMENT

Name ______________________________ Soc. Sec. No. ______________ Phone No. ______________
(Last) (First) (Middle)

Address ______________________________ Birth Date ______________________________
(No.) (Street) (City) (State) (Must be completed by applicant under 19 years of age)

Spouse's name ______________ No. & Ages of Children ______________ Other dependents ______________

What transportation can you use to get to and from work? ______________________________

What position are you applying for? ______________ Full time ______________ Part time ______________

EDUCATION RECORD		From		To		Did you Graduate?	Course
Type of School	Name and Place	Mo.	Yr.	Mo.	Yr.		
Last Grammar or Jr. H.S.							
Last High or Prep. School							
College or University							
Specialty Training							
Other							

EXPERIENCE—PLEASE ACCOUNT FOR ALL TIME SINCE LEAVING SCHOOL—LIST LAST EMPLOYER FIRST

Firm Name	Place	Your Position	Describe the Work you did	From		To		Salary or Wages	Reason for Leaving

May we contact the employers listed above? ______________ If not, indicate which ones you do wish to be contacted ______________

PLEASE COMPLETE REVERSE SIDE OF THIS SHEET

THIS OFFICE DOES NOT DISCRIMINATE ON THE BASIS OF AGE, RACE, COLOR, RELIGION, SEX OR NATIONAL ORIGIN.

Form 9877 Colwell Co., Champaign, Illinois

Give name, address, and business of each of two references:
(No relatives, but at least one former employer)

What special equipment have you used?

Describe previous experience you believe will help you in employment with us. ____

When could you start to work? ____ What salary would you consider to start? ____

Do you have any chronic ailments or other physical limitations which prevent you from performing certain kinds of work? ____

How many days have you been ill during the past two years? ____

Have you ever been hospital confined? ____ Where? ____ When? ____ Why? ____

Are you willing to submit to a medical examination? ____ Have you ever had any kind of industrial accident or occupational disease? ____

Would you agree to being bonded? ____

(Signature of Applicant)

Interviewed by: ____ Date ____

This Application For Employment is prepared for use throughout the United States. The Colwell Company assumes no responsibility for the inclusion of any questions which, when asked by the employer of the job applicant, may violate state and/or federal law.

Figure 16–1. (Courtesy of Colwell Systems, Inc., Champaign, Illinois.)

information whenever possible. Your comments on her answers should be neutral, and it's best if you do not take notes.

When you are finished with the application form, refer to a list of supplemental questions at hand and select the most appropriate. Here are some suggestions; once again, I'd advise you to have your attorney review your list before you use it:

1. Why are you applying for this position?
2. Tell me about your duties in your present or last position.
3. Have you had any associate or superior whom you particularly liked or disliked? Why?
4. What are your career goals? What would your goals be in this office?
5. What are your strong points as you see them?
6. What are your weak points?
7. Can you think of any personal problems that might interfere with the performance of your duties in this office?
8. Why do you think you might succeed working here?
9. Why might you fail?
10. What would you would bring to this office in terms of personality, education, skills, or other attributes?
11. Which aspects of your present or past positions did you like best, and which the least?
12. What accomplishments in your present or last position gave you the most satisfaction?
13. How do you feel about working late or under pressure?
14. Is there anything that irritates you in working with people?
15. What are your salary expectations?
16. The last question is usually an open-ended one: What else would you like to tell me about yourself?

Throughout the interview, be guided only by items on the application form and the questions on your list. Do not wander.

Allow enough time for her to reply to each question and to ask questions of her own. As you listen to the replies, use your "third ear." That is, listen not only with your ears and your mind, but tune in to your feelings.

The subject of salary will come up. When it does, inform her of the salary range and the benefits available, but avoid making a precise commitment. If you are pressed to give an exact figure, do so, but let her know it is negotiable. You would like to interview all of your top candidates before setting a definite salary.

When you are satisfied with the interview, tell her what happens next and when, determine the date she will be available, be sure that you have a current telephone number, stand up, thank her, and escort her to the door. Make no commitment at this time, but do promise to let her know your decision one way or the other as soon as possible.

Immediately after each interview, grade the candidate using a simple code. Assigning numerical values to half-a-dozen major qualifications and figuring a total for each candidate is a good way to put applicants on a relative scale. Items you might include are apparent health, energy, enthusiasm, dress, grooming, personality, education, training, and experience. Put your grading and general comments on the same sheet of paper you used for the telephone screening. Each application form must be kept on file for two years in case of legal action, so anything written on the form itself should be carefully considered.

Next it is time to check the references. Don't overlook this step. Always telephone at least two, speaking peer-to-peer. Never omit the last employer. Writing letters is a useless exercise that can cause legal problems at both ends. Suggested subjects to ask about are the dates she was employed, position held, promotions, salary, and raises, duties performed, ability at these duties, particular problems encountered, attendance record, punctuality, and the employer's version of the reason she left. The last two questions are: "Would you rehire her if she should reapply at your office?" and "Is there anything else you would like to tell me about her?" Prepare a simple list of questions for use ahead of time, have it at hand, and jot down the answers on that ubiquitous sheet of paper you have been using. Be alert for any hesitation or evasiveness, and pursue it.

Then it is time to make your decision. If two or more applicants are close, interview them a second time. Don't deliberate too long. The best candidate can be lost by a delay of half a day. Once you have decided, call her and offer her the position with a definite salary. This is the time for any final negotiations and adjustments to the salary and benefits. Don't let a few dollars' difference stand in the way, but cut short any attempts at manipulation. Choose a date for her to report that will allow time for thorough orientation and instruction. Do not reject the second candidate on your list just yet. Wait a few days to see how the first choice performs under office conditions. You can send rejection letters to the others, however.

Now review all the application forms before they are filed to make sure they bear only those notes that you wish to be part of the record. State clearly on each, in the space allowed, the reason for acceptance or rejection. Be certain that this reason complies with the law. For example, "lacks recent experience" is legal, but "too old" is not. As stated before, keep these applications on file at least two years, or as long as your attorney advises.

When your new employee reports, sit down with her and go over the employment agreement form (see Fig. 16–2). You will both sign each copy. One is for her and the other for your personnel files.

The orientation of a new employee should follow a plan. It is advisable to schedule the first few hours for a time when no patients are to be seen. The first part is usually a more thorough tour of your office. The second might be a discussion of the job description with amplification and illustration. The third could consist of her reading the office manual and signing the face sheet, acknowledging that she has read and understands it. Then assign simple tasks that can be monitored easily.

Be available for questions during the first few days, and set aside time at the end of each morning and afternoon for a quiet discussion. Praise her whenever possible, even if only for her attitude and spirit. As soon as you can, have a name tag prepared to help her feel she belongs. Gentle reminders on some of the requirements in your office manual—such as your rules on smoking, personal telephone calls, jewelry and makeup—should be given early. Have her fill out a W-4 form. Start her attendance record (see Fig. 16–3). Setting up her personnel record will be described later in this chapter.

Have her become familiar with the front office reference books and the other manuals and instruction materials you have assembled there as soon as possible. Ask your major insurance carriers to send representatives to talk to her. She should also familiarize herself with the office forms you will be using and with your patient information booklet. Have the accountant come in to explain your bookkeeping system and her role in maintaining it, and to answer any questions she may have. Arrange outside continuing medical education for her and encourage her to join the local chapter of the AAMA if there is one in your vicinity.

Many physicians avoid or delay setting up a system for performance review. But clear communication with employees about the quality of their work must be systematic if poor employees are to improve and good ones to be properly rewarded. It is actually much easier for you and fairer for them to utilize a system than to do without one. You can't put evaluation off for long. New employees should have their first review at the end of the first month and their second three months later, coinciding with the end of your probationary period. Thereafter it is conducted every six months on the same date for all employees.

Once again, it is best to use a prepared form. After each performance review, the completed form is filed in the employee's personnel record.

EMPLOYMENT AGREEMENT

(Complete in duplicate. One copy to employee, one for personnel records.)

NAME ______________________________ DATE ______________

JOB TITLE ______________________________ FULL TIME/PART TIME ______

DUTIES AND RESPONSIBILITIES (check appropriate space)

______ Listed on reverse side. ______ Copy of job description attached.

WORKING HOURS

Usual working hours are from ______ to ______; lunch ______ ; breaks ______.

Days per week: S ______ M ______ T ______ W ______ Th ______ F ______ S______

When working hours vary, you will be notified in the following manner:

____

____

____

____

SALARY AND BENEFITS

Starting rate: ______________________________

Provisions for increases: ______________________________

____

Paid: Vacation days ______ ; Sick days ______ ; Personal time ______;

Other benefits ______________________________

____

____

____

UNIFORM REQUIREMENTS (if applicable)

____

____

CONDITIONAL PERIOD OF EMPLOYMENT

For each new employee the first ______ weeks of employment are considered a conditional or probationary period. During this time the employee may leave, or be dismissed, with 24 hours notice.

TERMINATION

The employee is expected to give ______ weeks notice.

If dismissed, the employee will receive ______ weeks notice or the equivalent in severence pay. In the event of fraud, theft or unprofessional conduct, the employee may be dismissed without notice or severence pay.

______________________ ______________________

Employee's signature Employer's signature

Form 9876 Colwell Co., Champaign, Illinois

Figure 16–2. (Courtesy of Colwell Systems, Inc., Champaign, Illinois.)

PERSONNEL ATTENDANCE RECORD

EMPLOYEE ____________________ JOB TITLE ____________________ YEAR __________

Employee is entitled to

_______ sick days

_______ personal days

_______ vacation days

(*note time carried forward from previous year.)

CODE

S = sick leave

P = personal time

V = vacation time

L = late

A = absent for reason other than the above (if employee does not call in, circle in red)

MONTHLY TOTALS

	1	2	3	4	5	6	7	8	9	10	11	12	13	14	15	16	17	18	19	20	21	22	23	24	25	26	27	28	29	30	31	S	P	V	L	A
JANUARY																																				
FEBRUARY																																				
MARCH																																				
APRIL																																				
MAY																																				
JUNE																																				
JULY																																				
AUGUST																																				
SEPTEMBER																																				
OCTOBER																																				
NOVEMBER																																				
DECEMBER																																				
ANNUAL SUMMARY																																				

Form 9874 Colwell Co., Champaign, Illinois

Figure 16–3. (Courtesy of Colwell Systems, Inc., Champaign, Illinois.)

You can use a standard form from a cataloguer but it is best to prepare your own, based on the attributes *you* consider to be the most important in your practice (see Fig. 16–4). Decide on these attributes and list them down the left side with a column to the right for rating each trait, setting up a wider third column for comments. Monitoring improvement is made easier by assigning a numerical value to each rating, adding the ratings at each review, and comparing totals (see Fig. 16–4).

Suggested traits for inclusion in the first column are personal appearance, punctuality, knowledge of job, industriousness, adaptability, dependability, disposition, cross-training skills, quality of performance, judgment, initiative, leadership, politeness, ability to take constructive criticism, cooperation with other members of the staff, and efforts made to improve job skills. You will not need all of these—just pick a dozen or so that you believe to be the most significant.

Before the performance review, have the employee fill out the performance review form herself with a pencil or a different color pen than the one you will use. The review should be conducted privately in your consultation room at a time when you will not be interrupted. Allow about 15 minutes for this on job time. Have her personnel record at hand. Discuss her own ratings first. With the form on the desk visible to you both, enter your ratings and write your comments. Discuss the differences. Try to focus on problem areas and don't let the discussion wander. Determine the reasons for any problems and work out plans with her for their correction. Try to end the session with a positive statement about one or more attributes she has demonstrated.

The salary of each employee must be reviewed at least annually. The best time to do this is at the conclusion of a semiannual performance

PERFORMANCE REVIEW

Attribute	Rating	Comments
Total		Total Last Review

General Comments: ______________________________________

Recommended Action: ___________________________________

Employee's Signature   Date   Reviewer's Signature

Ratings:
1 = Unsatisfactory
2 = Requires Improvement
3 = Adequate
4 = Above Average
5 = Outstanding

Figure 16–4.

evaluation. This review is extremely important for employee morale. Too many physicians drift on year after year keeping their employees at the same salary, ignoring improved performance and the rising cost of living. Employees may be reluctant to raise the issue and become quietly resentful. If you establish definite dates for salary review and discuss the subject honestly, your employees' morale will be lifted, even if no changes are made. In a small office where automatic promotions accompanied by salary increases are not possible, as they are in large operations, a "cap" or salary ceiling is not advisable. If you do have one, it should be mentioned at each review, pointing out that neither the cost-of-living adjustment nor bonuses are affected by such a cap.

There are three types of salary increments—cost-of-living adjustments, merit raises, and bonuses. These three must be kept distinct. As a minimum, the salary is raised by a cost-of-living adjustment on a fixed date each year. This is the same date for all employees regardless of the date of employment, and should be based on *local* cost-of-living figures. The national Consumer Price Index may not be applicable in your area.

Merit raises are based upon performance reviews and should never be tied to seniority or to any index of practice productivity. They are given strictly for good performance on the job. If one is to be granted, it is discussed at the appropriate performance evaluation and instituted at the next anniversary of employment.

Bonuses, however, *are* related to practice productivity. If both fixed and variable expenses are deducted from the gross over a representative period, say 6 months, each employee could receive 5 per cent, or perhaps more, of the difference (which represents practice profit). The period must be representative, i.e., not span your vacation or an exceptional collection effort, yet short enough to be effective in motivating your staff. Employees should always know how the bonuses are calculated. Giving a bonus to one employee for a particular job well done is not recommended. It does boost the morale of that individual, but over time such bonuses tend to be inequitable and to have a bad effect upon the whole staff. They also foster unrealistic expectations on the part of other employees. Bonuses on birthdays, if not related to productivity, tend to be less appreciated over time and eventually are regarded as a right and so lose all effectiveness. It may be difficult to avoid one at Christmas, so make it clear if you do give one then, exactly how it is related to office productivity. Better a gift than a bonus. Instead of giving all bonuses in cash, from time to time give a uniform allowance or some other benefit that is deductible by you and not taxable to the employee. Your dollars will go farther this way.

Staff conferences are important and should be held every month. Although they may not be productive for the first few months, keep having them and they will be rewarding beyond your expectations. It is here you will learn about most of the problems in your practice *and* most of the solutions. A good time is on the day you usually take your afternoon off. Set an agenda for each conference and adhere to it. A week or so ahead of time, jot down the topics you want to discuss on a sheet of paper setting the date and time of the next conference. Post it in the office and invite employees to add their own topics. This is the agenda. The conference must start on time and all must attend. Encourage discussion and suggestions. Listen carefully, because early warning signs of employee disaffection can be detected at these conferences. Your own ideas should be brought forth as suggestions, not edicts. These conferences are an excellent arena for the education of your employees and also an opportunity for you to provide motivation.

By law, a personnel record must be kept for each employee. It is really quite simple to compile. Start with a manila folder and have the employee's name typed on the tab. The first item in each is the job description. The second is the resume and cover letter the employee sent in. Then comes the application form that was filled out at the time of hiring. Periodically, check the address and telephone number on it to make sure that both are current and correct. Next is the employment agreement, then the performance evaluations. Any oral warnings should be documented on these evaluations, and any in writing included as separate items. All written warnings should have the employee's signature under an acknowledgment that the two of you have discussed the matter. This acknowledgment is required as a precondition of termination under some state laws. The next component is the pay record. See Chapter 24 for the form. The initial salary and all raises, bonuses, and benefits are recorded on it, with effective dates. If you provide an annual summary, keep a copy here. The last component is the attendance record indicating vacation time, sick leave, and emergency leave, both earned and taken. It is advisable to keep personnel records in a locked cabinet or desk drawer to which you have the only key. They must be retained for at least three years after an employee has left your employ, or as long as your lawyer advises.

Let's talk a bit about attendance and overtime. By law, an attendance record must be maintained, but you certainly don't need a time clock. A suitable form is illustrated in Figure 16–3. The assistant who keeps it only needs to make the entries once a week from memory. Make sure this is done and spot-check for discrepancies at least once a month.

In private practice it is often necessary for employees to stay late when patient care requires it. Sometimes paperwork deadlines mean late hours as well. So the problem of overtime is a constantly recurring one. The point was made in the last chapter that if you cannot give compensatory time off during that same week, you are required to pay one and a half times the salary for any time worked in excess of 40 hours during any one week. Compensatory time in a subsequent week is not allowed. If you are ever found in violation of this particular point by the National Labor Relations Board, you may have to pay overtime to all employees over the past several years, including those who have left your employ. However, *administrative* and *professional* employees are exempt from these overtime regulations. The meanings of these terms are carefully set out by the United States Department of Labor, and your attorney will provide you with these definitions. The positions must truly be professional or administrative—assigning such a title is not sufficient. There is another reason to be careful. Pension law requires that all part-time employees working more than 1000 hours a year be covered by your pension plan, so the IRS may also come in to look over your attendance records for *their* purposes.

Of the four mistakes concerning overtime that most frequently result in legal problems for physicians, only one has been mentioned—failure to give either compensatory time in the same week or time and a half pay for overtime. The second has to do with the lunch hour. Since it is better practice of medicine to have the lunch hour covered by an employee in the office rather than by an impersonal answering service, and since some employees like to bring their lunch, it would seem to be an innocent thing to ask an employee to pick up the phone during the lunch hour if it should ring, or to talk to any patients who may come in. If she does this either on your instruction *or voluntarily*, the entire lunch time must be considered part of her working week, even if she does not perform a single task. For this reason, the assignment of employees to such duties during the lunch hour should be rotated so that no one employee exceeds a total of 40 hours per week.

The third overtime situation that frequently creates difficulties for physicians occurs on their day or afternoon off. An employee may dawdle when the physician leaves and then work after normal closing hours without his knowledge in order to accomplish her assigned work. This additional time also counts toward her work week of 40 hours. Clear instructions in your office manual, periodic reminders, and occasional unexpected visits can discourage this.

The fourth way you can get into trouble happens at the end of a typical working day. You leave the office, ask your employees to lock up when they are through, and assume that they will leave at the scheduled time. Sometimes one or more may stay late to catch up (or read a novel); that time counts in their work week also. The same remedies apply. Forewarned is forearmed.

Fringe benefits were discussed in Chapter 15, but one more suggestion is pertinent here. At the time the annual W-2 form is given to an employee each January, staple a sheet to it outlining the dollar value of all benefits received during that year. Items to select from, as appropriate in your practice, are cost-of-living adjustments, raises, bonuses, and overtime pay. Include your contributions to state and federal unemployment funds, state disability plan, and FICA, even though most of these figures are reported on the W-2. Add retirement plan contributions, premiums paid for health, disability, life, and workers' compensation insurance, holidays, vacations, sick leave, emergency leave, uniform allowance, lunches given them during conferences or on other occasions, refreshments, medical treatment you may provide, any petty cash that may be given them for various purposes, and allowance for continuing medical education, including time off with pay. For retirement plans, you might give a projection of retirement income at certain ages. After stating the dollar value for each benefit, estimate the total and point out any tax advantages to the employee. Benefits usually amount to a third of an employee's actual salary, yet may be taken for granted. If they are properly selected and presented, this will improve morale and job performance, and also favor retention when other employment is offered for which the benefits are not as clearly delineated. See Figure 16–5 for an annual benefit summary format recommended by **Rocky Mountain Professional Consultants, Inc.** which can be modified to suit your practice.

More on morale. Its maintenance is a vital consideration for any employer. The most important ingredient is the belief of employees in the value and quality of the service they render at your side. Next in order is the degree of compatibility that exists in the office, both with other employees and with you. Third is the recognition and praise they receive when warranted. Your expressed interest in their professional and personal welfare usually comes fifth. Believe it or not, salary and benefits follow these, in sixth place! Often, when complaints are made about salary, it is because the employee is not receiving sufficient reward and satisfaction in the first five nonmaterial job needs, which are more difficult to articulate.

Because of both the varying demands in a medical office and the increasing movement of women into the work force, it would seem that hiring part-time employees would have considerable advantages. Many women prefer such employment as a first step in returning to a full-time career after years of marriage and raising children. But certain factors militate against this choice. Chief among these is the poor

Rocky Mountain Professional Consultants, Inc.

10403 West Colfax Avenue, Suite 650A • Denver, Colorado 80215-3869 • Telephone (303) 233-4131

Donald L. Ankerholz, C.P.B.C.
Gary W. Thompson, C.P.B.C.
Roger J. Newton, C.P.B.C.

EMPLOYEE NAME________________

TOTAL SALARY REPORTING FORM

FISCAL YEAR__________

		EMPLOYEE BENEFIT	EMPLOYER COST
1.	TOTAL W-2 SALARY	________	
2.	SOCIAL SECURITY BUSINESS TAX	________	
3.	STATE UNEMPLOYMENT		________
4.	FEDERAL UNEMPLOYMENT		________
5.	WORKMEN'S COMPENSATION		________
6.	RETIREMENT PLAN _____%	________	
7.	HEALTH INSURANCE	________	
8.	DISABILITY	________	
9.	LIFE INSURANCE	________	
10.	MEDICAL SERVICES PROVIDED	________	
11.	BONUSES	________	
12.	SICK LEAVE	________	
	TOTAL	________	________

DAYS OFF - NON-PAID______
VACATION DAYS ENTITLED______
VACATION DAYS USED______

SOCIETY OF PROFESSIONAL BUSINESS CONSULTANTS
MEMBER FIRM

MANAGEMENT CONSULTANTS TO THE PROFESSIONS

SMD
SOCIETY OF MEDICAL-DENTAL MANAGEMENT CONSULTANTS
MEMBER FIRM

Figure 16–5. (Courtesy of Rocky Mountain Professional Consultants, Inc., Denver, Colorado.)

communication that you often have with such an employee. Frequently, also, she is not available on short notice when her services may be most required. Still another factor to consider is the tendency of your full-time employees toward "buck-passing." One or more of them may claim that a certain task was assigned to the part-time employee, and the latter is not there to clarify the situation. Still another problem is the possibility of office discontent over a wage differential, actual or perceived, because the part-time employee is paid by the hour at a higher rate without benefits than the full-time employees, who are paid by the month with benefits. This problem can be avoided if permanent part-time employees are paid a percentage of a monthly wage with benefits according to the time they work. One last disadvantage of part-time employees is that they may find it difficult to fit into the smooth cooperation and harmony developed among the full-time employees over the years.

Most of these disadvantages can be avoided with good management. Start by using part-time employees for certain assignments that occur regularly, such as the preparation of insurance forms, billing, collections, and correspondence or other transcription. Make it clear that whatever is assigned them is their responsibility alone. This works especially well with tasks that can be taken from the office, done at home, and returned completed the following day.

A dramatic recent trend is staff leasing. The **Tax Equity and Fiscal Responsibility Act** of 1982 appears to allow the "firing" of personnel by the physician and their immediate hiring by a company that leases them to the physician. The staff-leasing company then handles all administrative matters, pays salaries, arranges for vacations and sick leave, and sometimes even increases employee benefits. The advantage to the arrangement is that TEFRA only requires that such employees contribute 7.5 per cent of their salary to a pension plan, whereas the physician previously was obliged to make contributions for them proportionate to his own. Under a staff-leasing arrangement, therefore, the physician can contribute to a defined benefit plan for his own retirement at a much higher level than he could before because he does not have to include his former employees.

However, certain limitations of staff leasing were not perceived at first. If the employees are young and receive lower salaries, the savings are less significant. The physician also gives up the pension forfeitures that result from employee turnover. In a small office with only one or two employees, the purported advantages almost disappear. There are other, more subtle, disadvantages. Although low at the start, the fees of the leasing corporation have a tendency to rise to the point where the total cost is greater than it was before the plan was set up. A decline in employee morale and loyalty is frequently detected, for two reasons. If the staff sees that the motivation of the physician for participating in such a plan is greed, they may lose respect for him. And when the employees realize that they are actually hired by the leasing corporation and through it can obtain other positions easily, the authority of the physician is undermined.

These are minor objections. The major ones will probably eliminate these plans altogether. The Internal Revenue Service in 1984 issued its opinion that an employee working in a physician's office and taking day-to-day direction from that physician was in fact the employee of that physician under common law despite any staff-leasing arrangement. While there is a possibility that this ruling may be challenged in court, behind it lurks the probability of legislative action. Congress views staff leasing as an attempt to get around the intent of TEFRA to provide proportionate retirement benefits to employees, and there is legislation pending at the present time to prevent staff-leasing plans. My advice is to avoid them.

The subject of employing relatives in the office is a complicated one. They can be either a bane or a boon. If you are a man and your wife helps you, she has a dual role as wife and worker that creates difficulties both for her and for the other employees. Even the patients do not care to confide in someone, not a professional, whom they may see socially. So employing your wife is usually done only until you can afford to hire your first assistant. As long as she does work, ask your accountant about the tax and pension advantages. The **Economic Recovery Tax Act** of 1981 provides a tax credit for the cost of caring for children, as well as a tax credit on a joint return of 10 per cent of her salary up to a maximum of $3000. Under certain conditions, she may also contribute to her own IRA up to 15 per cent of her annual income, to a maximum of $2000, and her FICA contributions may raise her future social security benefits higher than they would be as your wife. For the physician near retirement there is another advantage. He can employ his wife the last year or two and set up a defined benefit plan for her that will give quite a boost to their retirement finances. It is usually advantageous to employ children during school vacations, because their income is taxed to them at lower rates. With any relative, as with all employees, personnel records must be kept and the salary has to be justified by the work actually performed.

A few comments on adding the second and third office assistants. The first indications that you need a second aide (and then a third) will arise in the business office, so keep an eye upon this area. You may compensate for short handedness in the clinical tasks without thinking much about it. Look over your appointment book. Check the reception room from time to time, and ask patients about waiting time. Review patient questionnaires. Check to see if statements are being sent out on time. Note the percentage of your time-of-service collections, because this is one of the first tasks to be neglected when your employees are overworked. The collection percentage is usually second to decline. The accounts receivable total is a rather rough indicator, but if it is steadily rising over a number of months, it may indicate an organizational or disciplinary problem in the office, *or* it could be because your present personnel are too busy.

The total number of employees you will have when working at full capacity is determined primarily by your specialty. However, secondary determinants can affect staffing considerably, especially if they operate in combination: your personal preferences as to patient volume, the time you spend with each patient, laboratory or other procedures that are done in your office, and how much clinical work you are able and willing to delegate. The total payroll as a percentage of gross receipts offers a rough guide. The assumption, of course, is that the gross itself is satisfactory and the salaries are fair. Annual, not monthly, figures are the best ones to look at. Most physicians in primary care have an annual payroll in the range of 15 to 20 per cent of the annual gross. Internists, OB-GYN specialists, and orthopedists are somewhat lower, in the range of 10 to 15 per cent. General surgeons are still lower, usually around 7 per cent.

The method for hiring the second and third employees is similar to that followed in hiring the first. Now, however, you want your present aide to participate in the process. She can offer you her impressions on the resumes, conduct the office tour, and do an informal interview herself. Before you make your final decision, treat her and the applicant to lunch—just the two of them—and go by her recommendation afterward.

Office organization is simple with one or even two assistants. Each is responsible directly to you. However, when you have three assistants, the question of delegating some authority to one as office coordinator comes up. If you do, you are relieved of many aspects of day-to-day management but you lose some of her help as an aide. It has to be an individual decision. If you take the step, record it in her personnel record, adjust her salary accordingly, prepare a new job description for her, and change the office manual and the other job descriptions as required.

The decision is easier if you have *more* than three employees. An office manager is almost always essential then. Bring in a person who has a business degree and background, with emphasis on management experience that is not necessarily medical. An office manager who has been an aide for a number of years tends to step in and take over various functions of other employees to the neglect of her managerial duties.

The termination of an employee is always a sticky situation, both emotionally and legally. But if the last performance review is conducted properly, the termination itself is much easier. The form completed then should reflect a reason for the firing that is in compliance with the law, and it should bear the employee's signature acknowledging that a face-to-face discussion of the problem was held. A warning letter is not necessary, but if one was given, a copy bearing the same acknowledgment and signature should be kept in the personnel file.

The strain can be further reduced if you prepare for the termination properly and conduct it calmly. First, decide how the tasks are going to be performed after the employee has left. Make a list of the items in her possession you want returned. Arrange for rekeying the outside locks—it is not necessary to change them. Review the individual's personnel record for completeness and accuracy. Pay special attention to the attendance record to be certain all overtime has been compensated. Review your attorney's summary to make sure you are complying in all respects with the law. Be sure to keep the personnel records secure once you have made your decision. Some employees seem to have a sixth sense about their impending termination, and an unscrupulous or angry one may alter or steal her record and cause you all sorts of difficulties. The last step before the termination is to decide if it is to be for one or more of the causes specified in your manual, without warning or benefits. If it is, the task is much simpler. The same is true if termination is during the probationary period. You may also consider requesting a letter of resignation. This has the dual effect of preserving the employee's reputation and of avoiding an increase in your contribution to the state unemployment fund. You can ask her for such a letter at the time of termination.

Now for the termination itself. Select an appropriate time. The best is at the end of the last day of the work week. Give no advance notice to anyone. Prepare the final check yourself, covering her pay period to that date, two weeks' severance pay in lieu of notice, and accrued vacation time, all with appropriate deductions. Ask another employee to remain in the front office to avoid charges of sexual harassment or physical abuse, but conduct the matter privately in your consultation room. Call the employee in, ask her to sit down, then get right to it. Tell her your decision and state the reasons for it in as few words as possible. This can be as simple as telling her that the improvements promised at the last review have not been forthcoming. Do not dwell on the problem any more yourself, but give her the chance to state her version and ventilate her feelings. Even if you disagree, say nothing—let her have the final word. Then collect the items you listed, hand her the check, and escort her to the door. Immediately afterward, document all details in her personnel record. At the next opportunity, inform the other employees of the termination, observing legal confidentiality restrictions in doing so. Assure them that your purpose was to benefit the office and to reinforce the standards that you have set. That's all there is to it.

17

Building and Maintaining Your Practice

Today physicians in private practice must devote far more time and entrepreneurial skill to building and maintaining their practices than was ever needed by earlier generations of physicians. One reason for this is the number of physicians in practice. In response to a perceived shortage of physicians in the 1950s, an influx of federal dollars starting in the 1960s increased the number of United States medical schools from 89 to 127, and expanded their capacity as well. From fewer than 7000 graduates per year in the fifties, our schools now produce nearly 17,000. Foreign graduates have come to our shores in greater numbers, and the ranks of United States citizens graduating from Caribbean and other foreign schools have also expanded during this time period. Meanwhile, the population has increased only fractionally. If a shortage did exist then, that shortage has now become a surplus. There are nearly 500,000 physicians in the United States today—twice as many as there were in 1960. Our country will soon have the highest physician-to-population ratio in the world.

There are other reasons for physicians to be concerned. Big business has entered the health care field. Hospitals are expanding their services and outreach programs. Ambulatory care centers have sprung up all across the country. Allied health personnel are increasing in numbers and becoming more competitive. Highly skilled nursing specialists in hospitals have quietly assumed responsibilities that were formerly the province of physicians. Less traditional practitioners—self-styled "nutritionists," exercise "experts," "stress counselors," "naturopaths," chiropractors, "holistic health" advocates, and herbalists—have moved aggressively into the field.

Private practitioners must also deal with new forms of competition within the profession: the prepaid health plans (HMOs) that have proliferated over the past two decades, and Preferred Provider Organizations (PPOs). Many groups have grown in size to achieve economy of scale, and have added satellite facilities.

As a result of this environment of intensified competition, the net income of physicians in private practice has begun to decline for the first time since such data have been compiled.

At the same time, there has been a continued spiralling of expenses, especially malpractice insurance and personnel costs. In addition, the government, insurance carriers, employers offering health plans, and patients themselves have become more actively involved in holding down medical expenses. The Department of Health and Human Services is now working on plans to extend payment by diagnosis-related groups (DRGs) to physicians' hospital-based Medicare charges.

As a result of all of this, we must make realistic and practical decisions about what we are going to do to survive in this increasingly competitive medical marketplace. Without doubt, we will continue to practice high-quality medicine in a concerned and caring manner. But doing so is no longer enough to ensure a physician's survival in practice.

Let's look at the solutions in two phases: (1) building your practice and (2) maintaining it.

If you are a young physician just establishing your practice, your most important step is to become known by your colleagues. Almost all your patients at the start will come from other physicians. First call upon those who practice nearby. During such a courtesy call, the established physician will get an initial impression of your personality and training that you can strengthen by offering a curriculum vitae. Leave one card with him and two or three with his receptionist. When he refers a minor problem, handle it well, and others of greater complexity will follow.

Then extend the range of your calls. Remember, you are not bothering these physicians—they want to meet you. Be sincere in your desire to get to know each one: any commercial concern will come through clearly to your detriment. At the hospitals, introduce yourself to colleagues at lunch, in the library, and in the doctor's lounge. Get active in staff functions and on hospital committees, and attend all general staff and departmental meetings. Give a talk on a subject in which you have special expertise. Do the same at the local medical society. If your specialty has a local chapter, join and attend meetings. If there is a medical school in your area, attend grand rounds and specialty clinics. Volunteer for a teaching position and a clinical appointment. Get to know the full-time faculty and other attendings.

Throughout, try not to become attached to a particularly strong figure or clique, but endeavor instead to establish good relationships with all the physicians in the community.

Don't overlook other health care professionals such as dentists, neighborhood pharmacists, optometrists, podiatrists, nurses at the hospitals, and the medical assistants of other physicians. These can be sources of referral as important as physicians.

Let me reiterate the reason for this emphasis on getting to know your professional colleagues before making any efforts in the direction of the public at large. Although over the long run most of your patients *will* come to you on the recommendation of other patients, at the start, you simply don't have many patients to do the recommending.

As soon as you can, get on the emergency room panel at each of your hospitals. Smaller hospitals staff emergency rooms with on-call rotation of generalists and panels of specialists, but others have full-time coverage by emergency medicine or traumatology specialists. Fit in however you can, but in any case become known by the physicians and nurses who work there. Many established physicians look upon their rotation on emergency room panels as a chore they would rather dispense with. If you develop a reputation for responding promptly and giving good care, the nurse on duty or the full-time emergency room physician will often call you rather than the physician next up on the roster. When this does happen, go—and once at the emergency room call the physician who would have been next. Tell him you are there, and ask him if he wishes to attend himself. Chances are he will tell you to see the patient and harbor no resentment at all.

Get on the referral lists of your hospitals and medical society. Ask the **Visiting Nurses Association** if you can assist them in some way. Join a busy voluntary call group. Most let you charge for the patients you see when you are on call, and this will be quite a boost to your income. Respond promptly and in person, charge the same fees, and you will find that the other members will send you their overflow patients.

It will soon be productive to entertain small groups of physicians in your home. During conversations at such get-togethers they are able to evaluate your personality, and to some extent your training. This may be sufficient for them to send you some patients with minor problems. Again, treat these patients well and others will follow. The entertainment costs are usually deductible, but consult your accountant.

Once you are known among your colleagues and other professionals, it is time to extend your efforts to the public. Join civic organizations such as the Chamber of Commerce and service clubs. Become active in fraternal and religious organizations. Volunteer to give talks on medical subjects at any sizable gathering. Look for opportunities in the community to be of service, such as giving free Boy Scout and pre-camp physicals, or volunteering as a team physician at the high school. Give physical examinations or advice on exercise at health clubs. Be active in organizations with a medical orientation, such as the Arthritis Foundation, the American Heart Association, and the American Diabetes Association, and join their speakers' bureaus. At your church or synagogue, become active in fund raising, study groups, and other activities. Take cultural courses at local community colleges with your spouse. Give free influenza injections at senior centers. If you think your colleagues might object, take blood pressures instead. If you or your spouse has an unusual hobby or past experience, have an article about it put in the paper. Write "health hints," "traveler's tips," or columns on medical subjects for the local paper.

The most important service you have to offer in the first months of practice is your *availability*—prompt and at all hours—for the first referral from whatever source. If you accept each call cheerfully and care for the patient competently, others will come from that same source. Although income from part-time employment may be important, do not allow your availability to be restricted because of it. If you cannot respond to the first referral from a particular source, you may never get another one.

Be careful to observe certain courtesies with physicians who refer patients to you for consultation. Establish first if you are (1) to consult, (2) to consult and manage, or (3) to consult and manage in concert with him. Explain your role and your fees to the patient. Call the referring physician immediately after you see the patient. Thank him, give your initial impression, and outline what your approach will be. If he is not clear on your fees, give him an estimate. When his patient requires hospitalization, ask him if he would like to admit the patient under his name or if he wants you to do it. If you do, ask the ward secretary to notify his office when the patient is admitted. He may want to visit his patient socially and check the chart in order to keep informed. Have copies of all hospital records and reports sent to him. A phone call, followed by an informal note upon discharge of the patient, are well-received. Your formal report should be sent him as soon as possible. Avoid having the patient visit his office before he has received your consultation report. And, above all, return the patient to him as soon as your role as consultant has been concluded.

Some of the traditional methods of building a practice are no longer effective today. The mailing of announcement cards is one. Another is publishing announcements in the paper. Patients will not choose you on this slender basis alone. Performing insurance or Federal Aviation Administration physical examinations is another. This gives only a brief contact with individuals, most of whom already have physicians. I won't go so far as to say you shouldn't use such traditional methods, but I do caution you against high expectations concerning the results.

In your practice, pay special attention to courtesies to your patients. Monitor the manner of your receptionist on the telephone and in greeting patients. See all patients on time. For the first few months, conduct new patients to your consultation room where you can take a few quiet moments to put them at ease and become acquainted. Be relaxed and confident yourself. Ask each patient how he prefers to be addressed. Note this preference in the chart and instruct your assistants. If you are a specialist, stick to your specialty. Later, when the patient becomes established, you can provide some general care as well. Be sure your fees are reasonable, and offer to discuss them upon request. Start out by preparing insurance forms at no charge. Later, if they become overwhelming for your staff, you may charge for all after the first one. Show a concern for the cost of the medical decisions you make, and explain these costs as carefully as you can.

Patients in the hospital frequently complain about the little time physicians spend with them. They are unaware of the time taken discussing x-rays with the radiologist, checking tests in the laboratory, conversing with nurses and reading their notes, consulting colleagues, doing research, and writing progress notes. Do as much of this as you can at your patients' bedsides, and let them know how the rest of your time in the hospital is spent on their behalf. They also complain when their family is not kept fully informed. Discuss with them what they want the family to know, and select one family member to whom you report daily.

Prepare an effective patient information booklet early on. (See Chapter 14.) Give two copies to each new patient. Put a bulletin board in your reception area and post items of health information on it. Patients also appreciate a suggestion box even if they don't take advantage of it.

Have a supply of Patient Survey Questionnaires (obtainable from the AMA) there and invite patients to fill one out. Each new patient should be given one by your receptionist, with a stamped return envelope. For now, just add your name and address to the questionnaire. Later, you will want to develop your own questionnaire. When you do, retain optional patient anonymity, and frame the questions as positive statements allowing a range of responses, e.g., "strongly agree +1, +2, +3," and "strongly disagree −1, −2, −3," with "0" for "neither agree or disagree." It helps if you alternate positive and negative statements and approach each subject from two or more angles. Tailor the statements to your practice and focus on the most important aspects as you see them. Leave adequate space for the patient's comments at the end.

As you set about establishing your practice, remember that, with the sophistication of medicine today, patients may not be able to judge the quality of care you render, but they can tell if *you* care.

Until the last few years, the advice given so far would have been sufficient, and the chapter could have ended here: once the physician had acquired a full roster of patients, the success and stability of his practice was almost assured. But, as I noted at the start of the chapter, changes are taking place that make the practice of medicine more and more a highly competitive business. The wise physician will not only be alert to these changes and adapt to them, but will do his best to *anticipate* them. If you wait until a downturn in your practice occurs, you may be too late. The remainder of this chapter will focus on methods for maintaining your practice.

"Marketing" is the buzz word currently in fashion. As used in the business world, the term *marketing* usually suggests a larger component of advertising than is acceptable to most physicians. But in marketing a medical practice, this component can be kept small, professional, and tasteful. If you wish to avoid having anything to do with marketing, you may want to employ a professional to do it for you. One of the best is HM and Associates, 702 Washington Street, Suite 178, Marina Del Rey, CA 90292; or telephone (213) 822–5430.

But you can do an effective job yourself. Marketing is divided into two phases—an analysis and a plan of action. Marketing *analysis* is quite simple:

1. Analyze the community your patients come from in terms of its dominant socioeconomic and cultural characteristics, and its medical needs.
2. Evaluate the health care providers that are in competition with you.
3. Estimate objectively how your services compare with theirs.
4. Examine the impact that personal factors—your philosophy, personality, and professional skills—have on the success of your practice.

These four steps form the basis of your marketing analysis. A marketing *plan* merely plugs the gaps you find.

Let's expand on the analysis itself. Look at Chapter 5 again to review the community characteristics you need to consider. Your analysis will be similar to that used to select a location, but somewhat more detailed, especially in its focus on community demographics and economic base. Nationwide information for comparison can be obtained from the **National Clearinghouse for Census Data Services**, Bureau of the Census, Washington, DC 20233. Write the **Census Bureau State Data Center Program** at the same address for the address of the Data Center for your state. Then write that Data Center to request whatever relevant material they can provide. Information on your county or city can be obtained from the **U.S. Department of Commerce,** Washington, DC 20230. Your local chambers of commerce, your banker, and your accountant are among the other available sources of information on your community. Inquire especially about economic indices, housing starts, the unemployment rate, and projections of recent trends. Study all this information, especially as it applies to the type of patients you want in your practice.

Next, assemble information on all the health care sources in your area. An excellent book entitled *The AHA Guide to the Health Care Field* can be obtained from the American Hospital Association, 840 North Lake Shore Drive, Chicago, IL 60611, or from your medical library. Another good source is *Medical Practice in the United States,* which gives information on physician services organized by specialty. You can get a copy from the Communications Office, Robert Wood Johnson Foundation, P. O. Box 2316, Princeton, NJ 08540, or look in your library. Check again the sources given in Chapter 5. In your own community, information on health care providers can be obtained from the public relations departments at the hospitals where you practice, as well as from the health department and local health systems agencies. Note especially all data concerning the newer types of competition such as HMOs, IPAs, allied health practioners, and ambulatory care centers. Determine the number of physicians and other providers in relation to the population, including those who would refer to you and those in the same specialty or otherwise in direct competition with you. Your specialty society, the state and local medical societies, and the state board of medical examiners may have additional information. Talk to local pharmacists, representatives of medical supply houses, and pharmaceutical detail men.

Then your attention will shift to your practice. Trace the path a typical patient takes in coming to see you. Look at your listings in the telephone directory. Are they easy to find? Do they communicate your qualifications and skills? Do you have enough trunk lines to your office? Have the telephone company do a busy signal and peak load study. Evaluate your telephone procedures and etiquette. Are appointments available at the times requested? Do your office hours conform to community patterns? How courteous and competent is your answering service? Are you promptly available when on call? Do the others in your voluntary call group render good medical care when you are not available? Next review your business cards, letterhead stationery, and forms. Are they attractive, appropriate, and functional?

Look again at the location of your medical building. Is it accessible by public transportation? Is parking adequate and close? If there is a parking charge, do you reimburse your patients? Are your medical building and grounds attractive? Are there any tenants who might detract from your prestige? Are public lobbies and hallways attractive and clean?

Go through your own office suite critically. Is it tastefully furnished? Is seating adequate and well arranged? Is it straightened up frequently throughout the day? Does the reception room contain an aquarium, potted plants, or fresh flowers, and if so, are they well maintained? Are your magazines interesting and recent? Do you have travel, art, or photography books on the tables? A bulletin board with items of patient interest? Is the ambient light pleasant and is reading light adequate? Is your smoking policy observed? Are there any unpleasant odors? Is the area quiet? Do you have large-print periodicals for the elderly? Is your patient information booklet available? Is it complete, up-to-date, and readable? How long do patients have to wait?

Inspect the rest of your suite in the same way, trying to view the facilities as they appear to the patient. Make notes on all features that could be improved.

Regard your assistants from the patients' perspective. Ask friends to phone the office and report to you on the promptness and courtesy with which they answer the telephone. Are they neat and appropriately groomed? Does the receptionist come out from behind her desk to greet patients and does she do so pleasantly? Does each wear a name tag giving her position? Do you have a "rose gallery" in the reception area with their pictures, names, and positions? Do they introduce themselves to patients and show an interest in them? Are they helpful and courteous constantly, even in collection procedures? How productive are they? Could you delegate more tasks to them? Do they provide you with helpful observations before you see each patient? Do they follow the patients preferences in addressing them?

Look at the scope of your professional services. Can the boundaries of your specialty be expanded? Could you add any appropriate procedures? Would wellness programs fit into your practice? Is there a nearby competitor who might be bought out? Are there prepaid programs, independent practice associations, or medical foundations that might be advantageous to join? Are there nursing homes, hospices, senior centers, or educational institutions with which you could become affiliated? Would home visits by your clinical assistant be advisable? Are your follow-up visits scheduled properly? Are patient recalls effective?

Do a zip code study of your patients. Determine how many patients come from heavily represented areas and why, then do the same for lightly represented areas. Note your primary drawing area. Do a patient analysis: age, sex, education, and socioeconomic status. In doing so, ask yourself which of their health care needs you may not be meeting. Look at the sources of all new patients over the last year. Note those that have not been as productive recently. Try to determine why patients who have left your practice have done so. Compare the number of patients who have left to the number of new patients for a representative period of time.

Read over your patient education materials. Study patient questionnaires over the past several months and note any recurring themes. Look at your questionnaire with a view toward improving it. Mail questionnaires with a cover letter to the last 100 or 200 patients seen. Consider having an outside firm conduct a survey of your patients. One that provides this service is Rocky Mountain Professional Consultants, Suite 650A, 10403 West Colfax Avenue, Lakewood, CO 80215.

Look over the financial aspects of your practice. Determine the number of patients per day compared to the prior year. Study your fees and analyze the procedural codes if you are on a computer, or the practice summary columns of your pegboard if you are not. Note those professional services that result in the greatest net and those that result in the least. Look again at your time-of-service collections and overall collection ratio. Age your accounts receivable. Total them to make sure they are no more than three times the average month's gross. Look again at adjustments made for professional courtesy and write-offs given for other reasons. Review how your staff handles insurance claims. If you charge for their preparation, is the charge reasonable? If you do not accept Medicare assignment, review this policy. Are your patients adequately advised of the cost of hospitalization? Are appropriate adjustments made in cases of hardship? Have one assistant use a stopwatch and do a time management analysis of daily office procedures. Discuss your fees, bookkeeping, internal control systems, and collection methods with your accountant. Ask him to analyze fluctuations and trends over the past year or two in your gross income, overhead expenses, and resulting net income. Request his advice based upon his experience with other physician clients.

Look into possibilities for supplemental income. One often overlooked is the Armed Forces Reserve. You receive adequate compensation for one weekend a month and two weeks a year. At age 60, you can retire with a pension, free medical care, and space-available travel anywhere in the world.

The fourth part of your analysis is a more personal one. Try to appraise your own personality and interaction with patients. Are your professional skills of the standard you wish? Review your relationships with other professionals, physicians, and the administrators of the hospitals where you practice. Look for any ethnic, cultural, or philosophical conflicts you may have with the community. Are your language skills appropriate? Review your community activities and visibility. Are there any unique services you may be able to provide the community? Are your hospital visits regular and long enough? Do you explain consent forms and procedures carefully? In the office, how do you greet each patient? Do you show an interest in each as a person? How much time do you spend with each patient? Do patients appear satisfied? Do they understand their illness and the treatment that you recommend? Are they aware of the length of the treatment and its cost? Do you conduct each patient to the door at the end of the visit?

After completing the four steps of the marketing analysis, spend some time studying your notes and discussing them with your staff. Decide which parts of your practice you would like to improve, then take action to do so. At the same time, lay out a program to monitor both the improvements and their effects.

In the business world, marketing involves four P's: *product, price, place,* and *promotion.* We have covered the first three as they apply to medical practice. This leaves promotion. Although the Federal Trade Commission has made advertising legal, and medical organizations have had to accept this decision, there is an ethical boundary that you should not cross. In the last analysis, patients will *not* be better informed by advertising: medical services are so sophisticated today that the patient cannot select those which best suit his needs on the basis of media spots or slogans. Any advertising as such should only call attention to your presence in the community. Beyond this, the quality of care you render and the manner in which you do so are what count.

Having said that, let's look at some of the things you can do in the way of promotion. The final judgment as to whether any one suggestion is in good taste must, of course, be left to you.

- Look over the ideas offered in the first few pages of this chapter—some of them are suitable for maintaining as well as building a practice. Now, however, your primary source of new patients will not be your colleagues but your present patients.
- For all referrals, write a brief note in your own hand, taking care not to violate the privacy of the new patient, thanking your established patient for the confidence shown in you by making the referral.
- Look at your listing in the Yellow Pages to see if it can be improved. If you are near other communities, a listing in their directories might be advisable.

- Offer free reviews of all medicines, including over-the-counter drugs, through a small announcement in the paper.
- Prepare a news release on any subject of current interest on which you can comment knowledgeably, then take it to the editors of local papers personally. You might also write releases noting the medical meetings you attend.
- Prepare regular newsletters on medical topics—do *not* use "canned" newsletters—and mail them to patients and other health care professionals. You might distribute them even more widely, to major employers, for example. Keep some in a binder in the reception room with the note "copies are available from the receptionist."
- Offer to assist nonprofit organizations such as crisis care centers, alcohol and drug abuse counseling services, marital and family counselors, senior citizen care centers, and other community services beyond the usual circle of hospitals and nursing homes.
- Take out dignified announcements—just your name, specialty, and address with telephone number—in school yearbooks, newsletters of community associations, Welcome Wagon materials, church bulletins, fraternal and alumni newsletters, and similar organs.
- Conduct free seminars—with panels of experts—on health topics of interest to your community in school auditoriums and other suitable locations.
- Organize free health screenings, and participate in your local health fairs.
- Sponsor entrants in golf or tennis tournaments, marathons, and other community events.
- Be sure that your credentials are clearly stated in your patient information booklet and always have a supply of booklets readily available. If there is a significant change, mail new ones to all established patients with a cover letter explaining the alteration.
- Send cards to your patients on birthdays and anniversaries.
- Give out stickers with your number and other emergency information to be put on telephones and in medicine cabinets.
- Provide a mailbox in your reception area with stamped stationery, and free pens bearing your name and number.
- Hold an open house when you acquire a major item of new equipment and invite city officials, community leaders, and others.
- Have an assistant regularly check local newspapers for mention of your patients. When appropriate, write each a congratulatory note and post the article on the reception room bulletin board.
- Hold small discussion groups on medical topics of current interest in your office after hours.
- Phone patients after office procedures, the institution of new treatment, or hospital discharge to ask how they are getting along.
- Itemize "no charge" services on your statements.
- Prepare medical travel kits and give them to patients, along with instructions and "travel tips."

- Notify the local newspapers of any scientific papers you publish or present at medical meetings. Do the same on the receipt of any professional honors.
- Consider a call-in program on your local radio or TV station.
- Sponsor a public service announcement on radio or television.
- Print "numbers to call in case of an emergency" on the back of your business card. This way patients will be likely to keep your card with them, which may encourage them to make referrals.
- Send a Thanksgiving card with your thanks to all referring physicians. They are more unusual than Christmas cards.
- Get your name listed in specialized directories, in addition to the local telephone directories.

These are just a few promotional ideas to start you thinking of more. Some do go right up to the line that separates ethical and dignified activities from those that are not, but the majority are acceptable in most communities. Such activities, if done in good taste, represent a change physicians must make in their practices because of changes the medical marketplace itself.

18

Telephone Procedure

This subject is dealt with in a separate chapter because of its immense importance in a medical practice. The telephone is the major conduit of information to and from your office. Most of your calls are from patients, who are often fearful, ill, or in pain. You are in the business of caring and curing, and the first contact most patients have in seeking your help is with your assistant on the telephone. Therefore, your assistant must answer *all* calls as if they were from patients.

Several sources are available to help assistants develop proper telephone technique. The **American Medical Association** offers booklets, as well as audio cassette courses with workbooks. The **American Association of Medical Assistants** conducts workshops and classes. Every book for medical office assistants includes a chapter on the subject. Your local telephone company may also have materials and courses.

The problem is putting the theory into practice. This is something you must initiate yourself. Take notes as you read this chapter, add your own thoughts, then try to put together the procedure you wish to be used in your office. When your points of procedure acquire enough coherence, insert them in your office manual. Urge your aides to take advantage of the sources named. Instruct them yourself, and monitor them to make sure they are carrying out your instructions. Have others call periodically and tell you how your assistants handle the telephone.

The best procedures won't do any good unless callers can get through. Don't try to save money here—have enough trunk lines for your practice. The telephone company will do peak load and busy signal studies at no charge as often as you ask them to. These are done automatically, without interruption of your incoming calls, and with no invasion of privacy. The number of busy calls must be kept below 10 per cent, but the ideal is zero. If only one caller a day gets a busy signal, this might be a patient with an emergency, a nurse at the hospital trying to report a sudden change in one of your patients, or a physician who wishes to send you a consultation.

Always be sure you have enough assistants so that the phone will be picked up promptly at all times. One aide can cover no more than two lines, even if not distracted by other duties. Designate your receptionist as the primary person to answer the telephone, and instruct her to do so on the first ring, if possible. A second assistant should be designated to pick up the phone after the third ring if the receptionist is occupied.

Before your receptionist picks up the phone for the first time, instruct her on the proper use of names and titles—yours and the patients'. The worst way to answer the phone is with the telephone number. The second worst is to say "Doctor's Office." The title "Doctor" is used only when the nature of the degree referred to is clearly understood, and then with the last name. Only if *both* the nature of the doctorate and the surname are known is it acceptable to use "*the* doctor." The same holds true in correspondence. Initially, it is "J. Q. Jones, M.D." or "A. B. Smith, Ph.D." Once the degree is known, "Dr. Jones" and "Dr. Smith" are correct. Obviously, using only "Dear Doctor" in the salutation of a letter is as bad as saying "Doctor's Office" when answering the telephone.

The European use of titles was altered in our country early in its history when we embraced the egalitarian ethic. Respect for individuals then emerged over respect for social position. Thereafter the use of titles continued primarily for pragmatic reasons in public life and almost ceased in private. This is because roles often predominate over personality in the former, but the reverse is more often true in the latter.

The only problem with this arises when the delineation between public and private lives becomes blurred. Until this century, physicians were the only doctors in town and were always on call. Their public and private lives were merged. But things began to change in this century. Physicians now are off call a substantial portion of their time and pursue activities then as *persons*, not physicians, for the most part. Today many pharmacists hold a doctoral degree—so do lawyers, educators, and ministers. Dentists are doctors, too. In many urban and suburban social situations, physicians are outnumbered by those who have a Ph.D. So the use by physicians of the title "Doctor" in such settings no longer makes sense, nor is it in good taste.

Assistants often make the mistake of saying, "Doctor is with a patient" or "Doctor will see you now." This is terrible. If they have trouble understanding correct usage, ask them to substitute another title, such as "reverend" or "judge" for "doctor" in these phrases. They wouldn't say "Reverend's Office," or "Judge is with the plaintiff."

Be circumspect in this regard. Any misuse of your title tends to lump you with those who use a vague "Doctor" when discoursing on a subject outside their field of expertise or with those who put "Dr. Adjust Bones, D C" on their signs and stationery.

Before I leave the subject, I should stress that patients have titles, too—*Mr.*, *Mrs.*, *Miss*, or *Ms*. These are always used in the office, with last names, as a sign of respect. Only when a patient requests that you do so should you or your aides use first names. Respect goes both ways.

Let's return to your receptionist who is about to pick up the telephone. As stated in your office manual, she will never be chewing gum. Nor will she be eating or smoking, except in the employee lounge when she is off duty.

She should have the telephone log nearby, and pen or pencil in hand. Her manner in answering should convey the impression that she is there to help, not that she was interrupted while doing something else. She has to put herself in the patient's position and realize that although she may be busy with other things, the person calling is concerned only with the purpose of his call. If she *smiles* as she answers, her voice will almost always be pleasant and will make the patient feel just a bit better hearing it.

She first identifies the office, then herself as follows: "Doctors Smith and Jones' office, Kathy speaking. May I help you?" She politely asks the caller's name as soon as she can if the caller does not volunteer it. Thereafter, the caller's name is used just as she has used hers, and yours.

Her first task is to find out what it is the caller wants; the second is to provide it. She has to allow the person calling ample time to tell her what he wants. He may have difficulty articulating it. Then, if she cannot provide what the caller wants, alternatives are offered so that he can choose among them.

Anyone telephoning a medical office should *never* be put on hold, if it is at all avoidable. When it is absolutely necessary, your aide must first be certain it is not an emergency, and then *ask the caller's permission*: "May I place you on hold for a moment?" Only after getting permission should she do so. She must come back on *every minute*, keep the caller advised as to how long the delay might be, and continue to request permission. If it turns out to be longer than two or three minutes, she should ask if she can call back, and do so.

This is why I advise against such gadgetry as "Music on Hold"—the caller should never have to wait long enough to hear more than a few bars.

Another horrible habit is interrupting a telephone conversation (more than the moment it takes to excuse yourself) in order to take care of someone entering the office. Or the reverse. First comes first, whether on the phone or in the office, unless an emergency or unusual circumstance dictates otherwise

It is likewise deplorable to carry on a confidential telephone conversation within earshot of patients in the reception room.

When patients are ill or worried, they easily misinterpret words or phrases, and your aide must bear this possibility in mind. For example, if she says, "Doctor Jones is busy," they may feel that you are too busy to care about their problem. Instead, she could say, "Doctor Jones is with a patient right now," or "Doctor Jones is at the hospital." Similarly, they would not appreciate being told you are on the golf course while they are suffering. Instead, she should say, "Doctor Jones is not in right now—may I be of assistance?"

Here are some more suggestions for your aides:

Don't Say	**Do Say**
He's all booked up. He can't see you until ______________ .	Doctor Jones is scheduled at that time but he *can* see you tomorrow at ____. (Emphasize the positive.)
I'm sorry. I can't fit you in today.	Doctor Jones can see you tomorrow at ______________ . (Ditto.)
We are running late.	Doctor Jones has had his schedule interrupted. (Well, it was, wasn't it?)
Remind.	Verify or confirm. (Patients are not stupid.)
Cancellation.	Change in schedule. (Why did the *other* patient back out?)
Recall.	Examination. (The patient is not a car.)
Checkup.	Follow-up visit. (The patient is not a *defective* car.)
Old patient.	Former, continuing, or established patient. (No one wants to be old.)
Convention.	Seminar or conference. (A convention calls to mind drunks with funny hats.)
You misunderstood.	There was a misunderstanding. (And it *may* have been our fault.)
Are you a patient here?	When did we last see you? (I've obviously forgotten your name.)

Are you on welfare (Medicaid)?	What type of health insurance coverage do you have?
What's your problem?	Can you tell me what the problem is so that we can schedule you properly?
Pay for.	Take care of.
Deposit.	Initial remittance. (You're not a bank.)
Discount (on your charges).	Courtesy reduction or professional services by courtesy. (You're not a store.)
Price or cost.	Fee. (You are a *professional*.)
New or modern.	Improved methods. (They may like the old way.)
Dr. Jones is out of town.	Dr. Jones is attending a postgraduate course in Chicago or attending a meeting in Boston.
Who's calling?	May I say who is calling? (Asks permission.)

You can add to this list and post it near your receptionist's station. Have her add her own ideas. They may be the best of all.

Every call that cannot be taken care of at the time must be recorded on a message log (Fig. 18–1), not on odd scraps of paper, nor even on separate "while you were out" message forms. The best system is to use a log containing message forms you design yourself. These can be

TELEPHONE MESSAGE LOG

Date ______ Time Of Call ______

Caller ______ Patient ______

Address ______ Age ______

Complaint ______

______

Medication Taken ______ How Long Sick ______

Cough ______ Productive ______ Temp ______

Vomiting ______ Diarrhea ______

Pain ______ Location ______

Bleeding ______ How Long ______ From ______ How Much ______

Nurse Return Call ______ Doctor Return Call ______ Phone No. ______

Appointment Made and Response or/Prescription given ______

______

______

Colwell Systems, Inc., Champaign, Illinois Form 3302

Figure 18–1. Courtesy of Colwell Systems, Inc., Champaign, Illinois.

printed three or four to a page, and bound together with a spiral binding. The top form is perforated for easy removal and NCR-treated so that a copy is made on an identical form beneath it. A firm surface inserted under the copy ensures that the impression will not carry through. The detached top forms may be misplaced, but the copies always remain in the binder to form a chronological telephone log. Final action is always noted on the copy. Review the telephone log two or three times a day to make sure all telephone messages have been taken care of.

A protocol has to be set up for reporting laboratory and test results. In general, abnormal or otherwise significant reports should be discussed with the patient by you during an office visit. If one is not scheduled, your assistant should set one up, making a bland statement that does not alarm the patient. Normal results can be reported to the patient by an assistant, but she should never attempt to interpret the findings.

Don't overlook the role your answering service plays. I have already cautioned on selecting a good one and monitoring its performance. But your aides must do their part. Have them use your front line rather than the back line occasionally "by mistake" to make sure the service answers "Dr. Jones' *Exchange*," not "Dr. Jones' Office." Have them check your instruction-and-location cards at least once a month. Train your assistants to ask you where you will be and to inform the answering service—even when you are not on call.

When you put your telephone procedure in the office manual, devise a classification system for the various types of calls commonly received, with the action you wish your assistants to take for each category. Here are some suggestions:

1. *Emergency calls.* Put through to me immediately. If I am not in the office, take the course of action specified in the office manual.
2. *Calls from other physicians.* First, ask if the call concerns a patient. If so, pull that chart and give it to me when you tell me about the call. I will decide then if I will take the call or call back later.
3. *Calls from registered nurses* about hospitalized patients. These should be handled the same way as calls from physicians. *Never* relay orders through your assistant to a registered nurse. This is a breach of professional ethics.
4. *Calls from pharmacists.* Your instruction here is based upon your office policy. It is best if you don't refill prescriptions on the phone as a rule, but instead indicate the number of refills on all prescriptions. Patients should be scheduled to return to the office before the refills have been exhausted. On occasion, small quantities of medication can be prescribed on the phone to suffice until a patient is able to come in to the office. The same prohibition holds for new

prescriptions. Remember, all phone prescriptions must be entered in the patient's chart.

5. *Business calls.* This category can be subdivided into three or four types. One type may be of sufficient importance to be put through to you at once, perhaps another can be handled during your call-back time, and the rest be taken care of by your office personnel.
6. *Personal calls* and *calls from professionals other than physicians.* Your family should not call during office hours unless the matter is important. If they do, it is put through to you at once. Your attorney and accountant are spoken to when they call.
7. *Calls from patients* about matters that your assistants cannot handle. Have your assistant pull the chart or correspondence, attach the message, and leave it on your desk in the consultation room for call-back time, or other disposition.

Make sure that *all* calls by patients on clinical matters, not just prescription refills, are entered in the chart with the action taken. Some physicians prefer to use a different color pen for this.

One important point: never have your assistant place a call to another physician, or to anyone else, for that matter. Doing so tells the person that you consider yourself to be more important than he is, by making him wait when he comes on the line. It is *extremely* discourteous. The error is even more serious if you are calling a physician who is older than you or senior to you in some way. One such telephone call can alienate that physician for months or years to come. If someone does this to you more than once, think about retaliating by putting your assistant on to tell the caller when he comes to the phone: "Hold, please, for Dr. ________. You may never do it, but the thought itself gives some consolation.

19

Scheduling Patients

Patients have mostly good things to say about their physicians, but leading the list of their complaints is the length of time they have to wait before being seen. This is unfortunate, because most of the waiting time could be avoided if physicians would take a little of their own time to implement and monitor scheduling systems appropriate for their practices.

Part of the problem is that many medical assistants—and even some physicians—are not quite clear about what a scheduling system is supposed to do. It should allow time for the provision of the optimum quantity and quality of medical care to each patient with the minimum delay. It is *not* designed to make the physician's day smoother, although that may be one result. Nor is it to suit the convenience of any particular assistant by fitting around other duties she has to perform. The scheduling system is *for your patients.*

Historically, four systems have been used in physicians' offices:

1. The oldest one could be called "first come, first served." With no appointments, there is really no system at all. The physician cannot render quality care, sees fewer patients, and makes those he does see endure long waits. This "system" is rarely found today, even in rural areas.
2. The second is "wave scheduling." In it, a number of patients are given appointments for the same time at the start of morning and afternoon office hours, and are seen in the order of their arrival. These two waves of patient influx gave this system its name. As established patients become impatient with the waiting involved in this kind of scheduling, they will either come in before office

hours or drift in later toward the end. Those who time it perfectly arrive just as you are finishing with the last patient. They won't have to wait, but you won't have lunch. Nor will you get home on time in the evening. This second system has a strong tendency to degenerate into the first.

3. The third is "stream scheduling." In it, each patient is given a specific appointment time, an attempt is made to predict the time required for each, and the patients are spaced accordingly throughout the day. The main problem with this system is that it relies on estimates of the time required for each patient based upon past experience. It makes no allowance for the unexpected, which, in a physician's office, is exactly what is to be expected. Another problem is that most physicians think they have an accurate idea of the time they spend on a patient or procedure, but few really do. The result is that instructions given to their scheduling assistant are based on faulty assumptions. Still another problem is that many patients in the office for one purpose bring up a second, or even a third.

   The stream system *can* work under certain conditions: *if* the physician is a subspecialist who spends the greater part of an hour with each patient; *if* the patient population is reliable, punctual, and considerate of your schedule; *if* time is allowed in the schedule for emergencies and "work-ins"; and *if* open "buffer" periods are scheduled to compensate for unpredictable delays. Even then, the physician and staff must be continually conscious of the schedule and able to alter the tempo of their work to keep to it.

4. The fourth system is "modified wave scheduling." Instead of having a large "wave" of patients first thing each morning and afternoon, smaller waves are created hourly. Two or three patients may be scheduled at the start of office hours, then perhaps one on the quarter-hour, one on the half-hour, and none at the three-quarter mark. The patient who arrives first is conducted directly in to the physician; the second may require laboratory tests or other procedures, or patient education may fill his waiting time. If a third patient is scheduled at the start of the hour, it is with the expectation that one of the three may be late. The first patient seen has tests, procedures, and explanations *after* being seen, not before.

   How the patients are scheduled during the hour depends entirely upon the practice. The important thing is that the total number of patients scheduled during that hour equals the number the physician customarily can see per hour. The second hour is usually the same as the first. A break, plus at least one open slot for walk-ins, is scheduled in the third, and a call-back time in the fourth hour.

   The two advantages of modified wave scheduling are that overall patient waiting time is reduced, and the inevitable and irregular gaps between patients that occur for the physician with stream scheduling are reduced as well. There may be gaps, but they are the end of each hour, and are both longer and more predictable, so the physician can use them productively for phone calls, paperwork, or reading journals. Modified wave scheduling is usually the best system for primary care practitioners. Whatever system is used, the schedule must fit the practice and not the other way around.

Now to the appointment book. The standard one obtainable from a cataloguer covers six days each week, with each day from 8:00 A.M. to 6:00 P.M. divided into 15 minute intervals. But other formats are available (Fig. 19–1), and I would advise getting one with 10 minute intervals, no matter what your specialty. This allows you greater flexibility in developing the system that suits your practice. The paper quality must allow repeated erasures, and the printing should be in a color that is easy on the eyes. The size when open has to fit your available desk space; the wire-bound (not three ring) type allows the book to lie flat when open. Those designed for solo practitioners have a column for the patients' names, followed by another for the purpose of the visit. Some also have spaces for telephone numbers or other information. After you have experimented with a standard appointment book for a few months, you may want to design your own and have it printed.

Before your receptionist makes the first appointment, you have to decide on the hours you will see patients. Do this in accordance with the customs in your community and of your specialty. Starting office hours one or two days a week at 7:00 A.M. may be convenient for commuters. Extending your hours until 9:00 P.M. one night a week allows those who work (or those with small children who must wait until spouses who work return) to come in. If you are a surgeon and the operating room schedule is tight, consider doing your procedures in the afternoon and seeing patients in your office mornings. A pediatrician might have office hours through late afternoon into early evening every day. Saturday mornings are more common now for primary care practitioners, because of increasing competition from convenience clinics with extended hours. Physicians just starting out might want to schedule Sunday hours to help build their practices.

When you have decided what your hours are going to be, have your receptionist "outline" the appointment book one month ahead. The hours you will not be seeing patients are first blocked out with a large "X" from corner to corner. She should use a moderately soft (No. 2) pencil for this and all entries. Days blocked off will include vacations, medical meetings, and holidays. The hours to be blocked off are before and after the hours you choose, lunch, hospital rounds or procedures, and so forth. Then she will set aside "buffer" periods as you direct. A

MONDAY

8 00			
00			
00			
20			
20			
40			
9 00			
00			
00			
20			
40			
10 00			
00			
00			
20			
40			
11 00			
00			
00			
20			
40			
12 00			
00			
1 00			
00			
00			
20			
40			
2 00			
00			
00			
20			
40			
3 00			
00			
00			
20			
40			
4 00			
00			
00			
20			
40			
5 00			
00			
00			
20			
40			

Figure 19–1. Courtesy of Colwell Systems, Inc., Champaign, Illinois.

good way to do this is to put parentheses on either side of the name column, with the purpose of each buffer period stated between them, e.g., (work-ins), (call-back), or (break).

Before we have her make the first appointment, something should be said about the purpose of each of these three types of buffer periods. The term **work-in** applies to patients who must be seen that day but are not true emergencies. Don't confuse them with "walk-ins" who show up without an appointment, which are best discouraged. You should define for your receptionist four categories of patients based upon the degree of urgency; (1) emergencies, (2) work-ins to be seen that day, (3) those who need to be seen within two days, and (4) those who can wait one or two weeks.

In the average practice, one hour of each day is never booked until the morning of that day, to accommodate work-ins. Appointment slots are usually provided in the late morning and late afternoon, with more time allowed on Monday mornings and Friday afternoons, which is when work-ins tend to cluster.

Call-back time for the physician to return calls from patients, pharmacists, and others is usually scheduled for the last time slots each morning and afternoon. The total time to set aside depends upon the practice. A busy pediatrician may need an hour or more each day.

It is wise to schedule a **break** of 10 minutes or so in the middle of each morning and afternoon. Some states require that these periods be set aside for employees, and the physician will also work better after a breather.

New patients are vital for any practice, and this includes referrals if you are a consultant. The one hour reserved for work-ins each day will not be enough to accommodate new patients too. Reserve a whole day in the latter half of each week until that week starts. New patients will not want to wait more than a week for an appointment. This will also benefit your regular patients. It is inconsistent with good practice of medicine to be booked up solid for two or three weeks ahead. As your practice becomes busier and the pressure on your time builds, stretch out the intervals between follow-up visits, have your assistant give more normal laboratory results and other information over the telephone, or add an hour or so to your daily schedule.

Now let's have the telephone ring, or a patient pause at the receptionist's desk to request an appointment. One aide should be designated to make all entries. If she is occupied at the time, have the patient wait until she is free whenever possible. You must keep your hands off the appointment book, also. About 90 per cent of scheduling problems are caused during the 10 per cent of the day that a second assistant has to make appointments. The assistant in charge of the schedule first determines the approximate date the patient desires the appointment, then offers just two time slots: one in the morning of one day and another in the afternoon of the day before or the day after. This tactic avoids "ping-pong" conversations in which she suggests one time, which is declined, then another, which is also declined, and so on. A patient offered two times tends to choose one of them. When an appointment has been set, your assistant should end the conversation with a clear reiteration of the date and time. When the scheduling is done in person, an appointment-charge slip or appointment card is given the patient *every time*. Reappointments are best made for the same time and day of the week as the present appointment.

She then (not later) prints the patient's name legibly, last name first, followed by first name, in the proper column, and puts the purpose of the visit in the second column. If no special space is provided, the patient's telephone number for *the day of the appointment* is printed underneath the purpose. With the stream system, an arrow pointed down blocks out the time you expect to take with that patient. Otherwise, she conforms to your modified wave system. Procedures that your staff will do by themselves can be entered by any method that does not interfere with the basic purpose of the appointment book, which is to schedule *your* time with each patient.

Your patient information booklet will make clear that you expect cancellations to be at least 24 hours in advance. A statement to this effect should be printed on your appointment-charge slip or appointment card, and reinforced with a pleasant reminder by your receptionist. You may reserve the right to charge for appointments not canceled in time. Even if you don't intend to do so, reserving that right will increase patient compliance.

The receptionist should keep a list of patients who already have appointments but would prefer earlier ones. When a cancellation occurs, she can fill it with a patient on this "cancellation list."

"No-shows," those who do not cancel yet fail to keep their appointments, can be a serious problem. It is not merely a matter of wasted time and income lost. Much more serious is the threat of a malpractice action for abandonment. The charts of all no-shows *must* be given to you at the end of the day for your review. Look them over and decide on an appropriate response for each one. If a patient fails a second appointment, call and talk to the patient yourself, explaining why keeping the appointment is important for his health. Document this conversation in the chart. If the patient then fails a third time, you should discharge him using the proper procedure.

Reminding patients of appointments is almost an art form. New patients, those who are to have long visits, and those whose appointments are made more than one to two months in advance should all be reminded by telephone two days before their appointments. The two days allow your receptionist time to fill the slot from the cancellation list if the patient cannot keep the appointment. Patients who cannot be reached during the day can be called by your receptionist from her home in the evening. A recall mechanism must be set up for contacting patients who do not require a follow-up visit within two months but who should be seen every few months or annually. Caution is to be observed because it is unethical to solicit patient visits. The best way to handle this is to have cards printed bearing the statement "At your request, we are reminding you of your appointment on ________ at ________ . Please call at least 24 hours ahead if you wish to cancel." The receptionist will fill in the date and time while the patient is still in the office and hand it to the patient to put his name and address on the reverse. By doing so, the patient is giving implied consent. The card cannot be stamped and sent as is, because doing so would be a breach of confidentiality; instead, it is placed in a window envelope with the address showing. These are then kept in a tickler file by the week they are to be mailed. When the week comes, the appointment is checked, the envelope sealed, stamped, and mailed so as to arrive two or three days before the appointment. When this mechanism is used for all appointments made more than two months in advance, it will reduce no-shows by up to 75 per cent.

Scheduling time to see pharmaceutical representatives is problematic. There was a time when detail men had one or more years of pharmacology behind them, and those with the major firms gave ethical and balanced presentations. Often, too, poorer patients could have an entire course of medication provided free of charge. Representatives would also obtain unbiased reference articles for you. Since the late 1960s the situation has altered dramatically. Most detail men today have little or no education in pharmacology and are trained as high-pressure salesmen. The information most have is limited to that furnished by their firms. Even the research articles they offer are selected for their favorable assessments of the firm's products. Some give gifts to your assistants and gadgets to you, or offer trips and other inducements—all of which is unethical. The final decision is up to each physician. Most see certain representatives (the ones who tell good jokes or fish stories) at breaks during the day, discard their materials and samples as soon as they leave, and ignore what they have to say about their products. I found it easier to avoid them entirely and to derive my information from more reliable sources. If you decide to see pharmaceutical representatives, each is given a 10-minute appointment at times you designate. Respect these appointments as you would any other. Your assistant should have instructions to interrupt you when the 10 minutes is up.

I'd like to pass along a few tips from years of experience. One is to begin your office hours *on time.* Starting even a few minutes late will only compound scheduling problems by the end of the morning or afternoon. The most tempting time to drag your heels is after surgery or hospital rounds. Discussion with your colleagues about new developments in medicine, fascinating cases and complications, or the latest gossip all seem to be more interesting than office practice. But your primary responsibility is to your patients, and you must honor your appointment schedule. Try to arrive in the office a half hour before the first patient is scheduled in order to get all the little administrative problems out of the way so you can see that first patient on time.

Book your patients close together when you are starting practice even if you have only a few. This trains your office staff in the system you have selected, accustoms all of you to working efficiently, and allows you larger blocks of time out of the office for other activities. And it does not do any harm for one patient leaving to see another arriving.

Have your aide review the patient schedule the afternoon before or early that morning and pull the day's charts to check them for completeness before you arrive in the office.

Set aside 10 or 15 minutes each morning before the first patient to hold "chart rounds." This is an opportunity to explain to your assistants what you plan to do with each patient, to allow them to bring up problems you may be unaware of, and to coordinate all your efforts throughout the day. It also is an opportunity to educate your staff and raise morale.

Have your receptionist run off two copies of the schedule for the day on the photocopier. One of these is placed on the desk in your consultation room and the other in a central part of the clinical area. Each must be readily accessible for alterations to be made. If changes occur that cannot be penned in at the moment, new copies are run off and substituted as soon as possible.

Have all new patients and consultations come in at least 15 minutes before they are scheduled to see you. This allows time for them to fill out the patient registration form and for your assistant to check it. It also provides a few minutes for them to read over your patient information booklet and to ask your receptionist questions.

Talkative patients or those who are infirm, confused, or habitually late are better scheduled late in the morning or afternoon so the disruption to your schedule will be minimal. One technique to use with those who are talkative is to give them your full attention without comment.

Most soon run down. If not, wait for a breath, give any instructions firmly, say goodbye without a pause, smile, and leave the room.

Schedule all patients to be seen during the last hour of the day at the beginning of that hour. This will reduce the impact on your closing time if one is late or requires extra time.

Emergencies throw your schedule completely out of kilter. One way to reduce their impact and still care for patients promptly is to send appropriate cases to a hospital emergency room that is staffed by a physician and registered nurses, with a full array of emergency equipment and medications. Often the initial care and studies can be begun there while the patient is under competent supervision. In this way, you may be able to put off seeing the patient yourself for half an hour or so until your next buffer period. When you do see him there, your time is used more productively with the initial studies done. Meanwhile, your receptionist rearranges the rest of your schedule so you can remain with that patient as long as necessary.

Check your scheduling system every month or so to see how it is working. Have one aide record the time when each patient arrives, when he is conducted to the examination or consulting room, when you see him, and when he leaves. Then go over the results at the next staff meeting to work out any kinks.

One way the day can be made lighter for all concerned is to vary your schedule as much as possible. Alternate a long visit with a short one, an old patient with a new one, or a complex case with a simple one. Grouping similar diagnoses or types of patients together does not work very well. While theoretically more efficient, it is difficult to arrange, and seeing more than two or three in sequence may dull your interest.

Once the appointment schedule is properly set up, most delays are attributable to the physician. You can help by being aware at all times of how well you are keeping to your schedule. An assistant can help with gentle, prearranged reminders. When you are running five minutes behind she might say, "Mrs. Jones is waiting." When you are ten minutes behind she would change to, "You have a telephone call from Doctor Smith, and Mrs. Jones is still waiting." At 15 minutes, she might actually take the chart from your hands and stand at the open door. Try whatever works.

Most patients will wait up to 20 minutes before they become irritated. If a delay reaches this length, the patients in the waiting area should be approached by your receptionist and asked if they wish to wait longer or would rather have another appointment. At the same time, the next one or two patients who have not yet come to the office should be telephoned and rescheduled. Then the patients scheduled for the remainder of the day can be seen on time.

You might look at it this way. The total time lost by your patients is arrived at by multiplying the average number of minutes that each has waited by the number of patients who have waited. The total loss over the weeks and months can be absolutely staggering. Their time is worth as much to them as your time is to you.

20

Medical Records

You have already taken the first step in setting up your record-keeping system during the design of your office. You will recall that, in Chapter 11, open-shelf chart storage was recommended. But that still left you with two choices. If you prefer patient labels along the bottom edge of the file folder, each chart has to be stored resting on its fold (Fig. 20–1). A vertical distance between shelves of 10 or 11 inches is then required for the charts to fit. However, if you wish to have the labels on the side of the folder, the chart will then be stored on its bottom edge, which requires a vertical space of about 13 inches. It doesn't matter much which arrangement you choose—there are slight advantages and disadvantages to either one. Just be sure your folders fit your shelves. The following comments will apply to both types of folders.

Some new physicians make the mistake of purchasing the standard manila file folders found in a stationery store. If you do, your charts will look old and weary long before you do. You need sturdier stock—14 point thickness—with a folder expandable to ¾ inch capacity. The tab must be full-cut style with a double-thickness backing using Mylar or other reinforcement. These folders can be purchased from any major cataloguer. If you are tempted to purchase an assortment of colored folders to use for color coding, let me warn you that you will always be running out of one color just when you need it. Choose a neutral color for all, and use labels for the color coding. These can be purchased and stored in such quantities that you will *never* run out. The standard folder size is 9½ × 12¼ inches, designed to hold 8½ × 11 inch sheets. You have three choices on the fasteners. Those attached by adhesive backing to the upper inside right of the file folder tend to pull loose over time or with rough usage. Those inserted through two holes punched in the same location tend to tangle when the chart is being filed or retrieved. The best are the ones

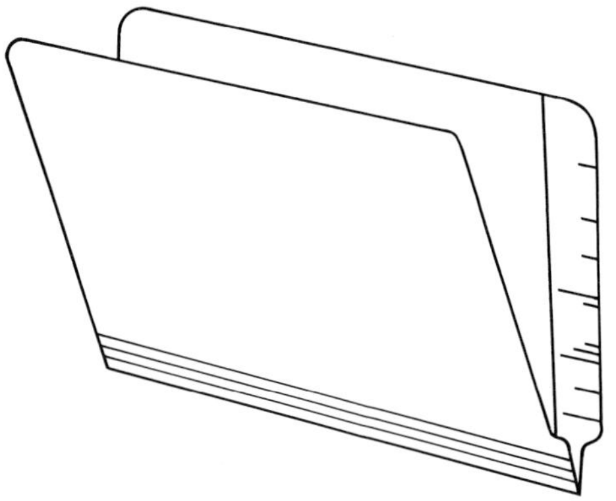

Figure 20–1. Double-edge file folder for storing files either horizontally or vertically.

built into the folder in a small depression. Whether the fasteners are plastic or metal is a matter of personal choice.

Those physicians who plan to use a *problem-oriented medical record* (POMR) can obtain file folders with columns printed on the inside left for recording problem number, date entered, problem description, and date of each occurrence. Below these columns is a space for a summary of medications and possible drug allergies. These folders have a patient registration form printed on the inside right (Fig. 20–2), but you may prefer to design your own and staple it to the inside left. It is also less expensive to have a POMR summary printed on a sheet and stapled

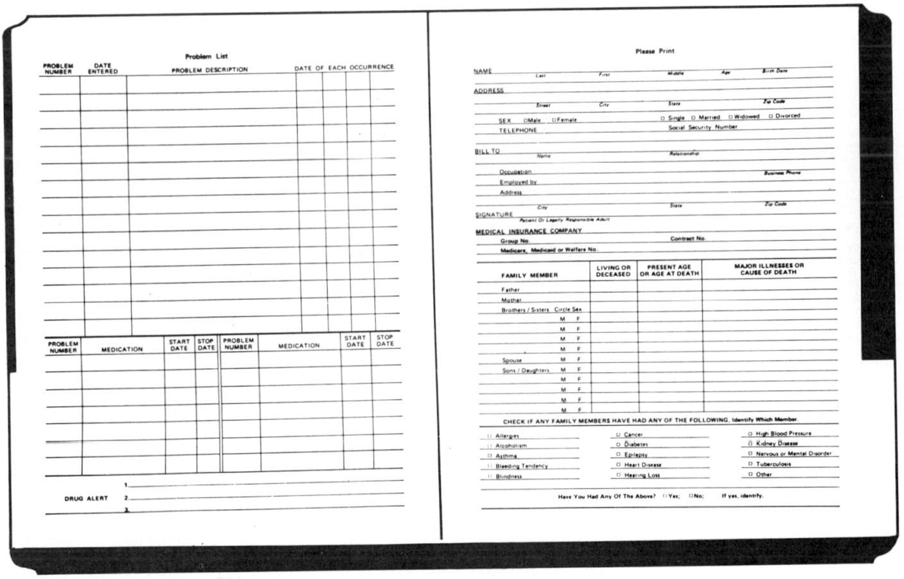

Figure 20–2.

TEST FLOW RECORD

NAME | DATE | AGE | S M D W

ADDRESS | PHONE | SEX

TESTS DATE										
WEIGHT										
BLOOD PRESSURE										
PULSE										
TEMPERATURE										
CBC										
RBC										
WBC										
HGB										
Hematocrit										
Acid Phosphatase										
Alkaline Phosphatase										
Blood Sugar										
Glucose										
Bilirubin										
BUN										
Calcium										
Cholesterol										
Creatinine										
Hb A1c										
Lipid Profile										
SGGT										
SGOT										
SGPT										
T3										
T4										
T7										
TSH										
Triglycerides										
1890 Series										
Uric Acid										
Sodium										
Potassium										
Urinalysis										
Albumin										
Calcium										
Uric Acid										
Pap Smear										
CHANGES										
Appetite										
Diet										
Medication										
Activities										
Physical										
Sleep										

FORM 8044 COLWELL SYSTEMS, INC., CHAMPAIGN, ILLINOIS

Figure 20–3. Laboratory flow sheet.

on the left than it is to buy these specially designed folders. It is not difficult to lift up the patient registration form to review the POMR summary, or vice versa. Some physicians like the file folders with pockets on the left side for miscellaneous items, but use of the pockets interferes with the placement of these two forms, and it is better if the miscellaneous items are filed in their proper places in the chart.

That is all that usually appears on the left when the folder is opened. The right side contains the clinical elements and constitutes the bulk of the chart. It is usually divided into four sections, but you can have as many as you wish. Tabbed section dividers are available, but they are only convenient when the contents become bulky.

Let's start with the last section of the clinical records on the bottom and work our way up. This section consists of laboratory data. Because the individual reports are small and of varied size, they are usually shingled on standard typing paper (using transparent tape for those that do not have an adhesive strip) in reverse chronological order so that the most recent report appears on top. These, or course, are not filed until you have initialed them. Lab flow sheets (Fig. 20–3) are included in the first section with the progress sheets.

The second section from the back consists of various reports from physicians: electrocardiograms with interpretations, pathology reports, radiology readings and reports of procedures or consultations.

The third section from the back consists of former physician's records and hospitalizations, each group arranged in reverse chronological order. Data pertaining to any one hospitalization are arranged either in the sequence that the hospital uses during the patient's stay, or the order used by the hospital when the record is permanently filed. The latter is recommended.

The fourth and uppermost section on the right is composed of your own office records. At the bottom is the history form filled out by the patient (Fig. 20–4), bearing your notes and signature if you have reviewed it. If the patient had a complete physical examination at that time, this will be next, also signed by you. Appropriate history and physical examination forms for any particular specialty are available from cataloguers, as was mentioned in Chapter 13, or you can design your own and have them printed.

Next come the continuation or progress sheets (Fig. 20–5) bearing a record of every contact with the patient: office visit, house call, telephone conversation, telephone prescription or refill, and hospital admission. The first contact is on the last sheet and the most recent on top. These sheets are tumble printed (on both sides) to conserve chart space. It's a good idea to have your clinical assistant keep one

Name	Age	Single / Married	Divorced / Widow(er)	Date
Occupation	All previous occupations			
Birth Place	Birthdate	List all States in which you have lived		

Education: ______years High School ______years College ______years Post Grad.

Date of last physical examination______
Please list all Symptoms
1. ______
2. ______
3. ______
4. ______
5. ______

Routine check-up—no symptoms ☐

P.I. Please do not write in this space.

	If Living: Age	If Living: Health	If Deceased: Age at death	If Deceased: Cause
Father				
Mother				
Brother or Sister 1.				
2.				
3.				
4.				
5.				
Husband or Wife				
Son or Daughter 1.				
2.				
3.				
4.				
5.				
6.				

Has any blood relative ever had:	Please encircle no or yes	Who
Cancer	No Yes	
Tuberculosis	No Yes	
Diabetes	No Yes	
Heart Trouble	No Yes	
High blood pressure	No Yes	
Stroke	No Yes	
Epilepsy	No Yes	
Insanity	No Yes	
Suicide	No Yes	

NOTE: This is a confidential record of your medical history and will be kept in this office. Information contained here will not be released to any person except when you have authorized us to do so.

PERSONAL HISTORY

ILLNESSES: Have you ever had

PLEASE ENCIRCLE ALL ANSWERS No Yes

Measles	No	Yes
German Measles	No	Yes
Mumps	No	Yes
Chicken Pox	No	Yes
Whooping cough	No	Yes
Scarlet fever or Scarlentina	No	Yes
Diphtheria	No	Yes
Smallpox	No	Yes
Pneumonia	No	Yes
Influenza	No	Yes
Pleurisy	No	Yes
Rheumatic fever or heart disease	No	Yes
Arthritis or Rheumatism	No	Yes
Any bone or joint disease	No	Yes
Neuritis or neuralgia	No	Yes
Bursitis, Sciatica or Lumbago	No	Yes
Polio or Meningitis	No	Yes
Nephritis	No	Yes
Gonorrhea or Syphilis	No	Yes
Gallbladder disease	No	Yes
Anemia	No	Yes
Jaundice	No	Yes
Bladder disease	No	Yes
Epilepsy	No	Yes
Migraine headaches	No	Yes
Tuberculosis	No	Yes
Diabetes	No	Yes
Cancer	No	Yes

High or low blood pressure	No	Yes
Colitis or other bowel disease	No	Yes
Hemorrhoids or any rectal disease	No	Yes
Nervous breakdown	No	Yes
Food, chemical or drug poisoning	No	Yes
Hay fever or Asthma	No	Yes
Hives or Eczema	No	Yes
Frequent infections or boils	No	Yes
Any other disease	No	Yes

ALLERGIES: Are you allergic to

Penicillin or Sulfa	No	Yes
Aspirin, Codeine, or Morphine	No	Yes
Mycins or other Antibiotics	No	Yes
Merthiolate or Mercurochrome	No	Yes
Any other drug	No	Yes
Any foods	No	Yes
Adhesive tape	No	Yes
Nail polish or other cosmetics	No	Yes
Tetanus Antitoxin or Serums	No	Yes

INJURIES: Have you had any

Broken or cracked bones	No	Yes
Sprains	No	Yes
Lacerations	No	Yes
Dislocations	No	Yes
Concussion, or head injury	No	Yes
Ever been knocked unconscious	No	Yes

WEIGHT: now____ one year ago ____
Maximum_____, when_____

TRANSFUSIONS: Have you ever had

Blood or Plasma transfusion ____ No Yes

SURGERY: Have you had

Tonsillectomy	No	Yes
Appendectomy	No	Yes
Any other operation	No	Yes

Type_____ Year_____
Type_____ Year_____
Type_____ Year_____

Do you smoke? No Yes
How many per day _____

Have you ever been advised to have any surgical operation which has not been done_____ No Yes

Have you been hospitalized for any illness _____ No Yes

Give details:

FORM 9878 COLWELL CO., CHAMPAIGN, ILLINOIS

Figure 20–4.

Illustration continued on opposite page

DO YOU NOW HAVE OR HAVE YOU HAD WITHIN THE PAST YEAR:

Frequent or severe headaches ____ No Yes
Fainting spells ____ No Yes
Dizziness on change of position ____ No Yes
Unconscious spells ____ No Yes
Blurred vision ____ No Yes
Double vision ____ No Yes
Spots before eyes ____ No Yes
Infected eyes ____ No Yes
Pain behind eyes ____ No Yes
Any change in vision ____ No Yes
Do you wear glasses ____ No Yes
When were they last checked ____
Earaches ____ No Yes
Discharge from ears ____ No Yes
Ringing in ears ____ No Yes
Decrease in hearing ____ No Yes
Recurrent nose bleeds ____ No Yes
Recurrent head colds ____ No Yes
Sinus trouble ____ No Yes
Hay fever ____ No Yes
Strange persistent odors ____ No Yes
Strange taste or loss in taste ____ No Yes
Persistent hoarseness ____ No Yes
Difficulty swallowing ____ No Yes
Enlarged glands ____ No Yes
Recurrent sore throats ____ No Yes
Recurrent sores in mouth ____ No Yes
Soreness or bleeding of gums on brushing ____ No Yes
Chest pain ____ No Yes
Angina pectoris ____ No Yes
Coughed up blood ____ No Yes
Pain in arm(s) ____ No Yes
Night sweats ____ No Yes
Chronic or frequent cough ____ No Yes
Chronic or frequent cough on laying down ____ No Yes
Wake up night short of breath ____ No Yes
How many bed pillows do you use ____
Shortness of breath on:
Walking several blocks ____ No Yes
One flight of stairs ____ No Yes
On laying down ____ No Yes
Purple lips or fingers ____ No Yes
Palpitations or fluttering of heart ____ No Yes
High blood pressure ____ No Yes
Swelling of hands, feet or ankles ____ No Yes
At what time of day ____
Leg cramps on walking or at night ____ No Yes
Enlarged veins in legs ____ No Yes
Recurrent stomach pain ____ No Yes
Belching or heartburn ____ No Yes
Relieved by food or medication ____ No Yes
Appetite — Good ☐ Fair ☐ Poor ☐
Nausea or vomiting ____ No Yes
Vomited blood ____ No Yes
Avoid some foods ____ No Yes
What kinds ____
Avoid spices ____ No Yes
Abdominal cramping ____ No Yes
Color of bowel movement ____
Any blood in BM ____ No Yes
Rectal pain with bowel movement ____ No Yes

DO YOU NOW HAVE OR HAVE YOU HAD WITHIN THE PAST YEAR:

Change in size, shape or texture of BM ____ No Yes
Describe ____
Pain on urinating ____ No Yes
Difficulty in starting urination ____ No Yes
Do you get up at night to urinate ____ No Yes
How many times ____
Urinate more than before ____ No Yes
Urinate less than before ____ No Yes
Any blood in urine ____ No Yes
How many times per day do you urinate ____
Full feeling of bladder, but only small amount of urination ____ No Yes

Lose urine on coughing or sneezing ____ No Yes
Discharge from penis ____ No Yes
Recurrent back pains ____ No Yes
Backaches ____ No Yes
Joint pains ____ No Yes
Swelling of any joints ____ No Yes
Redness or heat of any joint ____ No Yes
Tingling or weakness of hands or feet ____ No Yes
Muscle spasms ____ No Yes
Loss or change in sensation of hands or feet ____ No Yes
Trembling of any extremity ____ No Yes
Growth in neck or throat ____ No Yes
Hot flashes ____ No Yes
Tiredness without apparent reason ____ No Yes
Brittleness of nails ____ No Yes
Dryness of skin ____ No Yes
Easy bruising ____ No Yes
Inability to stand heat ____ No Yes
Inability to stand cold ____ No Yes
Change in hair texture ____ No Yes
Change in skin texture ____ No Yes
Any skin rash ____ No Yes
X-RAYS: Have you ever had x-rays of
Chest ____ No Yes
Stomach or colon ____ No Yes
Gall bladder ____ No Yes
Extremities ____ No Yes
Back ____ No Yes
Teeth ____ No Yes
Other ____ No Yes
EKG: Ever had an electrocardiogram? ____ Yes No
IMMUNIZATIONS: Have you had
Smallpox vaccination within last 7 years ____ Yes No
Tetanus shots (not antitoxin which lasts only 2 weeks) ____ Yes No
Polio shots within last 2 years ____ Yes No

DRUGS: Laxatives: never ☐ occ. ☐ freq. ☐ daily ☐
Vitamins: never ☐ occ. ☐ freq. ☐ daily ☐
Sedatives: never ☐ occ. ☐ freq. ☐ daily ☐
Tranquilizers: never ☐ occ. ☐ freq. ☐ daily ☐
Sleeping pills, etc.: never ☐ occ. ☐ freq. ☐ daily ☐
Aspirin, etc.: never ☐ occ. ☐ freq. ☐ daily ☐
Cortisone, ACTH: never ☐ occ. ☐ freq. ☐ daily ☐
Thyroid: never ☐ yes, in past, none now ☐
daily ☐ now on ____ gr. daily
Appetite depressants: never ☐ occ. ☐ freq. ☐ daily ☐
Have you ever been treated for drug habits ____ No Yes
Have you ever taken Insulin or tablets for diabetes ____ No Yes
Have you ever taken Hormone tablets or injections ____ No Yes
SEX — Entirely satisfactory? ____ Yes No

WOMEN ONLY — MENSTRUAL HISTORY

Age at onset ____
Regular? Yes ☐ No ☐ Varies
Cycle ____ days (from start to start)
Flow: Heavy ☐ Medium ☐ Light ☐
Number of pads used per period ____
Any clots passed ____ No Yes
Pains or cramps ____ No Yes
Date of last period ____
Date of last pelvic exam ____
Date of last Pap test ____
Results: Neg. ☐ Pos. ☐
Any discharge from vagina ____ No Yes
If so, color ____
amount ____
Any itching of vaginal area ____ No Yes
Do you take birth control pills ____ No Yes
How long have you taken them ____
Pregnancies:
How many children born alive ____
How many still births ____
How many premature births ____
How many Cesarean Sections ____
How many miscarriages ____
Any complications with pregnancy ____ No Yes
Describe ____
Other ____

Figure 20–4. *Continued.*

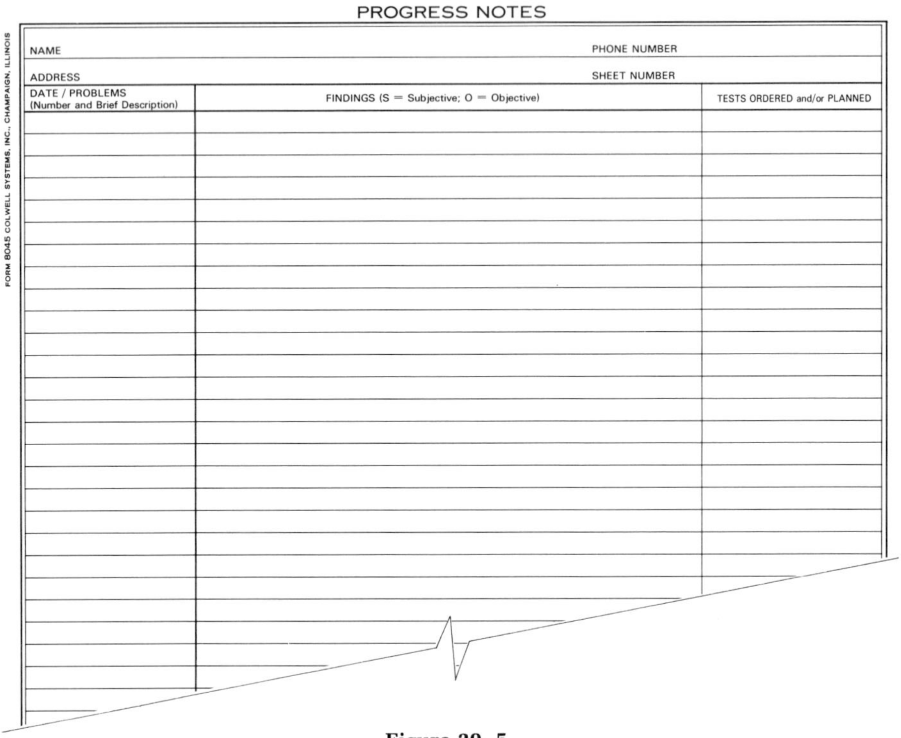
PROGRESS NOTES

FORM 8045 COLWELL SYSTEMS, INC., CHAMPAIGN, ILLINOIS

NAME — PHONE NUMBER

ADDRESS — SHEET NUMBER

DATE / PROBLEMS (Number and Brief Description)	FINDINGS (S = Subjective; O = Objective)	TESTS ORDERED and/or PLANNED

Figure 20–5.

or two blank progress sheets on the top folded back. You always seem to run out in the middle of an entry without blank sheets immediately at hand.

Most physicians use a simple lined sheet with the patient's name entered at the top such as the one used in hospital charts, although variations such as the one illustrated are available from catalogues. These normally come four lines to the inch, but those who write small may prefer six lines to the inch. Entries are always made in black ink, legibly. Dictated notes are typed in the same reverse chronological order on the sheets themselves, properly corrected and signed by you. Alternatively, they may be typed on labels that are permanently glued to the progress sheets. Do not use gummed labels that can be removed—these do not constitute a valid clinical record. All corrections are made by drawing a line through the erroneous entry, entering the correct information, then dating and initialing the change. Never scratch out or erase an original entry so that it cannot be read.

This is the time to discuss the problem-oriented medical record (POMR), introduced by Dr. Lawrence Weed over thirty years ago, as it applies to office practice. Taught today by all medical schools in the country, it is standard in most residency programs as well, and has demonstrated its usefulness in helping physicians in these clinical settings focus on the patient's pertinent medical problems. Yet only about 10 per cent of physicians in private practice use it for their office records. Most of these are in groups in which patient care is shared. Those few in solo practice who use it modify it to suit their preferences. The reason is simply that the pace of office practice, with its time demands and frequent distractions, does not lend itself to the use of a system so cumbersome and complicated, despite its obvious advantages. The best modification on the market is a "SOAP" progress sheet. It has four vertical lines, each of a different color, using the headings *subjective, objective, assessment,* and *plan.* The entries are made at the appropriate line, and the reverse side is printed the same way. These may be ordered from Bibbero systems. (Refer to the list of cataloguers in Chapter 7 for the address.)

Do not put financial, insurance, or other nonclinical material in the chart. Correspondence on medical matters is filed in the second section with physician reports. Correspondence on nonmedical matters is filed in the filing cabinet. Some physicians clip copies of current financial and insurance material together, and store it in the chart unattached to the record. When the chart is used for a clinical purpose, this material is removed and placed in a designated tray or basket in the reception area. Thus the chart contains only medical records whenever the patient is in the office. The material is then reinserted in the chart when it is refiled on the shelf.

Before we get to the labeling, color coding, and proper filing of medical records, something should be said about numerical as opposed to alphabetical filing. The only disadvantage of the latter is that it does not lend itself well to storing large numbers of charts because a missing or misfiled chart is difficult to find. For example, if you have 30 or 40 Smiths in a row, one Smith can be easily filed out of order and be difficult to locate. (Obviously, this is not as likely if you have only four or five Smiths.) For this reason, large clinics and hospitals instituted the numerical filing system about 50 years ago. In this system, each patient is assigned a sequential number at the time of the first visit. The charts are stored in that order and a cross-index (alphabetical to numerical) is maintained in order to locate the charts. A missing or misfiled number is easily spotted. Then, about 30 years ago, color coding was added to the alphabetical system, an improvement that invalidated many of the advantages of numerical filing. However, hospitals and large clinics stayed with the numerical system rather than convert, although most added color coding for further efficiency. An individual practitioner need not concern himself with the numerical system, because alphabetical filing with color coding becomes inefficient only when used for more than 4000 charts.

Color coding with an alphabetical filing system is really rather simple. The number of colors used depends upon the particular system you order. Five is usually enough, but 10 is not uncommon. Various combinations of color on white and white on color can be obtained to provide a maximum of 27 different color codes, if desired. Look over your catalogs—there are many systems on the market. One such system will be described for illustration.

First, take care of the labeling. Plain (or black border on white) name labels measuring approximately 1 × 3 inches are provided on sheets or in rolls. The patient's name is typed—never handwritten—on both halves of the wraparound label so that it can be read from either side of the folder. The surname is always in capital letters, but the given name and middle initial following may or may not be, as you prefer. The typed label is then carefully wrapped around the left or uppermost portion of the folder tab. Each patient, no matter how young, has his own chart. Never use "family charts." Names of family members change, so do addresses, and children become responsible adults. Contents are easily misfiled, and the charts themselves soon become excessively bulky.

Now, for one simple color-coding system: The frequency of occurrence of the first letter of the last name of the typical patient mix has been determined so that, barring any unusual ethnic preponderance, the alphabet may be divided as follows to give approximately equal numbers of charts:

A–C
D–H
I–M
N–R
S–Z

With this particular system, you will receive a roll of wraparound self-adhesive labels for each letter of the alphabet. Some systems, such as the one illustrated, have the letter on the name label, which bears a bar of the same color. Because *Q* is so rare it is often combined with *P*. *U* and *V* are usually combined, and *X*, *Y*, and *Z* almost always are. The letters themselves are colored, and the white label bears a bar of the same color (Fig. 20–6). In such a system, *A–C* might be red, *D–H* yellow, *I–M* green, *N–R* blue, and *S–Z* purple.

A label bearing the first letter of the surname is wrapped around the edge of the file folder to the left or just above the name label so it too can be seen from both sides. Then another label for the second letter of the surname is affixed to the right or below the name label. For common surnames, you may want to color code the initial or the first name also. If you do, be sure *all* charts with that surname are so coded. There is considerable variation from system to system, but the basic concept is the same for all. That's all there is to color coding.

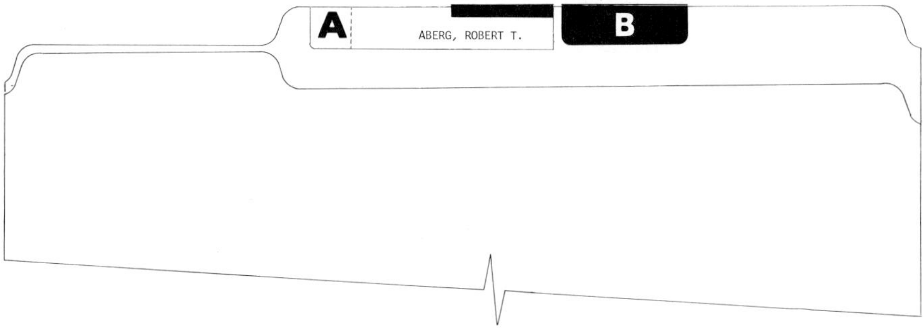

Figure 20–6. Colored alphabetical labels for file folders.

Although your assistants will be responsible for filing the charts, you should know a few rules so you can find a chart when you want to and will not return one to the wrong place:

1. No titles used before or after a name affect filing except two: "Junior" and "Senior" following the name. Only these appear on the labels.
2. Prefixes such as Mac, Mc, and O' are considered part of the surname.
3. Hyphenated names such as Smith-Jones or combination names such as Gonzales Chimichanga are treated as one surname.
4. A woman's legal name is always used. If she is married, it is her husband's surname first, followed by her first name and middle initial. If she has no middle name, then the initial of her maiden name is used instead. Whenever her legal name changes, *all* her records must be changed accordingly.
5. *Always* nothing before something. That is, if a person uses two initials for a first name, his chart would precede that of a person whose first and middle name begin with the same letters. The chart of a "Senior" or "Junior" would follow that of a person bearing the same name without such a designation. A "Junior," of course, is alphabetized before a "Senior" with the same name.

You will need to have one alphabetical file guide separating every 25 charts or so. I would suggest ordering a 100-division set at the time of your initial purchase, anticipating an eventual total of about 2500 active charts. If you do, the 26 letters of the alphabet will be broken down into 100 subdivisions, yielding, for example, *Aa–Alk, All–Am, An–Az* for the letter *A*, and so on for the other letters. These guides are of great assistance in filing and retrieval.

"Out" guides are also extremely useful. These are cardboard or plastic cards the same size as charts that are substituted for a chart when one is removed. In actual practice, out guides are not used to replace charts that are pulled for the patient's visit or for other brief uses. However, when charts will be absent from their proper place in the storage area for more than 24 hours, out guides should always be used. The name of the patient, the date, and the location of the chart are entered each time in the proper place on the card. Some out guides are provided with pockets for material that is to be filed in the chart, but I see no advantage to this. All such material will have a definite routing in the office, so it is simpler to leave it in the appropriate basket until the chart has been returned and the material can be filed properly.

The "golden" rule is that no chart should ever leave the office. If you violate this rule, no matter how careful you are, sooner or later a chart will be irretrievably lost. There are few exceptions to this rule, the principal one being when a chart is subpoenaed. It is so easy and tempting to drop by the office and pick up the chart of a patient you are called to see in the emergency room. Or to take two or three charts home to work on. Or to pick up a chart and walk to the office of a nearby colleague to discuss a case. Don't do it. Remember the rule.

The "silver" rule is that all medical records should be refiled in their proper place at the end of each day. This is a bit harder to observe. There are always a few charts having incomplete insurance forms, pending important lab reports, awaiting your progress notes, or having other problems that prevent their refiling. Have a few wire baskets or trays clearly labeled, put the charts that cannot be refiled at the end of each day in the appropriate one, and insist that all others be refiled.

One last rule—I hesitate to call it the "bronze" rule—is never put a chart in a drawer. Drawers are dangerous for any documents, but some seem to be especially voracious in regard to medical records. Every chart placed in certain drawers is mysteriously consumed and never seen again. Sometimes drawers develop appetites for other types of documents, such as insurance forms. Medical offices would be much better off without any drawers at all.

As long as your total number of charts does not rise much above 2000, there is no need to worry about "active" versus "inactive" charts. Sorting them out is just not worth the effort. When you get close to 3000, however, both time and trouble will be saved over the long run if you purge your charts periodically. The first thing, of course, is to decide on your definition of an inactive chart. Most physicians arbitrarily define it as that of any patient who has not been seen for three years or more. Then, because purging interferes with office routine, you must pick a good time for it. The best is when you are attending a medical meeting or on vacation. Then leave instructions with your senior assistant to remove all charts from the files that are older than three years (if that is how you choose to define inactive). The easiest way for her to do this is to open each one and glance at the top progress note. She will know at least half of the patients and will not need to look at their charts. Then the corresponding ledger card is pulled and attached to the chart, *not* placed in it. All insurance forms, other financial data, and any particular problems connected with the case are noted and this material is also attached to the chart. When you return, sit down with her and review each one. Ask yourself the following questions:

1. Is the record complete? This may be the patient who initiates a malpractice action, or, more commonly, requests that a copy be forwarded a few years hence. Think how much more difficult it will be to complete the record then. A good assistant will have obtained the missing items already.
2. Was the last appointment a no-show? If so, the chart should document the efforts that were made to contact the patient and should show that the proper discharge procedure was then followed. Otherwise you may be liable to a charge of abandonment.
3. Was a clinical endpoint reached? If so, then the patient can be left to his own judgment about returning to your office or seeking care elsewhere. But if a condition requiring further care is indicated, the chart should show that the patient was advised in writing and that clear instructions were sent him. This is best done by certified mail, return receipt requested.
4. Were the correct fees charged? If not, you should decide whether to request complete payment, write off the amount owed, or send a refund.
5. Was the insurance claim form paid in full? If not, consider pursuing this with the carrier.
6. Is there still a balance due? If so, then instruct your assistant to take the appropriate action.

A check-off list for these six points may help. Only when they have been checked should the chart be stored. Put the financial material in your inactive financial file. The best site for inactive chart storage, if you have open-shelf filing to the ceiling, is on the topmost shelves, which are awkward to use for active charts. A stable footstool helps here—some can be rolled about easily on castors but lock in place when they are stepped on. All inactive charts should be arranged alphabeticaly, because about once a month an "inactive" patient will come in and you will need to have the chart right then. Although the office storage closet or another similar site in the building can be used, the tendency with these is to tie or box each group of charts when they are purged. After several purges, retrieval of any chart on short notice is almost impossible. If you must use such a space, at least arrange the charts alphabetically in each box or bundle, and label each batch with the names of the patients whose charts are contained therein.

Management consultants have come up with other purging systems that I cannot recommend. One way is reviewing the ledger cards instead of the charts. This is somewhat easier than reviewing the charts themselves, but the time saved, relative to the total required by the task, is so slight that I do not see any significant advantage. Another way is to label the chart with the year the patient was last seen. Numerical labels for this purpose are obtainable from most cataloguers. However, this system requires periodic updating of all charts so the labels will accurately reflect the date the patient was last seen. This entails much more effort than the simple system I suggest.

The charts themselves, the physical elements of the medical records, belong to you. The information contained therein, however, is legally the property of your patient. The patient is within his legal rights when he requests to see the chart or to be furnished with any information contained therein. The patient's freedom is only subject to restriction if, in your opinion, that information would be detrimental to the patient. Then the information requested must be given to a designated responsible party. Consult your attorney in doubtful cases. A properly executed request to forward medical information must be honored, even if it is to a swami who cures cancer by mystic chants, a chiropractor, or a "naturopath" south of the border who uses exotic herbs and enemas for all ills. Be sure to observe the inclusive dates specified on the request. When no dates are given, request them. If you send information pertaining to other periods, you may be held liable for invasion of privacy.

The legal requirement for retention of medical records varies with the statute of limitations for legal actions in each state. Ask your attorney. For a child treated at age two it may be six years past his eighteenth birthday—a total of 22 years! Beyond the legal requirement, keeping records indefinitely may be beneficial to your patients. I once had an electrocardiogram on file that became crucial 30 years after it was taken. All of us are aware of the problems resulting from the administration of DES to pregnant women in the 1950s and 1960s. The detrimental effect of DES upon their female offspring was not discovered until much later. When you turn over your practice to another physician or retire, consult Chapters 9 and 34 for suggestions on the proper disposition of your medical records.

21

Establishing Fees

Time was, according to legend, when a physician could get by without charging his patients at all. According to this legend, grateful patients now and then would bake him a pie or drop off a chicken for his pot. In my own time, and this is *not* a legend, one could concentrate on the practice of medicine without giving much thought to financial matters. If assistants wanted to get paid, they made sure that enough money came into the office to go around. Although no truly reputable physician ever got rich from his practice, all or almost all were certainly comfortable. Even up to a few years ago, there was not much to worry about.

Not so now. The "physician shortage" of the 1960s has become a surplus. Patients are more conscious of the cost of medical care. HMOs are charging less and looking to federal funds to make up the difference. Cost-cutting convenience clinics are springing up all over. More IPAs and PPOs are being set up that offer substantial discounts on professional fees. Paraprofessionals such as emergency medical technicians, physicians' assistants, nurse practitioners, and midwives are doing more for lower fees. Medicaid has always been tight, and Medicare recently imposed prospective payment on hospitals. The CEOs (no longer administrators) of hospitals are transmitting this pressure to staff physicians. Something resembling payment by diagnosis-related groups (DRGs) may soon be extended to office practice by Medicare and other third-party carriers. Meanwhile, overhead costs for the private practitioner continue to spiral. Professional managers with MBAs, computers, and sophisticated business systems have taken over the financial affairs of the larger medical groups. This is no longer a world in which physicians in private practice or small groups can ignore the business side of medical practice.

What are we going to do about it? Well, we certainly can't just grumble to ourselves or gather together to toast the "good ol' days." It is said that physicians lack business sense. That hurts, perhaps because it's partly true. It may well be that those with the *most* talent in business gravitated toward a business major while we were grinding our way through premed, but this doesn't mean that physicians are *completely* lacking in business sense. We do have brains, and the principles involved are amazingly simple. This brings us back to the major theme of this book: physicians need to learn a few fundamental principles, put them into effect, and monitor their application. That is really all there is to it.

In our practices, we have to become familiar with every step of the trail, from the dollar charged to the dollar spent. That is what this and the next four chapters are about.

Setting your fees is the first step along this trail. But this requires some thought. Consider a couple of examples. An injection given by your clinical assistant takes only a minute or so of her time and perhaps 50 cents worth of medication. If you don't see the patient as well, you might think a suitable charge would be around one dollar. But look into this further. Calculate the time taken by your assistants in setting up the appointment, pulling the chart, greeting the patient, conducting him to the examining room, asking about allergies, preparing the injection, giving it, observing the patient for a possible adverse reaction, and documenting the injection in the chart. Then charges must be apportioned to include staff time required for ordering supplies and paying for them, the costs of billing and collecting, office rent and utilities, the expense of purchasing and maintaining emergency equipment, the value of time you gave to training your staff to take care of possible adverse reactions to the injection, and the premiums paid for your malpractice insurance. Once you have considered all of these, it is evident that even a ten dollar charge would not cover the costs, let alone allow a fair return.

Or, let's say you spend time consoling distraught relatives, watching at the bedside of a seriously ill patient in the intensive care unit, calming an emotionally upset patient in your office, or making a diagnosis in an exceptionally complex case. When it comes right down to it, all you have to sell is your time and skill. You might expect compensation for your time comparable to that received by a psychiatrist. To your dismay, you find that neither patients nor third-party carriers will compensate you adequately. This is one factor that has led to the depersonalizing of medical care. But if you had billed for a *procedure* requiring less time and skill, you would have received generous compensation. What you are up against here is a mind set that insurance carriers and patients developed around the turn of the century. Health insurance came into being to help patients pay for catastrophically expensive medical care. In those days, most illnesses of a grievous nature soon ended in death, except those requiring surgery. These ran up large bills, and health insurance was instituted to take care of them. The result is that today the time and skill spent in counseling and cognitive pursuits receive only a fraction of the compensation they would if they were invested in a mechanical procedure. There is no way you as an individual can alter this mind set, but changes are taking place—slowly. If all fees were made fair and proportionate at a stroke, there would be more compassion in medical care at much lower cost.

Perhaps the single greatest advance in helping establish appropriate fees started in 1956 with the studies undertaken by the **California Medical Association** (CMA). These resulted in a report known as the **California Relative Value Studies,** which was revised and reissued every few years up to 1974. Although no dollar amounts were given, the studies gave numerical unit values for each service and procedure that allowed accurate comparisons to be made. Each physician, having established one or two appropriate fees, could compute a conversion factor that could then be applied to the unit values of other procedures and services to determine fees for them. Physicians who were exceptionally skilled or eminent in their fields were free to use a higher conversion factor. Many other states subsequently produced their own *Relative Value Studies* (RVS) based upon these efforts of the California Medical Association.

To appreciate the worth of these studies, let's see how they would help in the two examples above. All the ancillary costs of a simple injection were determined by experience and incorporated into its unit value, so that the fee is fair. Some steps were taken to recognize the value of cognitive services by providing different unit values according to the time spent in an office or hospital visit.

However, in 1979, the Federal Trade Commission brought an action against the California Medical Association claiming that publication of the relative value studies was in restraint of trade. Rather than contest it, the CMA voluntarily ceased publishing the studies. Other states followed suit. The CMA publisher, Sutter Publications, Inc., 44 Gough Street, San Francisco, CA 94013, now offers the **California Standard Nomenclature,** which is similar to the AMA's *Physician's Current Procedural Terminology*.

The discontinuation of the California RVS created an information gap that was experienced most acutely by physicians just beginning practice. Some of the more resourceful of them contacted established physicians who still had ragged copies of the 1974 RVS and photocopied those pages applicable to their practice. Others simply borrowed a fee schedule from a physician in the same specialty based on the

1974 RVS and modified it. Both of these methods of determining fees could be considered in restraint of trade, so I cannot recommend them. What I would recommend is looking in your medical library for *Relative Values for Physicians*, published by McGraw-Hill in 1984. Or you can order it from Relative Value Studies, Inc., P.O. Box 6431, Cherry Creek Station, Denver, CO 80206.

I'd also recommend that you write the **Professional Relations Department** of your Medicare carrier on letterhead stationery and request the *Customary Fee Profile* for your area. Under the Freedom of Information Act, the carrier must comply. This will provide you with a list of all procedures and services with their "customary" fees. Curiously, this is the same information offered by a relative value study. The fees are low, but they are accurate in relation to each other, so they can be used exactly as if they were unit values of the RVS. All you need is at least one fair fee. If you do not have one, the Government will help you here, too. Request a copy of *Determination of Reasonable Charges Under Part B of Medicare, BHI029* from your Medicare carrier or from the **Health Care Financing Administration,** Department of Health and Human Services, Baltimore, MD 21207. This is an outline of the steps Medicare uses in determining their allowable charges that you can follow and modify as you go along.

Most states still use the 1974 RVS to set their allowable fees for Workers' Compensation. If you request a fee schedule from the appropriate agency in your state, you will have yet another RVS. You can do the same with the Blue Cross and Blue Shield schedules. Most health insurance carriers will provide indemnity schedules that can be used the same way. It is curious that publication of this information by a medical association is held to be illegal by the FTC, but if done by another Federal agency, a state government, or an insurance carrier it evidently is not.

Each year *Medical Economics* publishes one issue that profiles fees throughout the United States by region and specialty. This too is apparently legal. Some of the rough edges on your fee schedule can be smoothed out by reviewing the last such issue in your medical library. Before you have your fee schedule typed up, discuss any fees you are doubtful about with three or four physicians in your specialty and one or two physicians from whom you receive referrals. You should be somewhere near the going rate. Make it clear that you are asking their *advice* on certain fees you have already determined, not requesting their fee schedule in order to charge the same. Word your question, "Do you think this is fair?" *not* "What do you charge?" If you have any doubts about the legality of this inquiry, ask your attorney.

One interesting fact discovered through patient surveys should be mentioned, whether you make use of it in compiling your schedule or not. The fees that end in *0* cause the greatest number of complaints; those ending in 5 are next. Those ending in other numbers cause the least. Strange but true.

Have your first fee schedule typed up, date it, and make four or five photocopies. One will be given to your receptionist for use in filling out charge slips and collecting at the point of service. Another is for the assistant who prepares insurance claim forms, and one can be placed in a plastic cover for use in discussions with patients. Two are placed in the files, one to be used as a scratch sheet for the next revision and one as a spare. The first fee schedule should be reviewed about once a month during your first year of practice. Thereafter, about every six months or so will do. This procedure is important. You don't have to *raise* fees, just *review* them. Such reviews result in small changes that are more acceptable to patients. If any large changes must be made, your patients deserve to be informed by letter or by whatever means you think best.

Even when your fee schedule is prepared, you are still not done with the subject of fees. Decide on a few guidelines concerning those patients whom you intend to treat without charge, adjustments to be made in cases of temporary financial hardship, discounts for prompt payment of large amounts, and so forth. Communicate these guidelines to your staff, and emphasize that the final decision in each case will be yours.

Another decision is needed on what to charge patients for the preparation of an insurance claim form. The customary solution is to do the first one free, then charge your calculated cost for each thereafter.

Sometimes charging for laboratory tests performed by an outside laboratory can cause confusion. You are entitled to bill the patient for obtaining and processing the specimen. The charge for interpreting and explaining the results is included in the office visit. The laboratory bills the patient directly for the test itself. It is unethical, and in certain circumstances may be illegal, to include a charge for the test on your statement and to pay the laboratory yourself. Doing so may also raise questions in the patient's mind about a possible markup.

Large fees for substantial services or procedures should be discussed ahead of time with the patient, and a payment method worked out. The more elective the reason for the charge, the larger the portion that should be collected in advance.

You will have to establish a policy on professional courtesy almost as soon as you start practice. Setting aside the admonition of Hippocrates for a moment and looking at things as they really are, it is apparent that this ancient tradition is slowly dying. But there is a great deal of regional variation, so you are best guided by the customs prevailing in your community.

Three guidelines that can be followed by physicians in most areas are: First, recognize that only your time and skill are available to your colleagues as a courtesy, not your supplies and medications, or laboratory tests done outside of your office. So you may charge for these if you wish. Second, if a physician has health insurance, treating him without charge would benefit the insurance carrier, not the physician. Since this is not the intent of professional courtesy, the portion paid by insurance should be accepted. The third part of this tripartite policy: write off everything else. Remember as you do so that this is a *professional* courtesy, applicable to your colleagues [and their dependents], whether active or retired, local or foreign, able or unable to reciprocate. It is an honor to the profession of which you are a member.

The question always arises, what to do about psychiatrists? They *are* physicians, of course, but their specialty began to withdraw from the medical community a few decades ago. Try to remember the last time you saw one at a medical meeting, or even a hospital staff function. I think about this every time I attend a meeting on a psychiatric subject, trying to learn a little more about their field. Decide as you will. Magnanimity may be the better part of professional etiquette, so you may want to give them professional courtesy as if they were true colleagues. Do not assume, however, that they will reciprocate. Few do.

There are others in the health professions who are not included in the above courtesy policy: employees of nearby physicians, pharmacists, audiologists, hospital employees you work with, physiotherapists, registered nurses (active or retired), and so forth. Occasionally, physicians even include priests, ministers, and rabbis. Some professionals are more deserving than others. Rather than make an individual decision in each case, it is simpler to pick a percentage, such as 25 per cent, and give this discount to all. Health care professionals at the doctoral level (such as dentists, podiatrists, and optometrists), however, are on a straight reciprocity basis if you use their services. If not, they receive the same discount.

When these fee policies have been decided upon, summarize them in your office manual. Don't put your fee schedule there, because it will change too frequently. Explain as much as you wish in your patient information booklet, but cover at least these points: how your fees are determined, that payment at the time of service is expected, that a fee schedule is available, and that you and your assistants are happy to answer questions or discuss any problems.

22

Charges and Collections

With your fees established and your policies set, the next step is to put them into operation. This and the following chapter will guide you in doing so. A physician today has two choices for his bookkeeping system: a pegboard or a computer. Since those just starting out in private practice are already $50,000 or more in debt, adding another $5,000 to $10,000 for a computer system usually proves to be too much. It is, however, an attractive alternative for many physicians once their practices are established, and it will be discussed in Chapter 31.

A few years ago, there was a third choice. But computerized billing by an independent "service bureau" was found to be too cumbersome and expensive, and has fallen into disuse.

This leaves us with the pegboard system as the subject of this chapter. It is inexpensive, simple to operate, reduces errors with the "one-write" feature, and has several checkpoints to detect theft. It is the system used by more than 90 per cent of physicians in private practice today.

Your next choice may be harder—which cataloguer to contact for the components. Refer to the list of major cataloguers in Chapter 7, and look over samples from at least three. The entire system should be ordered from one because components of one system may not work in another. Select a firm with a local representative. All of the pegboard systems come with clear instructions, and major cataloguers provide toll-free numbers to call with questions. Business office suppliers in your locality may carry pegboard systems, but it is advisable to order yours from a major medical cataloguer. If you obtain *all* your business supplies from one, the local representative will be more helpful with a larger account to look after; he can adapt the system to suit your practice; he will take the time to train your personnel now and, in the event of turnover, later; he will have many helpful suggestions; and you will be sure that all the products can be used together.

Some physicians never go near the front office, and many of those who do really don't know how a pegboard system operates. The description and discussion that follow are sufficient to allow a physician to understand the system. They are not detailed enough to guide an assistant, who should consult the instructions that come with the system.

The materials consist of the following:

1. **The pegboard itself.** (See Fig. 22–1.) This is made of two pieces of aluminum bound together with vinyl. When folded, it fits into a filing cabinet easily. When opened on the desk, it is approximately 1 × 1½ feet and offers a good writing surface. The pegboard gets its name from the row of pegs down one side that hold the forms in alignment.
2. **The day sheet,** or daily log of charges and receipts. (See Fig. 22–2.) It is slightly smaller than the opened pegboard and has precision-punched holes along the edge to fit the pegs. Three larger holes are for use when it is placed in a three-ring storage binder for permanent storage.

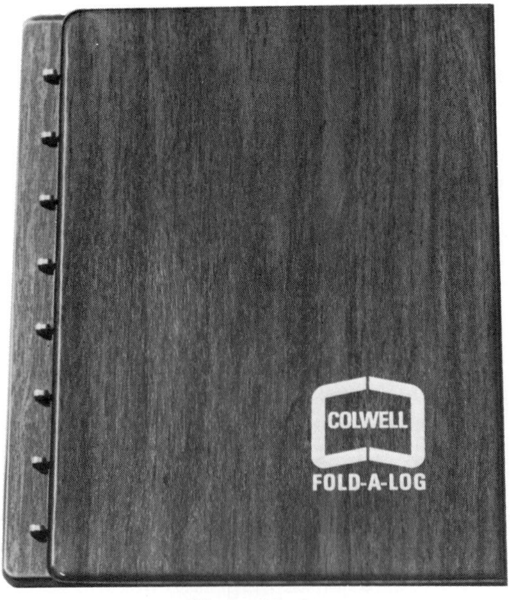

Figure 22–1.

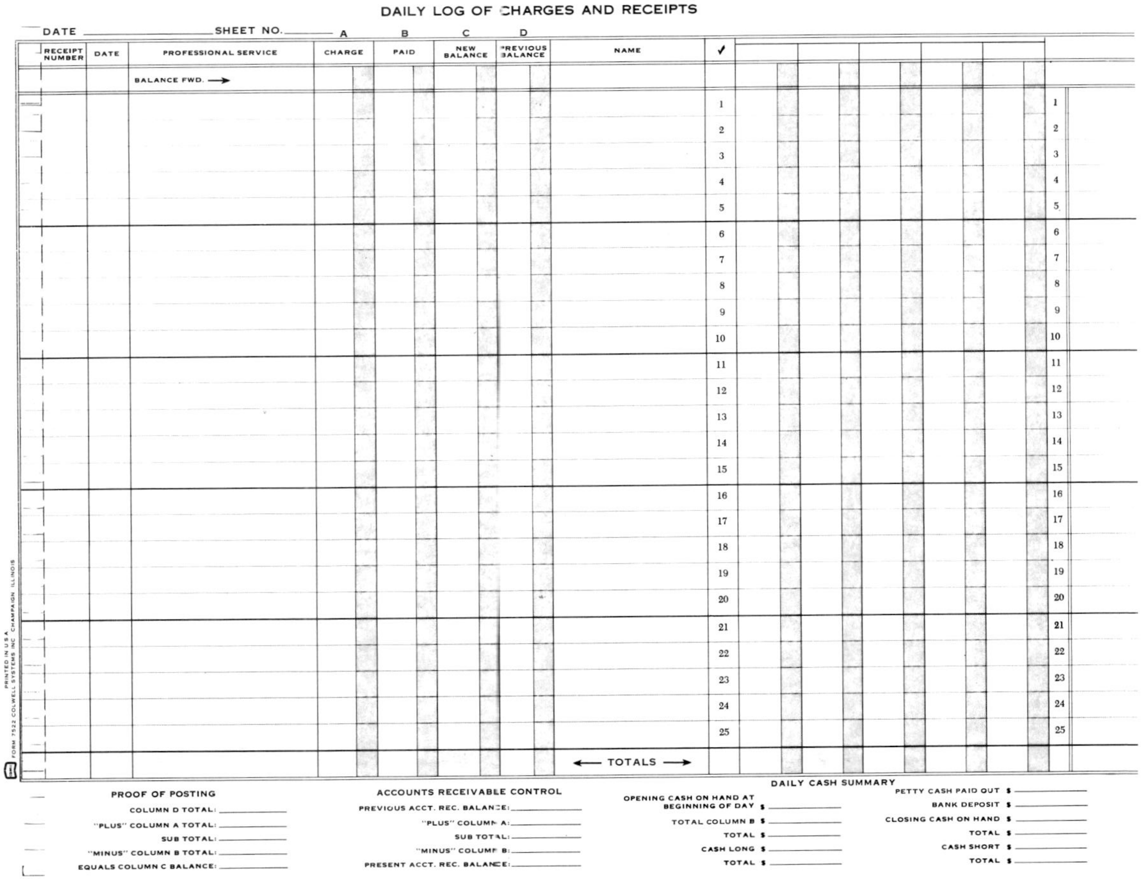

DAILY LOG OF CHARGES AND RECEIPTS

DATE ________ SHEET NO. ________

RECEIPT NUMBER	DATE	PROFESSIONAL SERVICE	A CHARGE	B PAID	C NEW BALANCE	D PREVIOUS BALANCE	NAME	✓						
		BALANCE FWD. ⟶												
								1						1
								2						2
								3						3
								4						4
								5						5
								6						6
								7						7
								8						8
								9						9
								10						10
								11						11
								12						12
								13						13
								14						14
								15						15
								16						16
								17						17
								18						18
								19						19
								20						20
								21						21
								22						22
								23						23
								24						24
								25						25
							⟵ TOTALS ⟶							

PROOF OF POSTING
COLUMN D TOTAL: ________
"PLUS" COLUMN A TOTAL: ________
SUB TOTAL: ________
"MINUS" COLUMN B TOTAL: ________
EQUALS COLUMN C BALANCE: ________

ACCOUNTS RECEIVABLE CONTROL
PREVIOUS ACCT. REC. BALANCE: ________
"PLUS" COLUMN A: ________
SUB TOTAL: ________
"MINUS" COLUMN B: ________
PRESENT ACCT. REC. BALANCE: ________

DAILY CASH SUMMARY
OPENING CASH ON HAND AT BEGINNING OF DAY $ ________
TOTAL COLUMN B $ ________
TOTAL $ ________
CASH LONG $ ________
TOTAL $ ________

PETTY CASH PAID OUT $ ________
BANK DEPOSIT $ ________
CLOSING CASH ON HAND $ ________
TOTAL $ ________
CASH SHORT $ ________
TOTAL $ ________

FORM 7522 COLWELL SYSTEMS INC CHAMPAIGN ILLINOIS PRINTED IN U S A

Figure 22–2.

3. **The ledger cards.** (See Fig. 22–3.) Each card is of heavy stock and measures 5½ × 8½ inches. It is printed only on the front in black ink for clear photocopying.

   The columns of the ledger card correspond to the first six columns on the day sheet and also to the top strip on the receipt-charge slip and the "superbill." Entries made in the professional service column are abbreviated according to the code you have printed at the bottom of the ledger card. There is room to list 15 of your most frequent services. The ledger cards of some systems are perforated along the left edge so that they fit against the pegs of the pegboard and stay properly aligned while entries are made.

STATEMENT

LEONARD S. TAYLOR, M.D.
2100 WEST PARK AVENUE
CHAMPAIGN, ILLINOIS 61822

TELEPHONE 367-6671

RECEIPT NUMBER	DATE	PROFESSIONAL SERVICE	CHARGE	PAID	NEW BALANCE

1631

PAY LAST AMOUNT IN THIS COLUMN

OC - OFFICE CALL
HC - HOUSE CALL
HOSP - HOSPITAL CARE
L - LABORATORY
I - INJECTION
INS - INSURANCE
OB - OBSTETRICAL CARE
PAP - PAPANICOLAOU TEST
OS - OFFICE SURGERY
HS - HOSPITAL SURGERY
PE - PHYSICAL EXAMINATION
EKG - ELECTROCARDIOGRAM
XR - X-RAY
M - MEDICATION
NC - NO CHARGE

Figure 22–3.

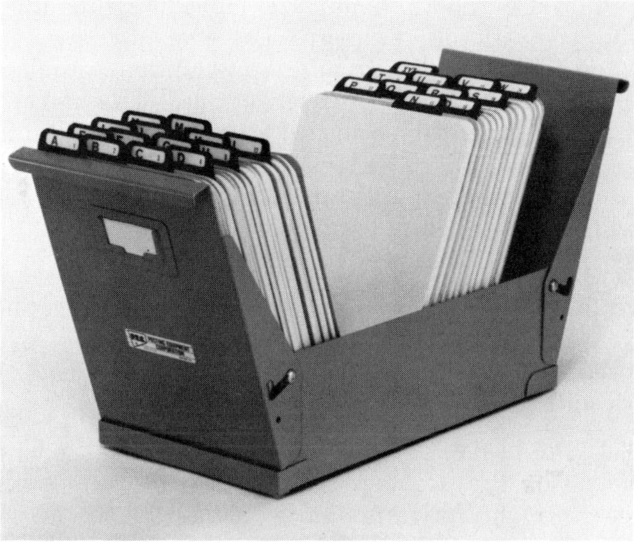

Figure 22–4.

The ledger cards are kept in a specially designed metal tray between the two end plates. (See Fig. 22–4.) The cards themselves are separated by alphabetical index guides that have sturdy metal-tipped tabs. The front plate tips forward to allow easy access to the cards. It is tipped back when the cards are not in use, which compresses the cards and locks them in the tray. The dimensions of the tray allow it to be placed sideways in a drawer of a filing cabinet.

4. **The receipt-charge slip.** (See Fig. 22–5.) This is perforated so that it can be separated into two parts—a charge slip on the right and a receipt slip on the left. The receipt portion also has a space for

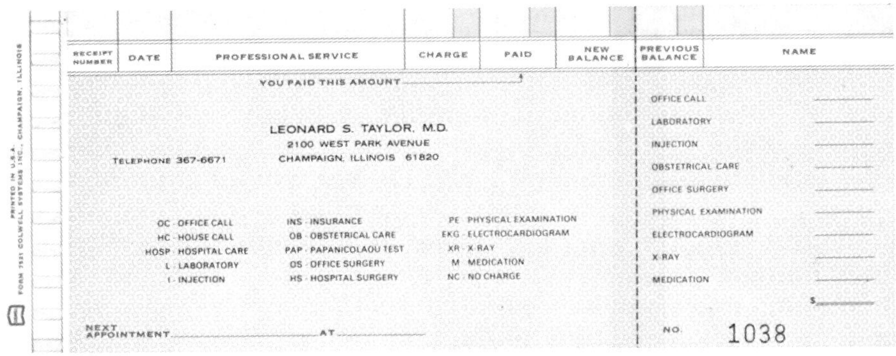

RECEIPT NUMBER	DATE	PROFESSIONAL SERVICE	CHARGE	PAID	NEW BALANCE	PREVIOUS BALANCE	NAME

YOU PAID THIS AMOUNT $

LEONARD S. TAYLOR, M.D.
2100 WEST PARK AVENUE
CHAMPAIGN, ILLINOIS 61820

TELEPHONE 367-6671

OC - OFFICE CALL
HC - HOUSE CALL
HOSP - HOSPITAL CARE
L - LABORATORY
I - INJECTION

INS - INSURANCE
OB - OBSTETRICAL CARE
PAP - PAPANICOLAOU TEST
OS - OFFICE SURGERY
HS - HOSPITAL SURGERY

PE - PHYSICAL EXAMINATION
EKG - ELECTROCARDIOGRAM
XR - X-RAY
M - MEDICATION
NC - NO CHARGE

NEXT APPOINTMENT ______ AT ______

OFFICE CALL
LABORATORY
INJECTION
OBSTETRICAL CARE
OFFICE SURGERY
PHYSICAL EXAMINATION
ELECTROCARDIOGRAM
X-RAY
MEDICATION
$

NO. 1038

FORM 7521 COLWELL SYSTEMS INC., CHAMPAIGN, ILLINOIS
PRINTED IN U.S.A.

Figure 22–5.

recording future appointments. The holes along the left border fit over the pegs of the pegboard. The receipt-charge slip comes preprinted with your name, address, telephone number, and the same procedure coding as the ledger card. The entry line has a carbon strip on the reverse so that all entries made are transferred through to the day sheet and the ledger card. The slips are sequentially numbered and come shingled in banks of 25 to match the number of lines on the day sheet.

That is about all there is to the pegboard system. Other components—the "superbill," single-window envelopes for mailing the photocopied ledger card statements, return envelopes, the summary log, and permanent storage binder—will be mentioned in passing as the use of the system is described.

This is what your assistant does. At the start of each day, a new day sheet is placed on the pegboard. It is dated and numbered, and the balances are brought forward. Only one day sheet is put on the pegboard at a time in order to have a firm writing surface for the "one-write" feature. Then a bank of shingled receipt and charge slips is aligned over the day sheet.

When a patient comes up to your receptionist, she removes his ledger card from the tray, and prints the name and previous balance (taken from the ledger card) on the entry strip of the uppermost charge slip. She should use a black ball-point pen and press firmly so that the day sheet beneath will be easy to read. The ledger card is immediately returned to the tray. The charge portion of the receipt-charge slip is torn off along the perforated line and clipped to the patient's chart to be passed along to you. From it you will be advised of the outstanding balance and can discuss it with the patient if you wish. Even if you do not, the patient knows you are aware of it.

When you are finished with the patient, indicate the services provided on the charge slip using your code, and hand it to the patient with instructions to take it to the receptionist. The patient is thus made aware of his charges for that day.

When the patient returns to the receptionist, she again takes the ledger card from the tray and aligns it on the day sheet under the receipt portion of the slip. The date, the services rendered, the charge for those services, the amount paid, and the new balance are written on the slip. This is transferred through to the ledger card and day sheet—black on the former for photocopying and blue on the latter through NCR treatment. If the NCR-treated form is not transmitting a clear impression through to the day sheet, a sheet of carbon paper may be positioned on top of it. The ledger card is immediately returned to its proper position in the tray.

The receipt portion of the slip is then removed and given to the patient. If the appointment line on the bottom of this slip is used, the date and time of the new appointment are entered *after* it is removed from the pegboard.

The columns of the day sheet to the right of those used to this point are for distributions according to categories of charges. Entries are made in these columns after the patient has left.

Payments received in the mail or from patients who drop in to pay are entered just as if the patient were seen that day, but no charges are entered.

At the end of the day, all of the columns on the day sheet are totalled. Accuracy is checked by the proof of posting at the bottom. Any error found must be corrected on *both* the day sheet and the corresponding ledger card. The deposit slip is then made out and the day's deposit taken to the bank. The total appearing on the deposit slip should equal the receipts for that day. The previous accounts receivable is brought forward, and the new accounts receivable balance is calculated and entered. Then the daily cash summary is completed. There is often some reluctance on the part of weary assistants to do all this, but it must be done at the end of every day. Spot check to see that it is.

The "superbill" was designed to save clerical work in preparing insurance claim forms. (See Fig. 22–6.) It may be used instead of the receipt-charge slip for all patients, or for just those covered by insurance, in which case the two forms will be used alternately throughout the day. It is considerably larger than the receipt-charge slip and contains much more information. Yours should be tailored to your practice. Have a list of diagnoses printed by the cataloguer, *with diagnostic codes included*. Each superbill consists of three copies that are NCR-treated. In use, all three copies are taken from the pegboard and clipped to the patient's chart. You make your entries, which carry through, and your receptionist makes hers while it is aligned on the pegboard. The superbill is then removed from the pegboard and separated. The top copy is retained for your records, the second is handed to the patient as his receipt, and the third may be sent with an insurance claim form either by your office or by the patient.

That is the record-keeping procedure each working day. Once a month, or on the day you send statements, your aide pulls all the ledger cards that show a positive balance in order to do the billing. Have her add these balances up before she proceeds with the billing. The total should match the accounts receivable figure carried on the day sheet for that day. This is called a "trial balance." If the two do not match, the error must be found and corrected. (The actual billing process will be described later in the chapter.)

FORM 7563 COLWELL CO. · CHAMPAIGN, ILLINOIS

RECEIPT NUMBER	DATE	PROFESSIONAL SERVICE	CHARGE	PAID	NEW BALANCE	PREVIOUS BALANCE	NAME

YOU PAID THIS AMOUNT ______
THIS IS A STATEMENT OF YOUR ACCOUNT TO DATE ______

Date of Service ______

CHART NO. ______

PATIENT: ______ ☐Male ☐Female

DIAGNOSIS: ______

ATTENDING PHYSICIAN'S STATEMENT

AMA Current Procedural Terminology, 4th Edition

DISABILITY: From ______ To ______

PHYSICIAN SERVICES		FEE
90000	Office Visit	
90017	Office Visit-Extended	
90020	Office Visit-Complex	
99050	After Hours O.V.	
99054	Saturday A.M., O.V.	
90600	Consultation	
99155	Conference	
	Accident-Evaluation	
	Admit · Routine	
	· Comprehensive	
	CPX · Male	
	· Female	
	· Pre-OP	
	· Pre-Employment	
	· VOC Rehab	
	· Insurance	
	· College Physical	
	· Executive Phys.	
	Pelvic · Routine	
	· Complex	
MINOR SURGERY		
	Incision & Drainage	
	Excision	
	Biopsy	
	Dressing	
OFFICE SERVICES		
	BP Check	
	Catheterization	
	Dietician	
	EKG	
	Ear Irrigation	
	Forms	
	Long Distance Phone Call	
	Nurse Visit	
	Patient Education	
	Patient Screening	

LAB PROCEDURES		FEE
82040	Albumin	
84075	Alkaline Phosphatase	
86060	ASO Titer	
82236	Bicarbonate	
82250	Bilirubin	
85005	Blood Count	
84520	BUN	
82310	Calcium	
85031	CBC	
82465	Cholesterol	
82435	Chloride	
82550	CPK	
82565	Creatinine (Serum)	
87181	Culture/Sensitivity	
86013	Differential	
85362	FDP	
86000	Febrile AGG	
86650	FTA	
83526	Glucose, Fasting/2hr. PPBS	
82951	Glucose Tolerance, 3 Hr./5 Hr.	
86285	HAA	
85055	Hematocrit	
83020	Hemoglobin	
86300	Heterophile AGG	
83550	IBC Iron Binding Capacity	
83540	Iron, Serum	
86006	Latex LE	
	Latex RA	
83615	LDH	
86300	Mono	
85580	Platelet Count	
84100	Phosphorous	
84140	Potassium	
85730	PTT	
85368	Protamine	
85044	Reticulocyte CT.	
90721	Rubella Antibody Titer	
85650	Sed Rate	
84450	SGOT	
83052	Sickle Cell Prep	

LAB PROCEDURES (cont.)		FEE
84295	Sodium	
87015	Stool-OCP/Occult Blood	
	T-3	
	T-4	
	T-7	
	Triglycerides	
84155	Total Protein	
86592	VDRL	
84560	Uric Acid	
81000	Urinalysis	
82996	(UCG) Pregnancy Test	
87210	Wet Prep	
85048	WBC	

X-RAY PROCEDURES		
74000	Abdomen	
72040	Cervical Spine	
71000	Chest	
73500	Hip	
72100	Lumbar Spine	
70160	Nasal Bone	
72190	Pelvis	
71100	Ribs	
70210	Sinuses	
70250	Skull	
72070	Thoracic Spine	

TOTAL FEE ______

SPECIAL INSTRUCTIONS:

INSURANCE CARRIERS— This form has been adopted to keep paperwork costs down. If any additional form or itemized bill is required they will be completed upon receipt of $ ______.

AUTHORIZATION TO RELEASE INFORMATION: I hereby authorize the physician (s) named in this form to release any information acquired during my examination or treatment.

Patient's Signature ______ Date ______

RETURN: ______ Days ______ Weeks ______ Months NEXT APPT. ______ Day ______ Month ______ Date ______ Time AM PM

LEONARD S. TAYLOR, M.D.
2100 WEST PARK AVENUE
CHAMPAIGN, ILLINOIS 61820
Telephone: 352-7658

IRS No. 123456
S.S. No. 000 00-0000

No. 1001

Figure 22–6.

When each day sheet is filled out, it is removed from the pegboard and placed in a storage binder. A pegboard summary log may be useful if your accountant does not supply monthly totals in his reports. It shows a monthly summary with charges and receipts for each day, expenses by category, and other information such as depreciation schedules and payroll. Since most physicians do not use one, an illustration has not been provided.

Nothing has been said about how to enter charges generated outside the office. At the start of office hours each day, have your assistant provide you with a 3 × 5 card listing your hospitalized patients (with room numbers), consultations requested, procedures scheduled, and house calls. She can also add medical meetings at the hospitals and other appointments you may have there. During lunch time, that afternoon and evening, and the next morning before office hours, note what you have done, including tasks that were not scheduled by her. Add dates and necessary details, then give the card to the same aide before office hours the next day in exchange for a new one for use that day. If you wish to handle any of the charges in a special way, indicate this on the card before you turn it in. On weekends and over holidays, she should give you a card for each day. Using your completed card, she makes the appropriate entries in the pegboard system, checking off each item on the card as she does so; then she puts the card in a designated file box in chronological order. Some physicians exchange cards the last thing in the afternoon, but quite often there is not time to enter the card into the system then, and *occasionally* one is overlooked the next day. Others hand a card in first thing each morning and receive a new one at the end of office hours each afternoon, but sometimes emergency calls to the hospital or work done during lunchtime are not entered. Some cataloguers provide booklets or forms to use, but there does not appear to be any particular advantage to either over cards. But if you are set up to dictate your records, carry a small recorder with you and turn in the cassette as you would a card.

With your charges recorded on the books, you are halfway there. Unfortunately, collecting is the harder half. Time-of-service collection—that is, collecting from patients *before* they leave your office—is the keystone of the rest of the process. Let me list a few reasons:

1. All charges collected at that time represent a 100 per cent collection rate. Once the patient leaves your office you will collect only about 70 per cent of what is owed you. The probability of collection continues to decline with time until it approaches zero 90 to 120 days later. Look at your collection rate, and calculate your financial loss.
2. The cost of sending out a statement depends upon many variables, but for purposes of illustration let us say it is two dollars. Multiply this by the number of statements you send out each month. Add this expense to the amount above.
3. Although each balance due may be small, in the aggregate your total accounts receivable can become quite large. Estimate the erosion of this total sum by inflation. Add this to the above.
4. Your accounts receivable represents a sum on which all overhead has been paid and which is rightfully yours for the services you rendered. It could be used by you in any number of ways if it were paid you. Assuming that you needed this amount for a certain purpose, what would a loan of that size cost you in service charges and interest? *All* year long, *every year*? On the other hand, if you had this money and could invest it, what would your return be at compound interest? To estimate this loss, take the difference between the cost of a loan and your return if the amount were invested. Add this to the sums above.

Look at this total. Then consider some of the less tangible advantages of an effective time-of-service collection: detecting and discharging "deadbeats" before they add more charges, making whatever arrangements you wish for patients whose finances are marginal *before* their balances overwhelm them, and avoiding the bother and aggravation of trying to collect overdue bills. Instead, you could be enjoying the satisfaction of rendering good medical care and the security of a well-run practice. There are other reasons, and I'm sure some occur to you. The important point is that once you have clearly in mind *how your practice might work* if the ideal of 100 per cent collection at the time of service could be realized, you have a model to which you can compare your collection process. However, exercise some restraint if you are just starting practice and no other physicians in the area are emphasizing time-of-service collection.

Here are some ways to improve time-of-service collection:

1. Inform patients of your policy in your patient information booklet, and add that it benefits *them* by holding down costs.
2. When your receptionist goes over the patient registration form with each new patient, she should remind the patient that this is your payment policy.
3. Although signs around the reception counter tend to clutter an otherwise dignified office, one requesting for payment at time of service might be an exception. Locate it where the patient cannot fail to see it when he returns to the receptionist. A reminder then by your aide reinforces the sign, especially if she offers a 5 per cent discount, which approximates your collection costs.
4. The charge slip and/or superbill must be designed so you can easily check the correct services and add others. Your receptionist must be provided with information that is rapidly and easily convertible into dollar charges.
5. The manner in which *you* use the charge slip is important. Make the entries *in the patient's presence* calmly, accurately, and completely, hand the charge slip to the patient in a confident manner, and request that it be taken to the receptionist.
6. The office should be laid out so that the patient naturally stops at the proper place to pay with his privacy protected there. See the suggestions in Chapter 11.
7. *One aide* must have time-of-service collections as her primary responsibility and be personally convinced of their importance. And she must *be there* when the patient approaches with the charge slip.
8. Her conduct at this time is crucial. She must convey confidence that payment will be forthcoming and that this is routine. As the patient walks up, she should take her pen, smile, and detain the patient a moment with a phrase such as, "I'll total this for you right now, Mrs. Jones." She then states the charges one by one as

she adds them up, gives the total for that day, the previous balance, and, finally, the new amount due. Then with a smile, looking directly at the patient, she should say, "Would you prefer to pay by cash or check?"

9. Assemble an array of effective answers for the most common ploys used by patients at this point. Certainly the most frequent is: "Just send a bill." A good reply is the rather firm "Normally, payment is expected at the time of treatment, but if there are unusual circumstances, I would be happy to discuss them with you." Rather than go into an embarrassing litany of woes, especially if they have to be thought up on the spot, the patient may pay.

   The second most frequent is: "It's covered by my insurance." You have the advantage on this one if your patient information booklet makes it clear that you do not accept assignment. But even if you do, your aide can counter with, "Your insurance is a contract between you and your insurance company that is separate from your relationship with Doctor Jones. Our relationship with you includes payment at the time services are rendered." If necessary, she can add, "We are happy to assist you in any way we can in preparing your insurance forms so that you can receive reimbursement from your insurance company." Notice the use of the words *your* and *you*.

   Probably the third most frequently encountered gambit is, "I forgot my checkbook," or one of its variants. The first reply might be that cash is perfectly acceptable, but the patient usually answers that he does not have enough with him. There are two possible strategies at this point. One is for her to take out a credit card blank with the statement, "We accept credit cards." I think their use is not in keeping with the dignity of the profession, but this reply may cause the checkbook to be found. The other is for your aide to reach for a stamped envelope addressed to the office, insert the charge slip, and give it to the patient with, "When you get home would you please place a check in this envelope and drop it in the mail? Thank you." She should add that she is making a note of this agreement, and then *do so* in front of the patient. This effectively concludes a contract with the patient, and people are more inclined to comply with a contract than to pay a bill—which many do not regard as a contract. A follow-up telephone call on the day the payment should have been received lends emphasis to the importance with which your aide regards the contract.

   Not all ploys can be foreseen, but it's fun collecting them and thinking up ways to deal with them. Over a period of time your aide will become quite skillful in her repertoire of replies. Some of the more spontaneous ones may turn out to be the best of all.

With all this effort expended on time-of-service collection, you have to set a goal with some system to check on the results. A monthly report from the aide responsible with a goal of 80 per cent time-of-service collection is the minimum.

One last comment on this. If your aide reaches only that 80 per cent, if your office overhead is around 50 per cent, and if you are in a hefty tax bracket, the amount uncollected may be *your entire after-tax income!* Think about that.

Let's return to billing and go into more detail. First of all, decide on the frequency with which you will send out statements. If you are vigorous in your efforts at time-of-service collecting, monthly billing is perfectly satisfactory. If not, give consideration to a "rolling" billing procedure, in which the ledger cards are not returned to the tray until they have been photocopied. Statements are sent in the next mail. This sytem is difficult to carry out and must be supplemented by monthly billing, so I would suggest rolling billing only if your time-of-service collection is ineffective.

Assuming you elect to have monthly billing, the next decision concerns the day of the month you will do it. Consider this in relation to the date other bills are received by your patients. If your statement arrives about the tenth, and your patient received most of his others by the fifth and has already paid them, you can imagine what he will do with yours. It is best to plan your billing date so that statements will arrive no later than the fourth of the month. Some physicians close out their books by the 25th so that statements will arrive *on* the first, but this causes a lot of bothersome questions in accounting for the period from the 25th to the end of each month, and is more trouble than it is worth.

With the frequency and timing decided, you have to ensure regularity. Too many physicians have statements sent out on their afternoon or day off following the first of each month. This results in a one-week fluctuation from month to month. Most consumers in this country do not pay all their bills. They let a few go and pay the "hard" ones first. These are the ones for essentials, or those with a high interest charge, or those that pose the threat of collection action. The ones with some "give" or softness are the ones they tend to set aside. Any variation in the day of the month your statements arrive gives just that impression of "softness." Your afternoons or days off *are* the best times to do the actual work, so have it done on those days off preceding the first of the month so that everything is ready to go on the first. Billing can then be completed in one or two hours by one aide. If the first falls on a weekend or holiday, send statements out *before* the first, not *after* it.

Sometimes the sheer number of statements precludes this degree of precision, and you may have to convert to "cycle" billing until the number is reduced. In this system, the first half of the alphabet is billed exactly on the fifteenth and the other half exactly on the first. To prevent an overlap or gap, have your aide put a divider in the ledger card tray separating the two groups.

Spot check your statements from time to time. They should be legible, accurate, and easily understood. The photocopying must be well done, the folding of the statement neat so that the patient's name and address can be read completely through the envelope window, and the envelope properly sealed. Patients tend to pay about as much attention to your statements when they receive them as you do when you send them.

You next have to come to a decision on what you regard as a delinquent account. Let's look at this for a moment. When a patient receives his first statement, he has already declined to pay in the office, even though he is aware that this is your standard policy. He was notified of the balance due then and had an opportunity to pay before receiving the first statement. By the time he receives a second statement, he could have paid at any time during the month between the two statements, but still did not do so. By then the balance has been owed for an average of one and one-half months. When anyone is that late with a mortgage or a car payment, he is considered delinquent. And well before then, department stores and credit card companies start charging their usurious interest rates. There is one other factor to consider. On receipt of the first statement, a majority of patients will pay. On receipt of the second statement, the majority *never* will.

So the second statement is a watershed. In my opinion, patients who do not pay within a few days of its receipt should be considered delinquent. But make your own decision. The following course of action is suggested for patients who fall into the delinquent category as you define it.

Prepare a series of four collection letters. Although these will need to be individually typed, prepare standard bodies that can be copied by your aide. If typing them becomes too burdensome, offset printing of the bodies is an acceptable second choice.

The first letter is an inquiry to see if you or your office might have made some error and serves to call attention to your statement. The implication is that payment would have been received by now from a patient of this caliber if there were not some error on *your* part. Suggested wording is: "We have not heard from you in response to our statement that $____________ is due on your account. Is there an error in your bill? If so, or if you have any question, please call us."

The second letter is sent after a telephone inquiry has been made, and refers to it. It continues to be courteous and to give the patient the benefit of the doubt. The theme now is that the *patient* must have some sort of problem (although you have not been informed of it), or payment would have been received. It might go as follows: "We have not received payment despite two statements, our letter of (date) and telephone call of (date), at which time you agreed to pay by (date). We are certain there must be a good reason. Please let us hear from you." It should be sent in a plain envelope addressed by hand without return address.

The third letter becomes firm, sets a deadline, and ends by stating the course of action you will take if payment is not received by the designated date: "You must have had a reason for failing to comply with your promise to pay by (date), but you have not advised us. We regret, therefore, that we will have to turn your account over for collection if it is not paid by (date)." The date selected should be approximately ten days after the patient receives this letter.

The fourth and final letter terminates your relationship. It should be sent certified mail with return receipt requested. "Because of your failure to pay your past due account, your relationship with this office is terminated and your account is being turned over for collection. Doctor ______________________ will be available for emergencies only until (five days after receipt), which allows you ample time to select another physician. Upon receipt of a signed release, we will forward a copy of your medical records to the physician you select." Although the first three collection letters are signed by your aide, you may wish to alter the wording of this fourth letter slightly and sign it yourself if you think this will be more effective.

In addition to the four collection letters, prepare an outline for your aide to use in a typical collection call. A suggested guide is:

1. Always talk to the responsible party. Do not continue if you cannot. Never ask that the call be returned.
2. Greet him or her pleasantly by name.
3. Identify yourself.
4. Inquire if the statement was received. If it has been, then ask the patient if there is some problem preventing payment.
5. If there is no problem, then ask when payment can be expected.
6. When the patient gives a date, repeat it back, state that you are making a note of it, and will look for payment then.

7. Conclude the telephone call with a polite "Thank you for your cooperation."
8. Always remain calm, confident, and pleasant. Do not get distracted by other matters or become drawn into arguments.

It isn't enough to present this guide to your aides. Train them in its use and rehearse with role playing. Then listen to them in action from time to time.

These are the tools you will need. Now for the method by which you will employ them. Until you have a large enough staff to permit an aide to do collections during office hours, you will have to confine these activities to your afternoon off. One aide should bear the primary responsibility. This not only increases her expertise and experience but ensures continuity of effort.

You may want to have her insert collection letter No. 1 in the envelope with the second statement, or send it separately a week or ten days later. If the former, this first step in the collection procedure is just part of your routine billing. If the latter, this starts your collection efforts which are thereafter kept entirely separate from routine billing activities.

If there is no payment in response to collection letter No. 1, have her follow up with a telephone call one week later, using your guidelines. If there is still no payment when promised, letter No. 2 is sent without a statement two weeks after the first letter. Letter No. 3 follows two weeks later, and letter No. 4 two weeks after that. Do not use stickers or message stamps on the envelopes, colored envelopes, fake telegrams, or other gimmicks. These are not only trashy, they are ineffective and some are illegal. Caution your aides to write nothing on the envelopes indicating that the contents are part of a collection action—this is illegal. Additional telephone calls may be interspersed at any time—they are especially effective when coordinated with the collection letters. A stratagem that is often successful, if the opportunity presents itself, is a person-to-person conference between your aide and the patient.

Notes on each step of the collection process and the patient's response are made in light pencil on the back of the ledger card or on pressure-sensitive labels attached there. Warn your aides not to make any entries about collection activities on the front of the ledger card, because the card may be photocopied and sent to the patient.

Consistency is the key. If you establish a positive pattern, with the mailing of the first two statements precisely on the first of the month, followed by the collection letters at exact two-week intervals, the patient will become convinced that you are serious and that in the end you will take whatever collection action you say you will take. This conviction is what you are striving for. Nothing will destroy it more rapidly and replace it with skepticism than flurries of activity interspersed with periods of inactivity. The worst thing you can do is threaten a course of action and not follow through. As a matter of fact, this is illegal under federal law.

There are other provisions in the federal Debt Collection Practices Act, the federal Fair Credit Billing Act, and related state statutes that you should know about and that your attorney should summarize for you. The federal Truth in Lending Act also applies if your aide agrees to a payment plan with four or more payments, even if no interest is charged. This requires a full disclosure as specified in that law, which is complicated to do. Your statements should always show the total originally owed, payments on the account, and new balances. There is no hint of a payment plan there. When a patient asks if payments of a certain number can be made, your aide must avoid a commitment to any such plan. There is one more legal snag you should know about. If a patient makes a partial payment by check and writes on it, "Payment in full," courts have interpreted this as an *offer* that is accepted if you cash it. Instruct your aide to hold all such checks and press for the balance.

For those patients who still do not pay after receipt of the fourth collection letter, there are three courses of action open to you, other than writing it off.

One is the use of a lawyer. Some specialize in debt collection. The first advantage sought is that the letterhead and signature on his demand letter will convince the delinquent patient that firm action will follow. But if you have been consistent in your efforts up to this point, the patient is already convinced. The second potential advantage is that an attorney is able to proceed one step further than a collection agency by instituting legal action. But you can do this yourself through small claims court if the amount is below the limit set in your area. A third possible advantage occurs when legal questions are involved, as in cases of bankruptcy, complicated estate settlements, or if garnishment is involved. In short, an attorney should become involved in your collection procedure only if the sum is over the small claims limit, or if legal problems such as these are present.

It is not quite as easy to make a decision on using a collection agency. The first problem is that you can be held legally liable if an agency takes any action in violation of federal or state statutes, and you have no reliable way of knowing what the actions of the credit agency are as they are taking place. The second problem is that even if their actions are legal, they may be unethical or in bad taste, and this will reflect upon you and your practice. A third is that if your efforts have been consistent up to this point, there really is not much more an agency can do without overstepping legal and ethical limits. Fourth, they will probably concentrate on the accounts judged easiest to collect according to the credit reports they receive, and may let the more difficult ones go, even though these are equally important to you. Fifth, they tend to concentrate on the largest accounts in order to obtain the larger fees. Doing approximately the same amount of work on each of the smaller accounts is often not worth the effort, although the aggregate of these small amounts may be much greater. A sixth and last problem is that collection agencies take approximately 50 per cent of what they collect, *including what patients may voluntarily pay to your office* once the accounts have been turned over to them.

If these points do not dissuade you, and you still want to use an agency, then take the following precautions.

1. Request a copy of *Harassment and Other Collection Taboos* from the National Association of Credit Managers, 475 Park Avenue, New York, NY 10016. Read it. Clip it to the legal summary from your attorney so you will at least take the step with your eyes open.
2. Select an agency with a good reputation. First, contact your local medical society. If it operates one, it is almost certainly ethical. If it does not but can recommend one, your chances are better than if you picked one on your own. If they cannot recommend one, check with the local Better Business Bureau, and ask your colleagues for their recommendations based upon their experience.
3. Visit the agency on site and examine their methods. Take their letters and literature with you to study.
4. Before you turn any accounts over to them, review the medical records carefully. Often the use of a collection agency stimulates a malpractice action or counterallegations.
5. Do not sign a contract with the agency until you review it with your attorney.

Then, when you have turned an account over, take no more collection action yourself. Report to the agency any payments received by your office.

The third choice is a small claims court. These exist in all states, but the local laws governing them vary widely, with dollar limits ranging from $300 in Arkansas to $5000 in Tennessee. Some states do not have a statewide system (Georgia is an example) but most counties in such states do have small claims courts. Still other states (such as Michigan) have municipal rather than district small claims courts.

There are several advantages to this course of action: (1) the fees are low, and if judgment is in your favor, the defendant must pay all costs; (2) you do not have to appear—an aide can represent you; (3) there are no attorney-generated complications or collection agency costs; (4) the payment performance when the patient receives the summons is about as good as a collection agency is able to achieve; (5) the hearing itself is simple, and in most cases you receive favorable judgment.

Claim forms and instructions are obtained at the small claims court. The form must be filled out and filed with a copy of your statement. The dollar limit must be observed, and there may be a restriction on the number of claims that can be filed at one time. A small filing fee of about ten dollars is required. Be sure the patient's address is correct, or the summons cannot be delivered. If your practice is incorporated, the corporation, not you, must be listed as the plaintiff, and the claim has to be signed by a corporate officer. Check to make sure there is no requirement in your state that a corporation filing a claim must be represented by an attorney. One copy of the claim form is sent by the court to the patient by certified mail, giving the date and time of the hearing. This is, in effect, a summons. For a fee, you may have it served by a uniformed sheriff or bailiff, which has additional impact.

When the summons is received, most patients realize that the judgment will be against them, so about half of the accounts are then settled in full. Some elect to sign a document stipulating that partial payments will be made, in which case the matter will come to trial only if they fail to comply. Most of those who do not take either action will fail to appear at the hearing. Nonappearance means you receive a judgment by default. Favorable judgment gives you the legal right to attach the debtor's assets. I do not advise doing this, but I do suggest that you record your judgment. Recording adversely affects the patient's credit rating and complicates his title to any real property he possesses in the county where the judgment is recorded. You may receive the amount owed years later when he attempts to sell his property.

If your patient does appear at the hearing and disputes your claim, he is entitled to file a counterclaim against you. If this happens, the court will refer the complaint to a higher court. This involves representation of both parties by attorneys. In actual practice, this rarely happens. In most states, if you receive judgment, the patient is entitled to appeal it, but very few do so. The normal course of events is that your aide presents your case and the patient presents his. If the service was indeed rendered by you and your charge is reasonable, the judgment is almost always in your favor. If your aide is not prepared with the right documents or the right answers, you usually lose the judgment. Once you lose, you have no rights of appeal, so review each case with your assistant to be certain she is prepared.

"Skip" tracing is another business skill you have to acquire that was not taught in medical school. A "skip" occurs when a patient with a delinquent bill moves in order to avoid payment. Some individuals are quite adept at this, and at hiding their trail when they do so. You don't have to do the detective work yourself—a designated assistant will do that and acquire considerable skill through experience—but you have to start her off and supervise her.

Before tracing a skip you should study the summary that your attorney prepared for you on the federal Debt Collection Practices Act and other pertinent federal and state statutes. This act prohibits revealing to a third party that any action of yours is in relation to a debt. When you make inquiries of a third party, merely identify the person you are seeking and state that you are endeavoring to obtain correct location information. This same legislation also prohibits contacting any third party a second time unless you have substantial information indicating that the first response was deliberately deceptive, erroneous, or incomplete, or that the third party has acquired new information in the interim. Telephone calls cannot be at unusual hours or in any other way harrassing. Confidentiality must be maintained in correspondence. It is illegal to use colored or coded envelopes, postcards with a text indicating that a debt is involved, or any stamp, sticker, or written notice on the envelope that indicates the nature of its contents.

You will be alerted to a probable skip when a statement is returned by the post office as undeliverable. Act at once, because from this point on the trail just gets colder. The worst mistake an aide can make is to fail to take action and send out another statement the following month. The second most serious mistake, one that causes a delay of a month or more, is to have "address correction requested" printed below the return address on envelopes used for statements. This directs the post office to correct the erroneous address and forward the statement, if a forwarding address has been left on file, and to send you a photostat of the corrected envelope.

Skips are surprisingly sophisticated. They rarely leave a forwarding address at the post office. If they do, it is effective for only a short time so they can receive certain pieces of mail they want. They discard other forwarded mail, including statements, while the physician and his staff naively wait for the check. It is far more effective to request the forwarding address at once from the post office. If one has been left there, it will be given you for a small charge. You can correct your records and either mail the statement to the new address or have your aide hand deliver it. When this ruse that fools so many has failed, some skips lose their starch. Yours is not the only debt he owes, so he may decide it is worth it to settle one bill and hope his other creditors are not as sharp. He is usually correct.

If no forwarding address was left at the post office, your success will depend entirely on the information you have on file. This starts with the accuracy and completeness of the information on your patient registration form. As was mentioned in Chapter 13, many of the items on the form are there for this purpose. It is of the utmost importance that your front office assistant verify the completeness and accuracy of this information at the time of each patient's first visit, and that she keep it updated. Some additional information may be on your history form if you have asked for a detailed family history, particularly the names and addresses of relatives. If the spouse is a patient also, there may be additional information on that registration form. Look over hospital admission records for additional data, and call each hospital for anything they may have that is more up to date on either the patient or spouse. Other physicians that cared for either one should be called, along with laboratories that bill directly, and providers of other medical services. The medical insurance information you have may provide contact numbers. If you have a space on your patient registration form, "Referred by ______________," you may have one more contact. Oftentimes your patient registration form will have, "Person responsible for payment ______________." If this is not the spouse, you may have another contact. If your form requests a bank reference, call the bank and ask if the patient or spouse still has an active account. Legally, they can give you no more information than this, but even this much is useful. An active account usually means that the person is still in the area.

The driver's license number on the patient registration form is extremely valuable. With it and the patient's full name and date of birth, you can call the State Motor Vehicle Bureau and ask if a valid driver's license is still held by the patient. You can request a copy of the vehicle registration if a vehicle is still registered in the state. The registration should have the new address. If not, try again later. Most states require that any change of address be reported within a limited time.

With the full name, birthdate, and social security number, you can obtain the information on file at your local credit bureau and at TRW Credit Data.

Most metropolitan areas have city street directories (reverse directories) that list street addresses followed by the names of the persons living at that address. Get one from the telephone company. Look up the address given by your patient and note the name of the person listed at that address. If this is different from that of your patient, then obtain the telephone number of this person from the regular directory or from information, and inquire about your patient. At the same time, the addresses of neighbors may be looked up and their names noted for a similar inquiry. If there is no city street directory in your area, it may be worthwhile having your aide drive to the address and make neighborhood inquiries.

It is always worth a try to have your assistant dial the home telephone number. Sometimes skips take the same one with them. Even if a telephone company computer should answer, it may give you a new number or other clue. The work number is usually more productive. Skips may change their residence but keep the same employment. Even if the person is no longer employed there, someone—the personnel department or a friend—may have a new address or new place of employment. If the patient had a highly specialized position, try calling other possible employers in the area. Have your assistant continue calling all possible contacts for location information until she is successful or has exhausted all possibilities.

I have never been sure if there is some sort of underground communication, or if skips develop a marvelous sixth sense, but it seems that those physicians who are lax in pursuing the first few skips suffer an epidemic over the next two or three years that, in marginal financial circumstances, can be fatal to their practices. On the other hand, those who are vigorous in pursuing the first few seem not to be troubled much thereafter. They also develop a staff that is more alert for possible skips and able to take effective action without delay.

This chapter on charges and collections has been a long one, but its length testifies to the importance of the subject.

23

Insurance Claims

Most physicians would far rather practice medicine and leave this subject to their aides. But medical insurance with its regulations, forms, and terminology is here to stay. Nearly 200 million Americans—88 per cent of the population—are now covered in one way or another. Insurers currently pay about 70 per cent of all health costs in the United States. Depending upon your specialty, between 60 and 90 per cent of your practice income will be from third parties, so it is something we all must learn to live with. As physicians, we do not need to know the details, but we must have some idea of what is going on in the front office. If we don't, chaos can occur. In one practice I helped with, all the "problem" claim forms had been stuffed into drawers for nearly two years. The total owed this physician amounted to nearly six figures, and much of it could no longer be collected.

There are about 2000 carriers in the United States offering some form of health insurance, with three or four times that many plans. But this variety can be simplified considerably. The types of health insurance fall fairly neatly into six categories: commercial, Blue Cross and Blue Shield, Medicare, CHAMPUS, Medicaid, and Workers' Compensation. This list can be trimmed a bit more by setting aside the last two, which are of concern mainly to full-time emergency room physicians and those who practice in an industrial area or inner city. CHAMPUS is almost identical to Medicare, and both were modeled upon Blue Cross and Blue Shield, so the subject is not really as complicated as it seems.

Let's look at the six categories more closely.

1. **Commercial** carriers offer contracts to individuals and groups, mostly the latter, under which payments are made to the beneficiaries (or to providers if they accept assignment of benefits) according to an indemnity table or schedule of benefits for speci-

fied medical services. The plans vary, but in general conform to one of these three types:

a. *Basic.* These pay total costs up to a maximum (usually around $5000) for all but a few exclusions such as cosmetic surgery and mental disorders. There may or may not be a deductible, which is a stipulated sum the beneficiary must pay. The costs may be incurred in the hospital, home, or office.
b. *Major Medical.* These policies are designed for catastrophic situations only, and there is no payment under such plans for minor health problems. They usually take up where the basic plans leave off, and almost always have a large deductible and copayment, which means that the beneficiary shares in the expense.
c. *Comprehensive.* These plans consist of combinations of Basic and Major Medical.

Group plans often have a provision that a patient covered by more than one carrier cannot receive combined benefits from all carriers of more than 100 per cent of the actual charges. For example, if both the husband and wife work and each has a different group policy that covers the spouse, the benefits must be coordinated. A formula has been developed among insurance carriers for determining primary and secondary carriers. In this example, the husband's carrier would be the primary one. The professional relations department of any insurance company will advise you in other situations. In general, the primary carrier pays benefits up to its maximum, and then the secondary carrier supplements these up to 100 per cent of the charges.

Prior to 1975, each commercial carrier required that its own forms be used for claims. But virtually all have come to accept the **Uniform Claim Form** introduced by the American Medical Association that year. CHAMPUS, Medicare, and most Blue Cross and Blue Shield plans do, too. These forms, with an instruction book, can be ordered in pads of 100 from the Order Department, American Medical Association, P.O. Box 10946, Chicago, IL 60610. (See Fig. 23–1.)

2. **Blue Cross and Blue Shield.** Blue Cross plans provide payment to hospitals, so your office will have little or nothing to do with them. Blue Shield is a nonprofit voluntary association, autonomous in each state, which provides subscribers (90 per cent are in groups) with coverage for certain medical expenses. Because policies and procedures vary from state to state, obtain information from the Blue Shield organization in your state. A *Directory of Blue Shield Plans,* No. 995-BSAA, is available from the National Association of Blue Shield Plans, 676 North Saint Clair, Chicago,

FORM APPROVED OMB NO. 0938-0008
READ INSTRUCTIONS BEFORE COMPLETING OR SIGNING THIS FORM
(CHECK APPLICABLE PROGRAM BLOCK BELOW)

HEALTH INSURANCE CLAIM FORM

☐ MEDICARE (MEDICARE NO.) ☐ MEDICAID (MEDICAID NO.) ☐ CHAMPUS (SPONSOR'S SSN) ☐ CHAMPVA (VA FILE NO.) ☐ FECA BLACK LUNG (SSN) ☐ OTHER (CERTIFICATE SSN)

PATIENT AND INSURED (SUBSCRIBER) INFORMATION

1. PATIENT'S NAME (LAST NAME, FIRST NAME, MIDDLE INITIAL)
2. PATIENT'S DATE OF BIRTH
3. INSURED'S NAME (LAST NAME, FIRST NAME, MIDDLE INITIAL)
4. PATIENT'S ADDRESS (STREET, CITY, STATE, ZIP CODE)
5. PATIENT'S SEX — MALE ☐ ☐ FEMALE
6. INSURED'S NAME ID NO. (FOR PROGRAM CHECKED ABOVE, INCLUDE ALL LETTERS)
7. PATIENT'S RELATIONSHIP TO INSURED — SELF ☐ SPOUSE ☐ CHILD ☐ OTHER ☐
8. INSURED'S GROUP NO. (OR GROUP NAME OR FECA CLAIM NO.)
   ☐ INSURED IS EMPLOYED AND COVERED BY EMPLOYER HEALTH PLAN
9. OTHER HEALTH INSURANCE COVERAGE (ENTER NAME OF POLICYHOLDER AND PLAN NAME AND ADDRESS AND POLICY OR MEDICAL ASSISTANCE NUMBER)
10. WAS CONDITION RELATED TO
    A. PATIENT'S EMPLOYMENT — YES ☐ ☐ NO
    B. ACCIDENT — AUTO ☐ ☐ OTHER
11. INSURED'S ADDRESS (STREET, CITY, STATE, ZIP CODE)
    TELEPHONE NO.
11.A. CHAMPUS SPONSOR'S STATUS — ☐ ACTIVE DUTY ☐ DECEASED ☐ RETIRED — BRANCH OF SERVICE
12. PATIENT'S OR AUTHORIZED PERSON'S SIGNATURE (READ BACK BEFORE SIGNING)
    I AUTHORIZE THE RELEASE OF ANY MEDICAL INFORMATION NECESSARY TO PROCESS THIS CLAIM . I ALSO REQUEST PAYMENT OF GOVERNMENT BENEFITS EITHER TO MYSELF OR TO THE PARTY WHO ACCEPTS ASSIGNMENT BELOW.
    SIGNED DATE
13. I AUTHORIZE PAYMENT OF MEDICAL BENEFITS TO UNDERSIGNED PHYSICIAN OR SUPPLIER FOR SERVICE DESCRIBED BELOW
    SIGNED (INSURED OR AUTHORIZED PERSON)

PHYSICIAN OR SUPPLIER INFORMATION

14. DATE OF ◀ ILLNESS (FIRST SYMPTOM) OR INJURY (ACCIDENT) OR PREGNANCY (LMP)
15. DATE FIRST CONSULTED YOU FOR THIS CONDITION
16. IF PATIENT HAS HAD SAME OR SIMILAR ILLNESS OR INJURY, GIVE DATES
16.A IF EMERGENCY CHECK HERE ☐
17. DATE PATIENT ABLE TO RETURN TO WORK
18. DATES OF TOTAL DISABILITY — FROM | THROUGH
    DATES OF PARTIAL DISABILITY — FROM | THROUGH
19. NAME OF REFERRING PHYSICIAN OR OTHER SOURCE (E.G. PUBLIC HEALTH AGENCY)
20. FOR SERVICES RELATED TO HOSPITALIZATION GIVE HOSPITALIZATION DATES
    ADMITTED | DISCHARGED
21. NAME & ADDRESS OF FACILITY WHERE SERVICES RENDERED (IF OTHER THAN HOME OR OFFICE)
22. WAS LABORATORY WORK PERFORMED OUTSIDE YOUR OFFICE? YES ☐ ☐ NO CHARGES
23. DIAGNOSIS OR NATURE OF ILLNESS OR INJURY, RELATE DIAGNOSIS TO PROCEDURE IN COLUMN D BY REFERENCE NUMBERS 1, 2, 3, ETC. OR DX CODE
    1.
    2.
    3.
    4.

B
EPSDT YES ☐ ☐ NO
FAMILY PLANNING YES ☐ ☐ NO
PRIOR AUTHORIZATION NO.

24.

A DATE OF SERVICE FROM	TO	B* PLACE OF SERVICE	C. FULLY DESCRIBE PROCEDURES MEDICAL OR SUPPLIES FURNISHED FOR EACH DATE GIVEN. PROCEDURE CODE (IDENTIFY)	(EXPLAIN UNUSUAL SERVICES OR CIRCUMSTANCES)	D DIAGNOSIS CODE	E CHARGES	F DAYS OR UNITS	G* T.O.S.	H LEAVE BLANK

25. SIGNATURE OF PHYSICIAN OR SUPPLIER (INCLUDING DEGREE(S) OR CREDENTIALS) (I CERTIFY THAT THE STATEMENTS ON THE REVERSE APPLY TO THIS BILL AND ARE MADE A PART THEREOF)
26. ACCEPT ASSIGNMENT (GOVERNMENT CLAIMS ONLY) (SEE BACK) — YES ☐ ☐ NO
27. TOTAL CHARGE
28. AMOUNT PAID
29. BALANCE DUE
30. YOUR SOCIAL SECURITY NO.
31. PHYSICIAN'S SUPPLIERS AND OR GROUP NAME AND ADDRESS, ZIP CODE AND TELEPHONE NO.
    ID NO.
32. YOUR PATIENT'S ACCOUNT NO.
33. YOUR EMPLOYER ID NO.

* PLACE OF SERVICE AND TYPE OF SERVICE (T.O.S.) CODES ON BACK
REMARKS

APPROVED BY AMA COUNCIL ON MEDICAL SERVICE 6/83
FORM HCFA-1500 (1-84) FORM OWCP-1500
FORM CHAMPUS-501 (1-84) FORM RRB-1500
APPROVED BY THE HEALTH CARE
FINANCING ADMINISTRATION & CHAMPUS

FORM 9380 COLWELL SYSTEMS, INC., CHAMPAIGN, ILLINOIS 61820

Figure 23–1.

IL 60611. Request the *Blue Shield Manual for Physicians* from your state office and any additional information available. With this, you can decide if you wish to participate or not. A participating physician is one who has signed a service contract with the state plan agreeing to accept its reimbursement as payment in full. There is automatic assignment of benefits, and payments are made directly to you.

Nonparticipating physicians may provide services to Blue Shield subscribers, but the payment method and schedule depend upon the individual state plan. In most states, there is no assignment and payment is made to the patient either according to an indemnity schedule or a "usual, customary, and reasonable" determination at 25 to 50 per cent of your usual fee. You are permitted to bill and collect your full fee from the patient, however, which is why you will not treat many subscribers unless you participate.

The compensation, whether you participate or not, is low so that most physicians elect not to. Participation for a time has advantages for a beginning physician, however. His name will appear in the directory given to subscribers, which will spread the word that he is there—and the additional patients will fill the blank spots in his schedule and help cover his overhead.

3. **Medicare** is a health insurance program under Social Security's Health Care Financing Administration (HCFA) that consists of two parts.

   Part A. This is hospital insurance (including skilled nursing facilities and home health care in certain cases) for almost everyone over 65, the disabled, and those with chronic renal disease. It is the part of the Medicare program that is in financial trouble owing to this extension of benefits by Congress, the increasing number of elderly and the greater costs of modern medical care. Prospective payment to hospitals by diagnosis-related groups (DRGs) was recently instituted as one attempt to save this part of Medicare.

   Part B. This is also known as *Supplementary Medical Insurance* (SMI). It covers physician services, laboratory tests, and x-rays. Although this part is voluntary, almost all who are eligible sign up. Those who are receiving social security benefits and some others have the low premium for Part B deducted from their monthly checks, while the rest pay it directly to the Social Security Administration. There is an annual deductible and a 20 per cent copayment. Processing of claims and payment is by private insurance carriers or nonprofit "Blues" under contract with Medicare. There are certain exclusions that you should be aware of. During the recent fee-freeze, physicians were urged to become "participating physicians" and accept assignment on all Medicare patients, but most chose not to.

Your office should have a copy of *Your Medicare Handbook*, available on request from local social security offices. This is intended for patients, but contains a great deal of information your assistants need to know and it will help them in counseling patients.

Payments to you under Part B are made on the basis of what the fiscal intermediary determines to be "reasonable" under HCFA guidelines. This word is defined differently under Medicare than by other carriers, so you should always think "allowable" when "reasonable" is used. There are *three* steps in determining a "reasonable" fee.

First, the assumption is made (unless your charge is buttressed by appropriate codes and procedure descriptions) that there was nothing complicated or unusual about the treatment that would justify more than the minimum payment.

Second, the lowest of the following three figures is chosen:

a. *Your actual charge*—this has a nice ring to it, but your fee is never the lowest of the three, so discount this possibility.
b. *Your customary charge* for that service or procedure. This is never the lowest, either, so let's go on.
c. *The prevailing charge* for similar services in your locality. Here is the rub. An accurate assessment of "similar services" would require comparison of your training, experience, and skill with those of other physicians in the community. In actuality, this is rarely done. Most Medicare intermediaries don't even use the same specialty or any other criterion such as certification in a specialty. Further, if there is any doubt about the level of the service, the lowest is always chosen. Then the *75th* percentile of the local charges for this "similar" service is used. Commercial carriers customarily use the *90th* percentile, and so do statisticians when they use any term comparable to "prevailing." But there is more. The 75th percentile is determined for a calendar year, yet not applied until July 1 of the following year. Even if a charge were determined correctly in the first place, its application an average of two years later would negate any validity it might have had as "prevailing." The *entire phrase* "prevailing charge for similar services" is meaningless and misleading.

Third, the **Medicare Economic Index** (which has little relation to the actual cost of providing medical services) is applied to limit fee increases from year to year.

At this writing, it appears that when the fee freeze terminates, it will be replaced by even greater restrictions on a physician's freedom of choice as to whether he will accept assignment or not.

He may have to accept prospective payment by DRGs for patients hospitalized under Medicare or a capitation system.

Currently, if you accept assignment, your office must file the claim, and 80 per cent of the "reasonable" charge is sent you directly by the carrier, less any deductible the patient might owe. The patient pays you the deductible and 20 per cent of what is determined to be the "reasonable" charge. You may collect your estimate of these two at the time service is rendered, but the "reasonable" charge must be accepted as payment in full *even if the patient has other medical insurance.* I would suggest that you select truly needy cases among the elderly and disabled and accept assignment only from these. You must bill the patient for the 20 per cent copayment and the deductible, or you will get into trouble with the carrier. But advise the patient to ignore your statement, then write off the copayment, deductible, and the remainder of your usual charge, and remember that in past years you would have treated the patient without charge. For all other Medicare beneficiaries, do not accept assignment, but instead send your statement directly to the patient who is responsible to pay it in full. The patient submits his Medicare form (SSA-1490) with a copy of your itemized statement to the intermediary and must accept whatever they pay him.

Keep an eye on your customary charge profile that the carrier maintains. Make any fee changes early in the calendar year so they will be reflected in your average charges for the year. Obtain your profile from the Medicare carrier as soon as it is available each year and review it. Errors are frequent and can be costly if you do not detect them.

4. **CHAMPUS** is the acronym for the **Civilian Health and Medical Program of the Uniformed Services.** This program provides health care services in the civilian sector to active and retired military personnel as well as their dependents. Because active duty personnel receive medical care at their assigned duty stations, except where facilities are not available, most of your contact with this program will be through retired military personnel and dependents. At age 65, all beneficiaries shift to the Medicare program. CHAMPUS is similar in most respects to Medicare, but there are differences in the deductible and copayment, and it is administered by different fiscal intermediaries. You may elect to participate or not by ticking the appropriate answer in box 32 of the CHAMPUS form 500. As with Medicare, I would suggest you accept assignment in cases of financial distress and write off any charges over the amount received.

   Request the *CHAMPUS Handbook* from the CHAMPUS carrier in your area or CHAMPUS Information, Aurora, Colorado 80045. This publication also gives the telephone numbers of CHAMPUS health benefit advisers who can provide additional information.

CHAMPVA is the acronym for the **Civilian Health and Medical Program of the Veterans Administration,** which is almost identical to CHAMPUS. This program is administered by the VA, and covers dependents of veterans who suffered total disability or death as a result of a service-related injury. You will rarely have anything to do with this program.

5. **Workers' Compensation.** The Workmen's Compensation program is still called that in many states, but because most have changed the name to "Workers' Compensation" to avoid the slightest sexist taint, I will use that name here. These programs started shortly after the turn of the century because of the hazardous working conditions resulting from industrialization. Before these programs were set up, an injured worker, or the family of one who had died as a result of injury on the job, had only one recourse—to sue the employer. In order for the suit to be successful, negligence on the part of the employer had to be proved. The hard facts were that the employee himself was often at fault, and about half the time *neither* was. The employer, on his part, had to contend with a large number of suits, and the awards for some of those that went against him were huge.

   Because of these problems on both sides, individual states set up programs under the Department of Labor or a special industrial commission. The programs are a compromise that respects the interests of both parties. Any work-related injury or illness is assumed to be no-fault, and the employer cannot be sued. On the other hand, medical care, rehabilitation, and partial compensation for lost wages are provided the employee. The benefits are low, but they are guaranteed.

   The problems for physicians who provide medical care under these programs are many. Special forms are required, filing deadlines and other regulations must be met, and the physicians have to accept the low compensation. Consequently, most avoid Workers' Compensation cases. Some specialists whose procedures receive fair compensation and others who practice in industrial areas have learned to fight fire with fire. They and their staffs have studied the regulations and have streamlined and specialized their practices to care for these patients, managing to do so at a modest profit. If you decide to accept Workers' Compensation cases, look in your telephone book for the appropriate local office, and request information and forms.

6. **Medicaid** is a state-administered program for which the federal government sets certain regulations and provides substantial finan-

cial support. It is designed to assist the poor with physicians' fees, hospital charges, medication costs, and other health care expenses. Policies and procedures vary from state to state.

The problems for the physician in the Medicaid program are the most formidable of all. The fees do not cover the paperwork, let alone the cost of providing the care. Many of the patients are inconsiderate of appointments, arrogant or abusive, unreasonably demanding of services, unaccepting of diagnoses, difficult to educate regarding their disease and its treatment, uncooperative in self-care and prevention, and, on the whole, hard to deal with.

But the patients are not the biggest problem. That award goes to the program itself and the way it is administered. Regulations limit the diagnostic procedures you can perform, the type of treatment you give, and the medications you prescribe. They even restrict your decisions on hospitalization. The claim forms used must be those provided by the carrier. They must be submitted within certain dates, complete in every detail, and routed first to all other possible sources of compensation. Payment, such as it is, is delayed interminably—sometimes forever without frequent follow-up inquiries. On top of all this, if you accept even one Medicaid patient, your are subject to an *audit* by their bureaucrats in your own office!

My advice is to select a few patients you can work with who are truly needy and deserve good medical care, and ignore the Medicaid program entirely. Treat these patients without charge. Provide their medications also. The only problem arises when hospitalization is required. Then you have to make a choice from the following alternatives: accept all the regulations and admit the patient under the Medicaid program; have another physician who takes Medicaid patients hospitalize yours; or refer the patient to the nearest public hospital. In this way you can do your share in providing care for the needy without the hassle.

The best instruction book on medical insurance and claim forms for your assistants is the *Medical Insurance Reference Manual* by Ann Ehrlich, obtainable from Colwell Systems, Inc., 201 Kenyon Road, Champaign, IL 61820. You should have one aide specialize in claim form preparation, since even one error can result in rejection. If she is ill or on vacation, the forms can wait a few days. Many communities have one or more experts, formerly employed in physicians' offices, who prefer to work at home. They usually have computers, will prepare your forms completely and accurately overnight and bring them to your office first thing each morning. In my opinion, this is the best way to go.

Either way, you will need two references in the office. One is the *International Classification of Diseases,* or *ICD,* often referred to erroneously as the "ICDA". Diagnostic codes are not *required* by carriers, but if you submit your forms with only a descriptive diagnosis, you are relying on a low-level clerk to translate it into the numeric code required by the carrier's computer. This slows down the process and may reduce the reimbursement if it is partially dependent on the diagnosis. If your descriptive diagnosis is not clear, the lack of the code may result in rejection of the claim. The second reference you will need is a book of procedure codes. The standard one is *The Physician's Current Procedural Terminology,* or *CPT,* published annually by the American Medical Association.

Once you have designated your "specialist," the rest is easy. She must get complete insurance information from new patients on your registration form and must keep it current. She must also photocopy the patient's identification card if the plan issues one, and she has to get proof of eligibility *each visit.* Rather than try to memorize the details of all the plans, she should learn what the most frequently encountered ones do *not* cover. Have her maintain an **Insurance Carrier Record.** (See Fig. 23–2.) This is invaluable as a ready reference for up-to-date carrier information. It will prove its worth if your specialist has an extended illness or leaves, and someone else has to take over insurance billing. It is always a good idea to have another assistant trained to take over in such circumstances. She should be familiar with the ICD, the CPT, and Ehrlich's manual, and work with your specialist from time to time.

An insurance log listing in chronological order all claims with their status may be useful. (See Fig. 23–3.) But you still will need to maintain a chronological set of carbons or photocopies of the forms in an accordion file, and status notes can be affixed to the copies with pressure-sensitive labels. Such a file works well if properly kept up, and if the copies are not misplaced in patient charts or elsewhere. Once you have confidence in your file and your personnel, you can dispense with the "back-up" log.

Go through this file about once a week yourself. All claim forms should be sent out within one week of the date the patient was seen. An inquiry by telephone is advisable if payment has not been received in one month. Such an inquiry works better than sending in a copy stamped "resubmitted."

Two tips. First, your patient registration form should have an information release block for your patient to sign. Even though the patient gives implied consent by supplying insurance information and forms, you should have a release signed before submitting an insurance claim. If you do not include one on your registration form, have the patient

Insurance Carrier Record

INSURANCE CARRIER Name and Address	PERSON TO CONTACT Relative To Claim Processing	EMPLOYER NAME, Address and Phone Contact	POLICY NO. or OTHER Identity No.	NOTES PERTINENT To Claim Processing
Blue Shield	George Victor	University Employees	123-45-678	standard form, attached
	Prof. Relations Dept.			statement OK
	Tel. 542-6600	Tel.		
Olympia Insurance Co.	Martha Ross	Ajax Construction	AJ 240	Schedule of benefits.
8941 S. Broad Street				Collect difference.
Metropolis, U.S.A.				
	Tel. 292-2242	Tel.		
Olympia Insurance Co.	Martha Ross	Telephone Workers	201-339	Does not cover routine
(same as above)		local # 201		office visits
	Tel. 292-2242	Tel.		
Medicare (Prudent Ins.)	Henry Douglass			
Prudent Bldg.				
Live Oak Blvd.				
Federal City, U.S.A.	Tel. 967-5590	Tel.		
Medicaid				check POE at each visit
State Office Bldg.				file claims first of month
Capital City, U.S.A.				use carrier's form
	Tel.	Tel.		
	Tel.	Tel.		
	Tel.	Tel.		

Figure 23–2.

Insurance Summary Log

PATIENT NAME	INSURANCE CARRIER	Accept Assignment		Claim Form Sent		Amount Received From Insurance		Other Coverage		Amount Patient To Pay	Date Patient Notified
		YES	NO	DATE	AMOUNT	DATE	AMOUNT	YES	NO		
HOUSER, GARY	BLUE SHIELD	xx		1/15	$175	2/12	$160		xx	--------	-----
WILLIAMS, PATRICIA	OLYMPIA		xx	1/16	$200	2/25	$150		xx	$50	2/25
REILLY, HAROLD	MEDICARE		xx	1/17	$50	2/28	deductible not met			$50	2/28
EDWARDS, JANICE	MEDICARE/MEDICAID	xx		1/17	$75						
TILLMAN, LAWRENCE	OLYMPIA		xx	1/18	$450			xx	submit again to Prudent		

Note – this patient has dual coverage with both Olympia and Prudent

FORM 9396 COLWELL CO., CHAMPAIGN, ILLINOIS

Figure 23–3.

sign a separate release. Second, remember to keep your accounts receivable accurate. Carrier payments usually fall short, and in some cases you are not permitted to collect the difference from the patient, so an adjustment must be made. If you fail to make these adjustments, over time the total of your accounts receivable will be grossly inflated.

One comment on superbills. Many offices have started to use them for all patients, insured or not, and do not use receipt-charge slips at all. There is no problem with this—in fact, it has some advantages. But difficulties may arise when a copy is given to patients to send with their claim form. Patients today expect better service from your office than this. They frequently find that they do not receive maximum reimbursement or that it is delayed because they are not familiar with the nuances of insurance billing. And when the patient pays up front, your assistant may be a bit careless about completing the superbill correctly. I would advise that your office submit all claim forms.

Let's try to summarize some guidelines on accepting assignment of benefits, because you will want a basis for making your decisions. Assignment means something quite different for commercial insurance than it does for Medicare, the Blues, and other plans. It is important that you know the differences.

The question does not arise with Workers' Compensation and Medicaid. If you see patients under Blue Shield all—or almost all—will be on a participating basis, so it will not arise much there, either. Your decisions on Medicare will be case-by-case as long as this is possible, as will those for CHAMPUS patients. I have given suggestions for this selection.

Most of the difficult decisions will be in regard to patients under commercial plans.

It is best to make a single policy and apply it to all such patients. To do so, you must consider several factors. First, some patients will pressure you to accept assignment so that they do not have to come up with the full fee right away, only a part of it. If you yield, it will fracture your "class policy," so you might as well not have one.

Second, ask yourself if you have strong convictions on the subject. Accepting assignment is a matter of principle with many physicians, in that it violates the concept of two separate contracts made by the patient, one with his insurance company and the other with his physician. You have to determine how you feel about this before you decide on one policy for all commercial carriers. This is the major reason assignments are accepted in only about 15 per cent of cases.

A third factor to consider is that acceptance may signal to some patients that you are willing to settle for the insurance check as payment in full.

A fourth is if you do not collect an estimate of the deductible and copayment portion up front, the patient may forget about his responsibility and resent receiving your unexpected statement for this amount two or three months after the service was rendered.

The fifth factor is the only one in favor of assignment. Some patients refuse to pay anything at all, even after they receive payment from their carrier, and you may then wish you had collected *something* directly from the insurance company. However, this problem can be limited to a great extent by selecting and educating your patients. You would probably want to discharge such patients anyhow as potential sources of other problems. Another argument in support of assignment is sometimes advanced, but I do not find it persuasive—namely, that it is better to accept assignment when large sums are involved to lessen the patient's financial burden. I believe it is more considerate to discuss such fees first, and to work out a plan suitable for each patient. For example, an amount approximating the deductible and copayment could be collected at the time of service, a moderate sum a month later, and the balance approximately a month after that when the patient receives the insurance check.

I would like to leave one last thought with you. No one likes to work with medical insurance claim forms. I have a hunch carriers don't either, and this is why they are developing electronic data processing systems. But if you accept the necessity yourself and indicate an interest in efficient handling of claims, your attitude will become apparent to your employees, and the entire process will go much more smoothly. If you do not, problems will plague you constantly.

24

Supplies, Disbursement, and Financial Reports

Supplies

Control of inventory seems to cause much more trouble than it should. Most of the time, this is because it is left to aides to take care of without any system being set up—or any supervision. It is actually simple. Designate one aide to be responsible, and order the five things you need for your system from any major cataloguer (see Fig. 24–1):

1. **Control cards**
2. **Alphabetical dividers**
3. **A control card box**
4. **Signal clips**
5. **Reorder tags**

Have the designated aide fill out one control card for each inventoried item. This does not mean everything in the office, just items that would cause a problem if you were to run out of them suddenly. The cards are filed alphabetically using the dividers in the control card box.

She may need a little help from you in filling out the two top blanks on each card (Fig. 24–2). The *order quantity* can be calculated from the rate of use, storage space available, and shelf life. Of course it may be modified on occasion to take advantage of discounts for large orders or special sales. The shelf life is determined by the expiration dates on drugs and vaccines and by the estimated duration of sterile

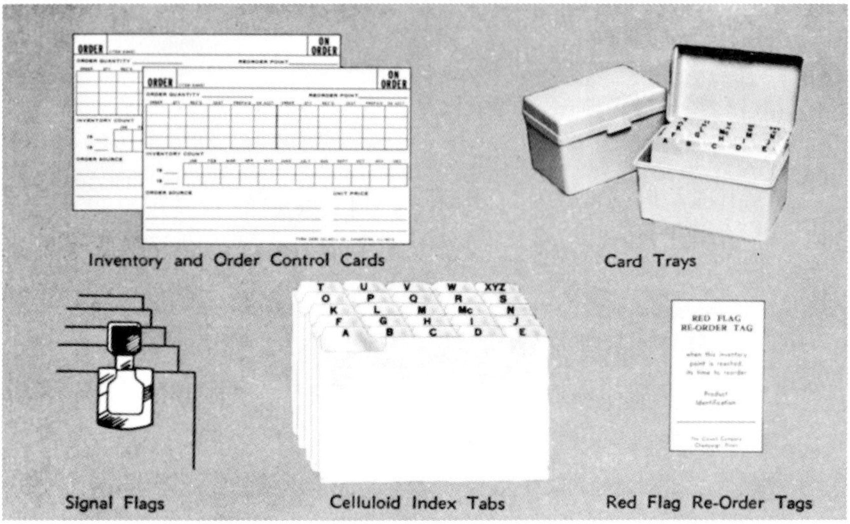

Figure 24–1.

ORDER (ITEM NAME) **ON ORDER**

ORDER QUANTITY ______ REORDER POINT ______

ORDER	QTY	REC'D	COST	PREPAID	ON ACCT	ORDER	QTY	REC'D	COST	PREPAID	ON ACCT

INVENTORY COUNT

	JAN	FEB	MAR	APR	MAY	JUNE	JULY	AUG	SEPT	OCT	NOV	DEC
19 ___												
19 ___												

ORDER SOURCE ______ UNIT PRICE ______

FORM 2450 COLWELL CO., CHAMPAIGN, ILLINOIS

Figure 24–2.

packages. The *reorder point* is approximately twice the time lag from placing an order to its delivery date.

Next, your aide indicates the reorder point in the stored supplies by placing a reorder tag at the proper place in the stock, using a pin, transparent tape, or other suitable means for keeping it in place. When supplies are used up to this tag, the last user removes the tag and gives it to the responsible aide. She immediately clips it to the control card in the file box under a signal clip at the upper left corner indicating "*order.*"

On the day that orders are placed, usually twice a month, all cards marked with a signal clip are pulled. Each order is placed and noted in the proper place on the card, the signal clip with the reorder tag is moved to the upper right corner indicating "*on order,*" and the card is replaced in the box.

She should not just mechanically reorder each time. Encourage her to bring you ideas she has obtained from catalogs, sales people, and meetings she has attended, along with her own suggestions and those of others in the office. Show some interest. Salesmen try to influence aides with blarney and gifts—this is about the only tactic you have to counter theirs. The time you take is a lot less than would be wasted talking to the salesmen yourself.

One supplier or several? I have tried the gamut from relying on only one supplier to ordering individual items in bulk quantities by mail from several suppliers. One time we got a tremendous bargain on toilet paper but didn't think about where we were going to store it. We stacked it to the ceiling in our restroom and had to use the patients' restroom for nearly three months. Even then, there was barely room in our own! The money saved using several suppliers—some of them by mail—never seemed to be worth the time and trouble involved. I would recommend a single large supplier if there is one in your area with a good representative. When we settled on one supplier for almost everything, we found that we enjoyed other benefits: we were never pushed for prompt payment; he would tell us about used equipment that could be purchased from other offices; we could return opened supplies if we decided to change to a new product; and we learned about new equipment and supplies suitable for our practice that were not listed in catalogs. But we made sure we were always aware of competitors' prices by checking catalogs and asking the office assistants of physicians who ordered from other suppliers. The representative of a single supplier is usually willing to negotiate—he wants to keep a good customer content.

Supplies should be stored in an organized way. The area must be cool, clean, and dry. Good lighting is necessary for finding supplies. Have your assistants think about ease of access when they put things away. Use adjustable shelves and label them. Heavy or large items should be stored near the floor, and lighter, smaller items higher up. Ask the assistant in charge to work out a convenient arrangement that can be used by others in her absence.

Usually, each package of supplies received in the office contains a packing slip. This slip describes the contents, but not the amount owed. Sometimes the slip inside is labeled "invoice," but this is an erroneous use of the term. If this "invoice" also requests payment, just ignore it. When a slip is in the package, it is a *packing slip*, period. Your designated aide should open the package and check the contents against the packing slip to make sure that the items are what you ordered, that the packing slip accurately reflects the contents, and that the contents are in good condition. If no packing slip is included, she should make notations on a piece of paper that thereafter will take the place of a packing slip. She then initials the slip and files it alphabetically in the *accounts payable* accordion file under the name of the supplier.

An *invoice* is just what the word indicates: a notice that an item or items have been sent. It arrives by mail, describes the items, and states the cost. Some firms request payment from the invoice; most do not. If they do, I ignore it too. Someone has to civilize the natives, right? All invoices are given to the same aide to match against the corresponding packing slips. She then clips them together and refiles them.

A *statement* is a monthly summary that shows the previous balance due, payments made, the amounts of purchases, with returns and credits during the period. It comes in the mail at the end of the month, and is your basis for payment. The aide checks each against the invoices received from that supplier during the month, at which time the packing slips are discarded. The statement is stapled to the invoices and refiled in accounts payable until the day you write checks.

Payment is customarily twice a month, unless substantial discounts make early payment worthwhile. The aide pulls all items from the accordion file and makes out checks for each statement. It is easier for you if the dates for taking care of accounts payable coincide with payroll so you can do both at the same time.

Disbursement

The word *disbursement* merely means making payments. Strictly defined, the term *accounts payable* applies to *all* of the bills that you owe, including personnel salaries. However, as commonly used in a physician's office, it pertains to such expenses as rent, supplies, laundry, insurance, and utilities, while *payroll* is used for salaries. This is the way I will use these terms.

Many physicians start practice using the large checkbooks supplied by banks with three or more checks to a page, and come rather late to the much more convenient "one-write" pegboard system designed for disbursement. The pegboard disbursement system reduces errors and facilitates organized record-keeping. These systems are obtainable from major cataloguers and consist of six elements:

1. **A folding pegboard.** This one is somewhat different in design from the one used for accounts receivable.
2. **The check register.** (See Fig. 24–3.) This has columns corresponding to the data on the disbursement checks, followed by other columns for reconciliation, the bank balance, bank deposits, and 12 to 15 columns for distribution of major expense categories. Some of these columns may have printed headings while others are blank for handwritten entries. Your accountant will advise you on the headings to use and may supply code numbers for them if he uses a computer.
3. **The checks themselves.** (See Fig. 24–4.) You have to decide whether to have two separate systems—one for accounts payable and one for payroll, or a combination system (as shown in Figure 24–4). The latter is the more sensible for a small business—it is simpler, and an accurate bank balance can be maintained more easily. The separate systems are more appropriate for larger businesses.

   The checks come shingled, 25 to a bank, usually precision-punched to fit the pegs, and are imprinted with your name, address, telephone number, sequential numbers, your bank's name, address, its ABA code number in the upper right, and the magnetic ink character recognition (MICR) number at the bottom. Your bank will supply a bank specification sheet for the cataloguer to make sure that these items are printed correctly. The cataloguer will offer you a variety of sizes, colors, and styles to choose from.

   The combination checks designed to be used for both accounts payable and payroll have a strip across the top for entering employee payroll information and another strip in the center of the check for recording accounts payable information. The former strip matches the columns on the employee payroll record, while the latter matches the columns on the check register. Both strips have carbon backing for automatic record-keeping.
4. **The employee earnings record.** (See Fig. 24–5.) One is needed for each employee. At the top are spaces for the employee's name,

Text continued on page 236

MONTH ______________________

PAGE ______________________

PAID TO	DISC.	DATE	CHECK NUMBER	AMOUNT	
BALANCE FORWARDED					
TOTALS (THIS PAGE)					
TOTALS MONTH TO DATE					
TOTALS YEAR TO DATE					

FORM 7548 COLWELL SYSTEMS INC., CHAMPAIGN, ILLINOIS

Figure 24–3.

Illustration continued on opposite page

CHECK REGISTER

√	EXPLANATION	BANK BALANCE	BANK DEPOSITS		PROF SUPPLIES	LABORATORY FEES	SALARIES	RENT UPKEEP
			AMOUNT	DATE				
1								
2								
3								
4								
5								
6								
7								
8								
9								
10								
11								
12								
13								
14								
15								
16								
17								
18								
19								
20								
21								
22								
23								
24								
25								

Figure 24–3. *Continued.*

Illustration continued on following page

√	ELEC. GAS WATER	TELEPHONE	OFC. SUPPLIES STAMPS	PROF INSURANCE	PROF TAXES		DUES MEETINGS	BOOKS JOURNALS	AUTO UPKEEP	LAUNDRY CLEANING
1						1				
2						2				
3						3				
4						4				
5						5				
6						6				
7						7				
8						8				
9						9				
10						10				
11						11				
12						12				
13						13				
14						14				
15						15				
16						16				
17						17				
18						18				
19						19				
20						20				
21						21				
22						22				
23						23				
24						24				
25						25				

Figure 24–3. Continued.

Illustration continued on opposite page

PAGE NO. ____________

TRAVEL	GOODWILL EXPENSE					MISCELLANEOUS		
						EXPLANATION	AMOUNT	
								1
								2
								3
								4
								5
								6
								7
								8
								9
								10
								11
								12
								13
								14
								15
								16
								17
								18
								19
								20
								21
								22
								23
								24
								25

Figure 24–3. *Continued.*

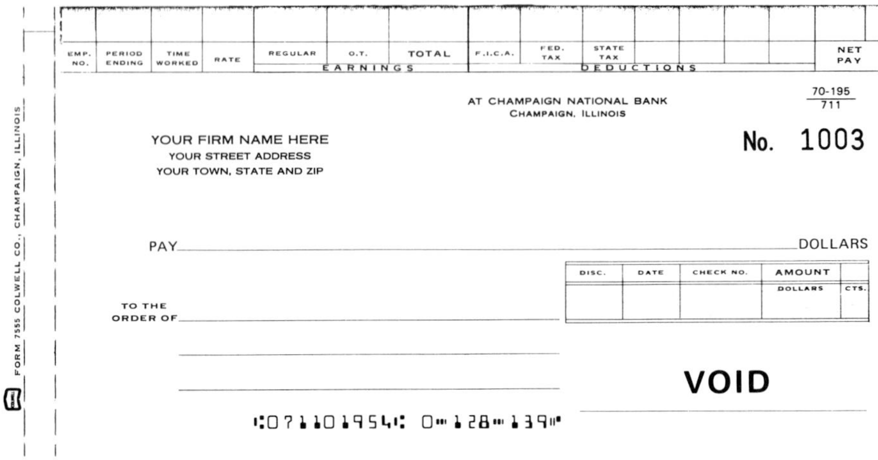

EMP. NO.	PERIOD ENDING	TIME WORKED	RATE	REGULAR	O.T.	TOTAL	F.I.C.A.	FED. TAX	STATE TAX					NET PAY
				EARNINGS			DEDUCTIONS							

AT CHAMPAIGN NATIONAL BANK
CHAMPAIGN, ILLINOIS

70-195
711

YOUR FIRM NAME HERE
YOUR STREET ADDRESS
YOUR TOWN, STATE AND ZIP

No. 1003

PAY ______ DOLLARS

DISC.	DATE	CHECK NO.	AMOUNT DOLLARS	CTS.

TO THE ORDER OF ______

VOID

FORM 7555 COLWELL CO., CHAMPAIGN, ILLINOIS

Figure 24–4.

address, social security number, and other payroll data. As stated earlier, the columns correspond to the spaces in the check payroll strip.

5. **The double window envelopes.** These are not the same as the *single* window envelopes used for sending out statements.
6. **The storage binder.** This holds the check registers.

The procedure for handling accounts payable is fairly straightforward. The check register is placed on the pegboard with a bank of shingled checks aligned over it. As each check is written by your assistant, the information on the strip is automatically recorded on the proper line of the register. As she completes each check, she extends the amount to the appropriate column of the register and calculates the bank balance remaining. Then on each statement she writes "paid," with the date and check number, and initials the entry. After all checks to be written at that time have been completed, she totals the amount column and each distribution column. The total across the foot must equal the total of the amount column. Then the register, checks, and statements with invoices attached are presented to you. Make sure her work is accurate first, then sign the checks. She puts each check in a double window envelope so that your address shows through the upper left window and the name and address of the payee are visible in the other. Although the *accounts payable* accordion file is arranged alphabetically according to supplier, the *accounts paid* accordion file is arranged by month. She files the statements (with the invoices still attached) in the latter under the proper month. At the end of each year, the file is tied with the string attached, labelled, and stored as is.

NAME	SOC. SEC. NO.		PAYROLL DATA
STREET	TELEPHONE NO.		RATE / DATE
CITY	STATE	ZIP	
SINGLE ☐ MARRIED ☐	NO. OF DEPENDENTS	DATE STARTED	DATE TERMINATED

EMP. NO.	PERIOD ENDING	TIME WORKED	RATE	EARNINGS REGULAR	O.T.	TOTAL	DEDUCTIONS F.I.C.A.	FED. TAX	ST. TAX					NET PAY	WEEK NO.	CHECK NO.
															1	
															2	
															3	
															4	
															5	
															6	
															7	
															8	
															9	
															10	
															11	
															12	
															13	
															14	
															15	
															16	
1st QUARTER TOTAL																
															1	
															2	
															3	
															4	
															5	
															6	
															7	
															8	
															9	
															10	
															11	
															12	
															13	
															14	
															15	
															16	
2nd QUARTER TOTAL																
YEAR-TO-DATE																

Figure 24–5.

Illustration continued on following page

NAME SOC. SEC. NO.

EMP. NO.	PERIOD ENDING	TIME WORKED	RATE	REGULAR	O.T.	TOTAL	F.I.C.A.	FED. TAX	ST. TAX					NET PAY	WEEK NO.	CHECK NO.
				EARNINGS			DEDUCTIONS									
															1	
															2	
															3	
															4	
															5	
															6	
															7	
															8	
															9	
															10	
															11	
															12	
															13	
															14	
															15	
															16	
3rd QUARTER TOTAL																
															1	
															2	
															3	
															4	
															5	
															6	
															7	
															8	
															9	
															10	
															11	
															12	
															13	
															14	
															15	
															16	
4th QUARTER TOTAL																
YEAR-TO-DATE																

NOTES

FORM 9354 COLWELL SYSTEMS, INC., CHAMPAIGN, IL 61820

Figure 24–5. *Continued.*

The method for making out payroll checks is similar. Your aide must first be familiar with the annual IRS publication, *The Employer's Tax Guide*, and the corresponding state publication. Your accountant will help her understand them, set up payroll records, and provide a calendar for state and federal remittances to remind her of the due dates. This is a backup system—the accountant will also provide completed forms prior to those dates, indicating amounts owed, with addressed envelopes for mailing.

Using the appropriate tables, the aide calculates the deductions for state and federal income taxes, and the employee's contribution under the Federal Insurance Contributions Act (FICA). These should be totaled and added to the calculated net to see if the sum matches the gross *before* she touches pen to the check. Then, the appropriate employee's pay record is inserted under the corresponding check and aligned. As the items in the top strip are entered, they are automatically transferred to that record.

After all checks have been written and signed, make sure you have enough in your checking account to cover them before they are sent out. Most physicians wisely keep their checking accounts "thin," so it is advisable to have a modest sum in a savings account in the same bank from which funds may be transferred to the checking account. A telephone call usually is sufficient, but if the bank requires written instruction, your aide can take it when your next deposit is made. Using the "float" is not worth the trouble. This involves keeping the maximum amount of money in accounts earning interest, and transferring funds to cover the checks just before the checks clear your own bank. This requires tricky timing, and the charges for overdrafts are higher now. One or two per month will more than cancel out any additional interest earned.

When the monthly bank statement with cancelled checks arrives, your aide should reconcile your practice account just as you do with your personal checking account. Always look at the reconciliation and cancelled checks to make sure it was done correctly and that no checks were altered.

Most of your disbursements will be by check, but a petty cash fund is required for small expenditures, such as postage due on letters or packages, and as a change fund for patients who make cash payments. There is no reason to have a separate change fund, because most patients have checking accounts and prefer to pay by check. If you keep $100 or so in small bills in your wallet or locked in your desk, you can rescue the petty cash fund on the rare occasion a large amount of change is needed.

The petty cash, in small bills and change not to exceed a total of $50, is kept in a locked metal cash box in the filing cabinet. The boxes designed for this purpose have a lower space for bills, receipts, and vouchers, and an upper removable half-drawer with compartments for change. Only one assistant should have a key, and she is responsible for seeing that a voucher or receipt is left for each withdrawal made. She enters all transactions in a notebook and balances the petty cash each month (or more often if necessary) on the day you will be writing checks. At that time the amount withdrawn should equal the total of the vouchers and receipts. These are stapled together with the sheet from the notebook for that period. She then prepares a check made out to *"cash"* for your signature to bring the total amount back to $50, and enters the sum of the check in the *office expenses* column of the check register. When you have signed the check, all receipts and vouchers, along with the notebook record sheet, are stored together in the "accounts paid" accordion file for that month.

If you have at least two assistants, one handles supplies and disbursements while another handles accounts receivable. The duties should be rotated periodically between them. If you have only one aide, let her handle the accounts receivable, and you can take care of the disbursements yourself.

Financial Reports

The preceding two chapters, this one, and the next cover the internal financial functions of your office but touch only lightly on the financial reports you should receive. This is because their frequency and content depend upon many variables: your interest and ability to understand them; your record-keeping system; your specialty; your practice organization; the number and expertise of your employees; the size of your practice; *and* the advice of your accountant.

Nonetheless, a description of the reports required in an average office would not be out of place here. I will suggest more, perhaps, than are feasible with a pegboard—yet fewer than are obtainable from a computer. There may be more than you have been getting, and perhaps fewer than you should. I have tried to strike a balance, and you can work with that as you will.

Reports are submitted to you weekly, monthly, quarterly, and annually. The annual has the same form as the quarterly report and basically sums up the contents of the previous four quarterly reports. In fact, almost all your accountant has to do to produce an annual report is touch one key on his computer to rework the information already in its memory. There is no need, therefore, to describe the annual report—only those received weekly, monthly, and quarterly.

The weekly reports are all yours to design and set up. Suggestions are: *time*—before office hours Monday morning; *place*—the consultation room; *persons* reporting—the receptionist and the clinical assistant in a small practice; the office manager in a large one.

Request three or four patient indices, such as:

Number of patient visits: office
Number of patient visits: hospital
Number of new patients
Number of no-shows
Number of patients requesting transfer with reasons

An internist might want to add the average number of patients admitted to the hospital, and a surgeon the number of procedures done that week.

Most financial information is contained in the monthly report, but you will want some "bare bones" indices in this weekly one:

Total accounts receivable
Number of insurance claim forms not submitted
Total accounts payable
Cash in checking account

The monthly report is the most important. Your accountant will work with you in designing a format. Smaller offices usually have an outside bookkeeper make it up under the accountant's direction. Rarely, the accountant himself prepares it. In larger offices, it will be prepared by the office manager. It is the principal management tool of the office; therefore, it must be given to you within a few days of the end of each month and be complete and accurate. It does not contain any information on your outside income or expenses.

The first part is a compilation of charges by services. This may be simplified into two or three categories if you use a pegboard, or expanded if you are on a computer to include percentage of total for each, comparisons with the prior month and the same month last year, and a year-to-date total. With either system, adjustments and write-offs are applied to the total charges to yield net charges.

Receipts are categorized as time-of-service, mail, insurance, and other. They are then totalled.

The collection rate is calculated and presented in percentage form.

Expenses are broken down into the categories established for your disbursing system and include payroll, deductions, and benefits. The total office overhead and net income are given followed by the total accounts payable.

The next section of the monthly report consists of the total accounts receivable, the totals resulting from aging the accounts, the action taken on delinquent accounts, and the insurance claim form status report.

Physician draw, contributions to your pension/profit-sharing plans, medical meeting expenses, and insurance premiums paid out of the office (e.g, malpractice) form the next portion.

The cash section is broken down to cash on hand, checking, savings, petty cash, and other.

The quarterly reports from your accountant are less valuable but much more impressive in their appearance. They may be presented in a form and jargon you will never fully understand, but some of the terms and ideas can be comprehended by a medical mind.

A knowledge of the difference between cash and accrual accounting systems is essential to start with. In the former, charges are counted as income when *received,* and expenses are recorded as such when they are *paid*. In the latter, each is recorded as *incurred,* never mind when received or paid. The former system is best for physicians; the latter apparently has advantages for merchants, although I don't know why. Be sure your reports are based upon the former.

Another set of useful terms is *single entry* and *double entry* as applied to bookkeeping systems. The pegboard in your office (and the computer) uses a variation of the single entry system. In its simplest forms, this consists of three elements:

1. *The journal*. This is a diary or day sheet on which all transactions are recorded as they occur.
2. *The ledger*. This indicates all accounts receivable with balance due. Entries are "posted" here from the journal. Physically, the ledger may consist either of a set of bound summary sheets or the ledger card file plus separate records of practice income from other sources.
3. *Disbursement record*. These are shown by category. Your check register (if it includes payroll and petty cash) is an adequate disbursement record.

Now for the double entry system, and here it may get confusing. Your accountant speaks the language; most of the rest of us do not. He takes your office information on charges, receipts, and accounts payable, including payroll tax liabilities accruing, and analyzes it according to this system. Its basis is the accounting equation:Capital *equals* Assets *less* Liabilities. *Capital* is equivalent to net worth. *Assets* includes your building, equipment, furniture, accounts receivable, checking and savings accounts, and cash on hand. *Liabilities* are what you owe.

Every transaction requires an entry on each side of the equation. Hence the term "double entry." The two sides must always be in balance.

A quarterly report to you based on the double entry system provides a comprehensive picture of the financial status of your practice, and the elements are arranged to facilitate the preparation of tax returns. However, in this form it has limited utility as a practice management tool, and usually comes too late anyhow. Don't be coaxed into having such a report monthly—quarterly is often enough.

The form in which it is presented depends upon your accountant, but it always consists of two parts:

1. *An income statement.* This shows income during the quarter from all sources, year-to-date totals, and comparisons with the same period the previous year. It also shows expenses by category for the same period, year-to-date totals and comparisons with the prior year. Grand totals of income and expenses are presented, with the resultant net profit.
2. *A balance sheet.* This refers back to the balance of the accounting equation and gives a "freeze frame" picture of the three elements at that point in time. **Assets** may be broken down to *current, fixed,* and *other,* with the total. **Liabilities** are *current* and *deferred,* with the total. **Capital** is broken down into several categories and totalled.

A summary of the changes in capital, assets, and liabilities over the accounting period may be appended.

25

Discouraging Embezzlement

Most physicians are aware that embezzlement is a potential problem in a medical practice, but are convinced it cannot happen in their own offices. This is an understandable attitude—the care of patients requires that you trust your assistants in many other ways. But let's look at the facts.

Embezzlements are reported in about 10 per cent of practices over any 10-year period. This is the figure often quoted, but it is only the tip of the iceberg. At least three or four times this many are strongly suspected or even *proven* but not reported. The employee is just let go. How many are neither suspected nor discovered? No one knows. The number can only be inferred through several approaches. If just one—what apprehended embezzlers tell of their activities for the years before they were caught—is to be believed, those that are never suspected or detected outnumber those that are several times over.

It can't happen here, you say. Well, let's see if it could. I'd like to describe a few of the more common methods used by embezzlers, and you can see for yourself if they could happen in your office.

"Lapping" is one of the most common. If an aide is running behind on posting the checks received in the mail, she can drift into this one quite easily. A few checks received the day before are finally entered on the proper ledger cards but not on the day sheet for the day they were received. The day sheet and deposit for that day look fine. Then she pockets cash on the second day totalling the same amount as the checks. The checks are entered on the day sheet the second day to cover this. Again the day sheet and deposit look fine. Patients never complain—they have either a cancelled check or a receipt from a dime store book. Their statements look fine, too, even if the aide has to photocopy dummy ledger cards to do it. The loss can amount to large sums when lapping is done repeatedly.

Almost as common is pocketing a cash payment either from a "walk-in" or from a patient you do not see but for whom one of your staff performs a service. These patients do not appear in the appointment book or in any other record.

A related trick is quoting a certain charge to a patient who pays cash, collecting it, recording a lesser charge, and keeping the difference.

Then there is the write-off or adjustment scam, with its variations. If an assistant is allowed to write off a balance herself she simply pockets all subsequent payments. If you insist on approving write-offs, she may present you with a list of "uncollectables," some of which are actually collectable. After you approve their being written off, she keeps the subsequent payments. The same thing can be done with adjustments. She can make them herself, or make larger ones than you have authorized, and pocket the difference.

In case you are wondering how an assistant can cash a check addressed to you, there are several ways. The easiest is to tell the patient, "I have a stamp for the doctor as payee" and then she writes in her name. Or she can open an account in your name at another bank with only her signature on the card. A post office box serves for an address to which statements are sent. She merely deposits your checks in the account and writes checks on it. If one bank balks at setting up such an account, she can usually find another that won't.

As long as we're on the subject of checks, let's look at your disbursement system and see if you would catch these schemes. An assistant opens a bank account under a fictitious name and presents you with a check for your signature, made out to that name, labelled "insurance refund." Would you catch this? A variation is opening an account under a business name similar to one of your suppliers. Or a check might be slipped into the stack for your signature made out to one of the assistant's own creditors. Or she might open a charge account in her name at one of the vendors used by your practice, charge items there, and include the amount in the check made out for your signature. All invoices are somehow "misplaced." Would you detect any of these schemes?

Then there is the "bounced check" routine. She takes some of the cash receipts with a plausible excuse in mind in case she is questioned, and substitutes a check of her own for that amount in the daily deposit. The balance in her account is kept low so her check bounces. Then all she has to do is intercept her returned check when it comes with the bank "NSF" notice, and remember to remove the carbon copy of the notice from the envelope containing the monthly statement and cancelled checks.

Would you notice a paycheck made out for a larger amount than the employee is owed?

We haven't touched upon altered or "kited" checks, outright forgeries, petty cash theft, or several other methods. But these few should be enough for you to see how effective your accounting control systems are. If they are a bit leaky, then you might want to strengthen them with some of the suggestions that have been presented throughout this book.

The most important of these are summarized here:

1. Check the references of employees at the time they are hired. Most embezzlements are not proved or, if proved, not reported. A question or two on the telephone may at least elicit the suspicions of prior employers and their basis.
2. An adequate pay scale and attention to staff morale are important. Listen for personal problems that might make an otherwise trustworthy employee yield to temptation.
3. Bond all employees. The principal purpose of a fidelity bond is to *deter*, not restitute a loss. The bonding companies require you to report all suspected cases of embezzlement to them or they will cancel your policy. When you are suspicious, their representatives come to your office to investigate, and employees know they cannot rely upon a tearful scene with you to win your forgiveness. The companies also require that you take the appropriate legal action if embezzlement can be proved.
4. Make sure your receptionist keeps an accurate appointment book. All patients seen in the office, even by your aides, are entered.
5. Keep the photocopies of the appointment book made for you each day under lock and key, or take them home.
6. See that the day sheet is accurate. All patients seen must be entered even if no charges are made, and all charges and receipts recorded promptly and accurately.
7. Charge slips should be numbered consecutively, with the numbers entered in the proper column on the day sheet. A charge slip is filled out for each patient, and the receipt portion given to each. All slips must be accounted for at the end of each day. Any with an erroneous entry should be voided, in the same way a check is voided and kept in numerical sequence with the others. They are retained in a binder for at least three years.
8. At the end of each day, the appointment book, day sheet, charge

slips, and deposit slip should be placed on your desk. This does not mean you have to check them every day—a spot check once a week will do. But if they are placed on your desk every day, and you indicate an interest in them, this practice will be a strong deterrent.

9. Bank deposits must be made at the end of working hours each day. If the bank closes before this, request a lock bag and use the night depository. Compare the amount of the deposit to the total receipts on the day sheet periodically.
10. Ledger cards should be removed from the tray for only three purposes and then replaced promptly: (1) to make entries on patient arrival and departure, (2) to adjust balances as authorized by you, (3) to be photocopied to prepare statements. Every now and then, pull four or five at random and compare them with your photocopy of the appointment book for that day and the day sheet. Have a trial balance run at least every month.
11. All receipts should be identified on the day sheet and ledger card as to source—cash, check, or insurance.
12. All checks received in the office should be stamped immediately on the reverse for deposit to your account. Don't have a "payable to" stamp in the office. All checks should be kept in a metal box in a locked filing cabinet until deposited. Any cash received is placed in the same box. The box is always locked, and only one assistant has the key.
13. All write-offs or adjustments must be authorized by you and bear your initial and the date. At least once a quarter your accountant should send out audit statements with the request that confirmation be mailed by the patients directly to him. Let your employees know he is doing this. Vary the groups audited. Include "uncollectables" before they are written off, and those that are already written off or adjusted, with the prior balance indicated.
14. Divide responsibilities as far as the size of your staff permits. If one aide collects receivables and handles the day sheet, another should make out deposit slips and take the receipts to the bank. Rotate duties from time to time at irregular intervals.

These steps are all on the receipt side, and are taken to establish an audit trail. This means that each patient seen, the service performed, the charge, and the payment received can be traced from the appointment book, through the day sheet and charge slip, to the deposit slip. Have your accountant come to your office from time to time to follow this trail, to see how well your systems are being carried out, and to make suggestions for improving them.

15. All disbursements must be made by check insofar as possible. Use petty cash only for small items when absolutely necessary. You, not an aide or office manager, must sign all checks. Although an assistant can make out the checks, you must match the invoices and statements against them. You also have to verify the accuracy of the payroll checks and deductions. Never make out a check payable to cash except to reestablish the petty cash fund, and *never* sign a blank check.
16. Keep an eye on your inventory of drugs and supplies. Thefts do not always involve money.
17. Bank statements with cancelled checks should always be given you with the envelope unopened. Examine the checks for alterations, make sure all signatures are yours, and that there are no missing checks. Either reconcile the statements yourself or check your assistant's reconciliation for accuracy. If time does not permit you to do this, have the bank statements mailed directly to your accountant instead.
18. Ensure that the petty cash fund is managed properly. It is here that embezzlement occurs most frequently. Although the amounts are small, repeated thefts can add up to large sums. An employee who is successful with small sums may be led to greater temptations.
19. Once or twice a month, gather up all incoming mail and open each item yourself. To check up on accounts payable, look for invoices and statements you have already paid or those for items that have not been ordered or received. On the accounts receivable side, there may be a letter from a patient complaining about improper account balances or other irregularities. Although you may not detect many abnormalities, your aides will be aware you are doing this. They do not have to think you are suspicious. Just tell them you are looking for a particular item, or want to give them a hand.
20. Have your accountant visit your office without warning from time to time to audit the books. This has a powerful effect as a deterrent.
21. Watch for certain warning signs. One is the indispensable "wonder woman" who works long hours, often alone, and who does not take vacations. She may be doing this to cover her tracks. Or the assistant who lives beyond her income and her spouse's combined. Or one with an alcoholic or gambling husband or a prolonged serious illness in her family, or one whose personality appears to change for the worse. Look for a decrease in your collection rate or a drop in your accounts receivable that is not due to an intensified collection effort. Or a decreased percentage

of cash receipts compared to check receipts. Or an unexplained increase in any expense category. Or photocopies substituted for original documents, odd alterations and erasures, missing records and other discrepancies.

Once an embezzlement is suspected, call your accountant first. Follow his advice. If his suspicion is strong, he will ask you to call the bonding company. The representative will work with your accountant. If the embezzlement is proved, call your lawyer. Avoid confronting the employee or calling the police until you are advised to do so. Do not discuss the matter with other office assistants or any outside individuals.

Note that the title of this chapter is "Discouraging Embezzlement," not "*Preventing* Embezzlement." No system is perfect, but if these suggestions are followed, the risk will be reduced as much as possible.

26

Personal Financial Management: The Early Years

One thing is certain—there is no shortage of experts who want to advise you on personal financial planning. But each represents a particular point of view and seems to have something to sell in his field. The one who would have you up to your ears in insurance usually has the letters C.L.U. or C.P.C.U. after his name. An investment advisor recommending outstanding opportunities in the stock or bond market happens to be employed by a major brokerage firm. And the one who advises you to invest heavily in real estate too often turns out to be a real estate broker.

You really have to be your own financial planner for the first few years. This chapter will start you off with basic advice, physician-to-physician, without any of the biases those just named may have. The best reference books and other information sources on each major subject will be named. Once you have acquired as much information as you can from them, turn to your practice management consultant, accountant, attorney, and insurance agents for additional advice. Later on, when your discretionary funds are substantial, contact the **International Association for Financial Planning,** 5775 Peachtree-Dunwoody Road, Suite 120-C, Atlanta, GA 30342 for the names of the area consultants on their registry. Or look for a *certified financial planner* who is fee-based. Get a list of his physician clients and check with them. Avoid any financial advisor who is commission-based: his advice tends to tilt toward his commission.

The preceding chapters dealt with professional financial management. If you continue to render high-quality, compassionate care and to follow the suggestions in those chapters, you will have a comfortable net income from your practice. This net is the basis of your personal financial plan.

Well, not quite. Uncle Sam steps in about here. Purchase a simple but comprehensive book on the subject, such as *Your Income Tax* by J. K. Lasser, available in most bookstores, and read it from cover to cover. You are the one who has to keep personal tax records and pay the (bleep) tax. It is in your interest to have a good understanding of the federal tax law. Then consult with your accountant. Ask him about state and city income tax. Develop a long-range tax strategy with him. If you don't have the time, ask your spouse to do this. Then follow it *throughout* the year, *every* year. A new issue of each tax book comes out annually and your accountant can give you a summary of the tax law changes each year. The changes that have been proposed this year (1985) are the most sweeping in history and may affect much of the advice in this chapter and the next. At this writing, however, it appears that special interest groups will nibble away at President Reagan's proposal so that the final version will not have the dramatic effect originally anticipated.

With that, you have taken your first step in personal financial management. The second is equally important. In your first few years of practice, try to keep your standard of living close to what it was during your last year of training. Pay off any indebtedness incurred during your education and training as soon as you can, with due regard to the interest rates on these obligations. Resist the almost irresistible temptations, after so many years of privation, to take advantage of the easy credit now obtainable, to move (finally!) into the home of your dreams, or to purchase (at last!) that new car before the old one falls apart. If you don't resist, you may have a fine plan but nothing to put into it. The dollars you invest now are much more valuable than those invested later. Look at any table that shows the results of interest compounding over the years. Your savings will also provide a measure of security during the early years of your career when your young children are totally dependent upon your efforts to make a living. These savings will be the wherewithal to use in investment opportunities, and will form the foundation for a secure retirement program. Saving 10 per cent after taxes is easy, but not enough; 20 per cent is a better goal. Don't ever fall below 15 per cent of your after-tax income. Underline *after-tax*. Remember, physicians are only hourly laborers. No matter how high your hourly income is, you will never be able to look forward to a life secure from financial disasters, to putting your children through the colleges of their choice, or to a comfortable retirement unless you have a good investment program. It is not your *income* that provides the standard of living you want for yourself and your family; it is your investment program. Capitalism means making capital work for you.

The next step in personal financial management is to prepare a plan. Sit down with your spouse and lay out your intermediate and long-range financial goals. Discuss the ways in which you can reach as many of your goals as possible. This is a large project, but the longest journey begins with a single step. Get some sort of folder, label it any way you wish, and drop in a copy of the net worth statement you prepared when you went to obtain your loan to start practice. Now you have *something* in your file. Next, put in the list of your financial goals. Then extract what applies to them from the remainder of this chapter, and add these notes and ideas to your folder. You are already well started on your financial plan.

Some of the best guides for setting up a financial plan are *Successful Investing: A Complete Guide to Your Financial Future* by Davis R. Sargent and the staff of United Business Service (Simon & Schuster); *The Lifetime Book of Money Management* by Grace J. Weinstein (New American Library); *Planning Your Financial Future* by Elliot Raphaelson (John Wiley); *The Intelligent Investor: A Book of Practical Counsel* by Benjamin Graham (Harper & Row); and *Personal Financial Planning* by G. Victor Hallman and Jerry S. Rosenbloom (McGraw-Hill).

Read these and other guides. Take notes and put them in your folder. Keep one thing in mind as you do so: those who fail to plan, plan to fail.

This chapter and the next are only an outline. Fill it in to suit yourself from these references and as you learn from your own experience. For reasons that will become apparent, I have divided a medical career into four phases. Special circumstances could easily place you between phases, but there is merit in considering your financial management plan in terms of these four:

Phase I. Starting Out
Phase II. The Growth Years
Phase III. The Peak Income Years
Phase IV. The Preretirement Years

PHASE I. STARTING OUT

Let's begin at the beginning. The main thrust during the first years is protection of your major asset—you, your education, skill, and potential earning power. Most of this protection is through insurance. But before we get to that, let's clear up some of the other items.

You have already set up a practice checking account at the bank that was your source of financing. A personal checking account has also been opened at the same or another bank near your home or main shopping center. You have looked into a NOW (or Super-NOW) checking account and found that the advantages are somewhat nebulous, and you have decided to stay with ordinary checking accounts. But you have also learned about the service charges and the balance that is necessary to avoid them. Keeping checking accounts "thin"—just above that balance—seems to be the best tactic. A small passbook savings account at the same bank is advisable so that you can shuffle funds back and forth easily (often with only a phone call) and so that you have a small cushion against unforeseen expenses. Because a savings account earns only 5½ per cent interest, no more than two or three months' income should be kept there. A savings and loan association pays ¼ per cent more, but this difference is usually not worth the bother. As your savings grow, you will want to keep the rest in a money market fund or in treasury instruments, options we will discuss later in the chapter.

The major protection against difficulties early in your career will be through insurance. But for minor problems that come along, you will need to establish credit-worthiness to be able to borrow what you need. Obtain at least two major credit cards, such as Visa and Master Card, along with a gasoline card and a few cards at local department stores. Make small purchases on each and pay the balance promptly. Your spouse should also get credit cards to establish credit in her name. Take out a small signature loan at the bank and repay it early. In this way, you can build up a credit-worthiness that will provide protection of $5000 to $10,000 in just a few months. Remember that Big Brother—the computer at the credit bureau—will be watching you. I don't agree with the standard advice of locking up six months' income in a liquid but relatively low-yield vehicle for protection. Good credit costs little or nothing, and you can put your money to work for you in better ways.

Get a safe deposit box at your bank. Keep documents in it such as birth and marriage certificates, passports, military records, contracts, leases, trust deeds, valuables, securities, inventory and photos of possessions, and a *list* of insurance policies, not the policies themselves. Place *copies* of your wills there, not the executed originals. Keep no cash unless you can prove income taxes on it were paid. Check whether your state has laws requiring that the box be sealed upon your death. Some do not; others do, but only for a few days.

Perhaps your first investment will be in an individual retirement account, or IRA. Try to do this your first year in practice. The present tax law allows you to set up an IRA even if you are participating in other retirement plans. You can contribute up to $2000 each year for yourself, and $250 more for your spouse if she is unemployed. If your spouse is employed, each of you can contribute up to $2000. These allowances will increase in future years. The amount invested each year, as well as the interest that accrues and compounds, are tax-deferred until withdrawal. This cannot be until age 59½ (except in the event of disability or death) without incurring a penalty of 10 per cent, plus the deferred tax, which is then due. An IRA also affords a degree of protection because you might be willing to pay the penalty to use these funds under certain circumstances. Or you can roll it over into another IRA and have a 60-day loan!

Find out all about IRAs by reading *The IRA Book* by Robert Krughoff, obtainable from the Center for the Study of Services, 806 15th Street NW, Suite 925, Washington, DC 20005. You can set one up at any bank, savings and loan, brokerage firm, or credit union. But look over the plans first and consult with your accountant. All IRAs are not alike. You can choose from among several plans at one institution, have IRAs at a number of institutions, or move funds from one to another, thus to some extent directing how your funds are invested. You are more interested in growth now and security later. Your principal purpose will be to lock in the highest possible return over a long period of time. Make your contributions *early* in the calendar year to take advantage of the income accrual in your account up to April 15 (or a later deadline), to gain the increased compounding effect, and to avoid the tax you would pay on the income from the funds if they were invested elsewhere.

That's about it for your investment plan during the first year or two. You will need all the money you can scrape together for an adequate insurance program. The purchase of a new car and home will be discussed in Phase II. Remember the rule—never go into debt for luxuries. During the first year or so, even these two are luxuries.

I could not find a good book to recommend on insurance, although I went through about a dozen. Medical Economics puts out *Insurance Strategies For Physicians,* but it is mediocre. Fortunately, the subject is not complicated.

The major item is life insurance, and the old saying is sad but true: "When you need it most, you can afford it least." There are six kinds of life insurance:

1. **Endowment.** This is an almost extinct type that pays out its face value after a certain number of years. It was designed predominantly as a savings vehicle. Most portfolios consist of older low-yield investments, which is why endowments are not around much anymore—and why they are not recommended.
2. **Whole-Life Insurance.** This is sometimes called "ordinary" or even

"straight" to make it appear more palatable. It combines investment and insurance features, but the investment return, although it accumulates tax-deferred, is in the range of 3 to 4 per cent. If interest rates ever drop down close to that, a whole-life policy might have one virtue—as a forced savings plan. Until then, it has none. The protection part costs up to ten times more than a comparable term policy. Keep in mind that insurance agents earn their highest commissions selling this type of insurance, so pressure will be brought to bear upon you. Just say no.

3. **Minimum-Deposit Insurance.** This is not really a type of insurance but rather a method devised to sell whole-life insurance with lower premiums by borrowing against accumulated cash value. You could do the same yourself and invest the difference, so forget it.
4. **Universal Life Insurance.** This is a newer type, with somewhat better portfolios than either of the above, plus certain flexibility features. But the 1984 tax law limits the amount of cash value build-up; you can do better investing on your own; and you still do not come close to the protection per dollar you get with term insurance. Avoid this one, too.
5. **Variable Life Insurance.** With this kind of policy, you are able to direct the investment yourself, but because of this, the cash value is not guaranteed. The only exception I know of is the Prime Plan of Merrill-Lynch, which does guarantee the funds at a future date. This sort of risk does not belong in an insurance program. Both universal and variable also have high sales loads and prohibitive administrative costs. My advice on variable is the same as for all of the above: stay away from it.
6. **Term Insurance.** This is straight protection for a specified premium over a certain period of time, hence the name "term." There is no savings feature. The usual terms are one, five, or ten years, at the end of which time the premiums are adjusted according to your age. Renewal may or may not be guaranteed at these times, so you may want to have at least one of your policies "guaranteed renewable," and pay the extra cost. One-year term is a better buy (despite the annual adjustments) because of the greater competition. If you compare a five-year term policy with five one-year policies including adjustments, you will see. Term life insurance is the type you should have. Get quotes from different companies through your life, health, and disability agent and contact your professional societies. If you do part-time teaching, you may be eligible for the **Teachers Insurance and Annuity Association** policies. Write the association at 730 Third Avenue, New York, NY 10017. In all probability, you will end up taking out one policy through your agent to keep him happy, and purchasing one or two larger group policies, which are about 25 per cent less expensive for the same

coverage. Watch out for one thing—the larger insurance companies sometimes "load" their term insurance to make their other offerings appear more attractive. Get additional quotes from smaller companies that handle *only* term insurance.

Some riders are offered with term insurance, but the only one that is actuarially sound is a waiver of premium if you are disabled. Get this and ignore the others.

The big question is how much term life insurance to carry. A rough rule of thumb for a beginning professional is about $500,000 if you have few assets, are married, and have (or expect to have) children. But it is better to tailor the amount to your particular requirements. This really isn't difficult. Start with the cost of supporting your family now. Figure 40 per cent of this will be needed for the support of your spouse alone, add 15 per cent for one child and 10 per cent for each additional child. Now you have to decide how long you would like this support to continue. Is your spouse likely to remarry? If your spouse is employed now, will that employment continue? If not employed now, is your spouse likely to learn a skill and be employed later? No one can know the answers to these questions, so a general guide is to plan coverage until your last child reaches maturity. Then major financial burdens are added in, such as large debts, home mortgage, and college costs for your children. The last expenses to add are burial expenses and death taxes. Summing all of these up will give up an estimate of your survivors' potential liabilities, but you are not done yet. You have to consider your assets: any assistance that your family might receive from parents or an employer, social security benefits for the time you have one or more children under 18, pension/profit-sharing death benefits, and other assets that you could convert. Subtract these from the liabilities, and you have the amount of life insurance you need.

More than you thought? Well, if you are not married and have no dependents, you may need no life insurance at all. If you are married, but have no children and your spouse is self-supporting, you may need only a fraction of this. Bear in mind that this burden will ease in the future. As you accumulate other assets, you can reduce your life insurance coverage accordingly. When your mortgage is paid and your children have graduated from college, you can reduce your protection even more. As you approach retirement, you may need only enough to cover burial expenses and death taxes.

Before closing the subject, give some thought to the financial drain or loss of income that would result if your spouse were to die. You might want to take out a separate policy for your spouse, or make one of your policies a joint-life that pays its benefits on the first to die. Life insurance on children is not worthwhile.

Death (and taxes) may be more certain than disability, but only a little more so. Almost half of all physicians have a significant disability at some time during their careers. You think it can't happen to you—but it can. Don't cut corners here. At age 35, a physician faces a greater risk of disability than death! The income stops just as certainly from disability as from death, and there is one more to provide for—you.

There are six things to consider in choosing disability income insurance:

1. *Your financial need.* Calculate the monthly income you would need from insurance if disabled. Remember, if you pay the premiums personally, the payout is tax-free. Use as a rough rule of thumb approximately one half of your present after-tax income, or calculate a more accurate figure if you wish. If you do become disabled, one of your major sources of assistance will be social security, after a waiting period of five months, if you meet the rather stringent requirements. You may be eligible for workers' compensation if you are covered and if the disability is work-related. Some salaried positions have salary continuation plans. As with life insurance, you can look forward to reducing the amount of protection as your other assets increase. Two cautions. Don't count on an office overhead policy to help with personal expenses in the event of your disability—these policies cover only the actual office expenses incurred. And allow for a lag of three or four months to build up your income again when you return to practice.
2. *The elimination period.* This is the time you have to wait before benefits start. It is best to take the longest waiting period possible in order to reduce the premium and/or increase the disability income. The premium is reduced about 10 per cent for every month the waiting period is increased. Your accounts receivable will come in on a declining curve for three or four months, and you have that small cushion in the bank, plus your credit-worthiness. It is wise to have two or three different policies, with one policy becoming effective in two months, another in three months, and another in six months.
3. *Renewability.* At least one major disability policy should be noncancelable and guaranteed renewable. Almost all individual policies are. A group policy may state that it is, but insurance companies offering group policies can cancel the group, or the group can change carriers. Even though individual policies are more expensive, you should have one that provides at least a third of your coverage, and reinforce this with one or two group policies.
4. *The definition of disability.* There are three basic definitions: unable to pursue "any occupation," unable to pursue "own occupation," and a split application of these two. Your policy must specify your own occupation at the start of disability as, "unable to practice

your specialty,'' with the word *specialty* emphasized. This definition should hold for a period of 24 to 36 months, after which it can drop to a looser formulation of your occupation as ''unable to practice medicine'' for the duration of the benefit period. Avoid policies with an ''any occupation'' phrase in the definition, such as, ''unable to engage in any occupation for which your education, training, or experience qualifies,'' even in a split form where it does not apply until after several years, because these definitions are often interpreted to your disadvantage. Decline partial disability benefit clauses unless they are ''up front''—that is, effective at the start. Partial disabilities that follow total disabilities seldom last long enough for you to achieve significant benefit.

Some newer policies have a ''loss of income'' provision that bypasses *any* definition of disability. They also cover you for partial disabilities if your income drops due to one, and solve the problem of picking a waiting period. About 95 per cent of all disabilities are resolved one way or another within 90 days—you are either dead or back to work. Ask your agent about these income replacement policies. I recommend them over the standard disability policies, all else being equal.

5. *The length of the benefit period.* This must be at least to age 65, at which time your retirement plan will presumably take over. Accept nothing less. If your retirement plan is not adequate, select a lifetime benefit period.
6. *A waiver of premium provision.* This means that the premiums for your disability policies will not have to be paid during the time that you are disabled. It is essential: be sure you have it.

Although group policies are less expensive, most of them come up short on one or more of the above points. Those sponsored by the AMA are a notable exception. Group policies usually have a coordination of benefits provision that reduces benefits available by the amount received from social security, workers' compensation, or other group coverage. At least one of your policies will be an individual one, and if the premiums pinch, stint somewhat on the *amount* rather than the *length* of payout.

Health insurance is the next consideration. The goal here is protection against catastrophes only. Professional courtesy and your assets can cover minor medical problems. The best for most physicians is a major medical policy with a high maximum (or no limit) obtained through a professional society. Get a large deductible and high copayment. It is better to have only one good policy that covers you and your family. With more than one, you run into coordination of benefits problems.

Whether you own your own home or not, a homeowner's policy is next. Even if you rent, you want coverage for your personal property.

Originally, these were in two major forms—"specified risk" in which the risks covered are stated (e.g., fire and theft), and "all risk," which specifically exclude certain risks (e.g., flood and earthquake). But these two major forms have become further refined and so standardized that your casualty agent may refer to them as "HO–1," "HO–2," and so on. There are now seven standard forms:

Homeowners 1 (basic specified risk form): Fire, lightning, extended coverage, vandalism and malicious mischief, theft, glass breakage on dwelling buildings and personal property (contents), and comprehensive personal liability.

Homeowners 2 (broad form): All the above, and additional extended coverage that provides coverage for other specified causes of loss.

Homeowners 3: "All risk form" on buildings and broad form on personal property.

Homeowners 4: Personal property coverage only (broad form) for tenants.

Homeowners 5: "All risks" on buildings and personal property.

Homeowners 6: Personal property and loss of use coverage (broad form) for condominium unit owners.

Homeowners 7: Coverage on buildings and personal property somewhat more limited than basic form; used to provide coverage on homes that may not meet the insurer's underwriting requirements for other homeowner's policy types.

Always insure for the *replacement cost* of the structure and contents. The amount of coverage must be for at least 80 per cent of the actual replacement cost or your reimbursement will be drastically reduced despite this provision. Increase the amount of coverage as property values appreciate, and don't be caught short.

Limits are placed on protection for items of unusual value. I would recommend a safe deposit box for small items such as jewelry. Larger valuables and those that have to be kept in the home should be covered by an endorsement to the basic policy, or by a floater, which is essentially another policy. This coverage is expensive, so you may want to reduce it and rely on other security precautions. In any case, prepare an inventory of all your possessions, take photos of them in your home, and keep this evidence in your safe deposit box.

The second major part of homeowner insurance is personal liability. Because physicians are prime targets for suits, the limits on bodily injury and property damage should be high enough to meet the lower limits of your umbrella policy. Be aware of the exclusions in your homeowner's policy. Some of these are aircraft, most watercraft, motor vehicles, business pursuits, rented premises, and professional actions. These must be covered under other policies.

Group homeowner policies are perfectly satisfactory and much less expensive. Check into the organizations to which you belong. The best policies obtainable are those of United Services Automobile Association (discussed in the next paragraph). If you are employed part-time, ask your employer about group policies available through your enrollment.

Although your automobile will be used mostly for professional purposes, the policy comes under personal protection. Because this insurance is expensive, ask your insurance agent for quotes from two or three companies while looking for group policies. Look into **AAA** rates. **GEICO** (Government Employees Insurance Company, GEICO Plaza, Washington, DC 20078) may cover you if you have been in government or military service, or if you have a good driving record. Any physician who has ever been an officer in the Public Health Service, the armed services (active or reserve) or the National Guard is eligible for coverage by the **USAA** (United Services Automobile Association, USAA Building, San Antonio, TX 78288). Grown children of members may belong to a subsidiary organization of USAA. Inquire of all companies about their rates for safe drivers, limited usage, and two cars on one policy. It may be expedient to insure an expensive car only for the one safest driver in the family or to limit its use in order to reduce premiums.

There are four parts to a typical automobile policy. The *first* covers damages due to almost all types of peril, regardless of who is at fault. This part is broken down into three sections: comprehensive (theft, vandalism, fire), collision, and towing costs. This is the most expensive part, so request high deductibles to reduce the premiums.

The *second* part is liability coverage. This provides payment for bodily injury and property damage sustained by others. It protects you in your own automobile as well as those not owned by you, and protects all members of your household or anyone else who may be driving your automobile with your permission. Obtain the same limits you have for personal liability.

The *third* part of an automobile policy pays claims for medical expenses incurred by any occupants of your automobile at the time of an accident. There is usually a $5000 limit per person and per accident. Accept the standard.

The *fourth* part is uninsured motorists protection. This covers you if you are injured (whether in a vehicle or as a pedestrian) by any motorist who does not carry liability insurance. This is usually limited to bodily injury only. If you already have a major medical policy, you may wish to have the minimum required by your state financial responsibility law.

Notice that nonowned automobiles used in your profession are *not* covered by a standard automobile policy. This is an item that must be included in your professional insurance program.

The last item of personal insurance is an umbrella policy for liability. This is relatively inexpensive, considering the amount of coverage obtained. The lower limits start where your basic liability protection ends, and upper limits extend to as high as $3 or $4 million. Get at least $1 million, and be sure to match the lower limits with your existing (automobile, homeowner, watercraft, and other) liability protection. When you calculate how much you save by lowering the usual limits on the other policies, the cost of an umbrella is surprisingly low.

Have your insurance agents carefully coordinate all of the above policies. Avoid gaps and overlaps. Their advice and coordination are the major reasons you place policies through them.

There is only one last item to touch upon relating to the first few years in practice. If you have not made out a will yet, sit down with your spouse and attorney, discuss all aspects of your financial situation, and have one drawn up for each of you. Doing so will also help you to tie up any loose ends in your financial plan. If you should die without a will, your estate is distributed according to state law, not your wishes, and you lose all the tax advantages of proper estate planning.

PHASE II. THE GROWTH YEARS

This period sees growth not only in your practice, but in your income, taxes, assets, family, and almost every aspect of your life.

This is a much more interesting phase than the first. You move from passive protection to an active investment program. There is also a greater complexity, and more challenge in trying to keep what you would like to think is yours in the face of opinions the Internal Revenue Service may hold to the contrary. Increased thought is also given to your children's future education and your own retirement.

The insurance part of this phase is the simplest. After all the time, effort, and money you put into setting up your insurance program, all you need to do now is review it annually with your insurance agents and make any alterations required because of inflation, additions to your family, the assumption of major new debts, and other significant changes.

Now for the investment part. With only a little inattention, the "cushion" of about two months' income in your passbook savings account will grow during the first year or two in practice. The easiest solution for a busy practitioner is to ask at the same bank (or at a nearby savings and loan association) for a "better deal." They are just waiting for you to ask. You will be told about plans with names such as "Money Market Certificates," "Thrift Certificates," and "Certificates of Deposit." The interest rates are much higher than that of your passbook account, there may be a starting bonus, and you will be assured that these plans are protected up to $100,000 by an instrumentality of the federal government (the FDIC for commerical banks and FSLIC for savings and loan institutions). The sales pitch may be difficult to resist, but I'll tell you how. Just thank them and walk out of the door.

There are several problems with these plans. A large initial investment is required. The service fees are substantial. Interest rates are often quoted on the basis of compounding interest daily, which makes comparisons with other investments difficult. You can't add new funds at will, but must purchase a new certificate. At the end of the period you have to be attentive or they will roll over your funds into a low-yield account. The greatest problem is liquidity, or the lack thereof. The shortest duration is approximately one month, and you *may* need your money even faster than that. You will be told that the interest rate is even higher if you leave your funds in longer, say three months. Then you may get greedy because six months or a year brings an even higher rate. If you yield to temptation and lock your money in for that long, you will almost certainly encounter a good investment opportunity or need money urgently during that time. Then you not only have to pay three to six months' interest as penalty but lose the starting bonus just to get your own money back! Their "money market deposit accounts" were created to overcome some of these disadvantages, but are only a little better.

If you want a certificate of deposit, see your stockbroker. Large brokerage houses purchase CDs from savings institutions (which are carefully canvassed nationwide for the best rates) in huge blocks at a discount. Even though the brokerage house may take ½ or 1 per cent off the top, they still give you a better rate than your local bank or savings and loan by at least 1 per cent. In addition, your minimum investment is lower, there is no sales charge, and the annual fee is only $50 to $100. You can add to your investment as you wish, and you are covered up to $100,000 by FDIC or FSLIC. But here is the real kicker. What you purchase are *shares* in the huge block, and these shares are readily salable on the secondary market, so you can get your money back on one day's notice without any penalty! It's as good as money in the bank—better.

There are about half a dozen other ways to accumulate your money with safety, liquidity, and a high return, but a busy practitioner needs only to know about two more.

When you have sufficient investment capital to work with, look into *United States Treasury bills,* or *T-bills.* These are backed by the "full faith and credit" of the federal government and come in minimum denominations of $10,000 with $5,000 increments, for periods of three, six, nine, or twelve months. You can purchase them for a small service fee ($50 or so) at any commercial bank, brokerage, or other financial institution. Or you can participate directly in the weekly auction in person or by mail through your nearest federal reserve bank and save the fee. The interest you earn is on a discount basis, so you can take this money and put it to work right away. The interest is also exempt from state and local income taxes. Best of all, you are not bound by the maturity date initially selected, because T-bills can be sold on the secondary market through any bank or broker for a small sales fee. For more information on T-bills, write: **Bureau of the Public Debt,** Department of the Treasury, 15th Street and New York Avenue NW, Washington, DC 20226. Ask for the proper forms and the free booklet, *Basic Information on Treasury Notes and Bills.*

If you don't have a lot of reserve capital, want reasonable safety, complete liquidity, checking (and sometimes credit card) privileges, and a higher return (¼ to ¾ per cent above T-bills), ask your broker about a *money market mutual fund.* Almost every major brokerage house has one. There are also several independent ones. A complete list can be found in Donoghue's *Money Market Fund Directory,* obtainable at P.O. Box 540, Holliston, MA 01746. The *Wall Street Journal* will tell you how the various funds are doing. Obtain a prospectus on each one that interests you. Some funds concentrate on higher yields with a correspondingly greater risk, some emphasize safety with portfolios consisting exclusively of treasury securities, and some have tax-free portfolios. The usual portfolios consist of T-bills, banker's acceptances, large certificates of deposit and commercial paper of major corporations, so although money market funds are not insured by the federal government, they are almost as safe as if they were. Select the one that suits you. A minimum initial investment of $1000 to $10,000 is required, depending upon the fund you select. But there is no minimum balance that must be maintained, so you could even borrow to get set up and repay your loan right away out of the fund. Insiders tell me that brokerage houses lose money on these funds—they are maintained only to encourage investment in other securities they sell.

Although there are others you may wish to investigate, these are three good ways to accumulate your money. None of them is considered a good long-term investment, however, because they are tied to prevailing interest rates. But they let you continue to look for better investments. If you think interest rates are starting down and you haven't found a better place to put your money, lock in present rates with treasury notes or bonds for a year or more.

During Phase II you will want to purchase a newer automobile and perhaps a second one. You will be guided by personal taste as well as more practical considerations—depreciation, safety, mileage, price, maintenance needs, and insurance costs. I would like to add one word of advice. In times past, some physicians purchased large, sleek, expensive cars and were accused of nothing worse than being ostentatious consumers. At least no one doubted their sanity. Today, especially among the younger physicians, there is a tendency to own something that looks as if it just came off the track at Indianapolis. These cars do at least 120 m.p.h., and look as if they are moving that fast even when sitting in the parking lot. They are outrageously expensive to purchase, cost much more to operate and maintain, and raise your insurance rates. But worse, they are more dangerous to you, your passengers, and others. This is a poor example for a physician to set. He is supposed to be wiser than most and dedicated to the health of all. In replacing the old car that served you so well through medical school and training, my suggestion is to go for the more modest, more reliable, and safer models. And now that you have accumulated the cash, you can do a better job of bargaining and avoid the usurious interest rates of the time purchase plans.

The next major investment is your own home, or moving up from the one you own to a better one. This can be a fee-simple house, a condominium, or a cooperative apartment. Look at this not only in terms of the plans and dreams that you and your spouse have been cherishing for all these years, but also impartially as an investment. This is your largest investment, and for some years may be the only large one you can manage. It can also be one of your better ones. Although mortgage interest rates remain high, the appreciation of a carefully chosen home can offset them. Despite the "flat tax" movement, home mortgage interest will probably remain deductible. The interest rates will not stay high forever, and you can refinance when they come down.

Look ahead, so that the size will be suitable as your family grows. Try to foresee the direction of the neighborhood and the quality of the schools. Consider the location in relation to your office and principal hospitals. Make some sort of estimate of the repair and maintenance costs. Find out about property taxes. Look at your prospective home with an eye toward its resale value some years down the line and the appreciation you can expect. This is a good example of the "invest only in what you know and can control" rule.

Stocks and bonds are almost always in violation of this rule unless you are a expert in the field and can devote full time to it. Nothing has been said so far about this type of investment and little will be. Most of the minor investment disasters that happen to physicians happen here. The major ones, of course, are in tax shelters. Most physicians do not have the time or expertise to investigate individual stocks or bonds carefully, and instead follow a hot tip from a colleague, or a first-, second-, or third-hand one from an "expert." You will earn enough over the years—you do not have to gamble.

The route that I would advise in this area is mutual funds. A wide variety of mutual funds, from speculative to conservative, is available. You can diversify. They are convenient and save you time. The unit size is reasonable. Purchase plans provide discipline as well as dollar-cost averaging. Your funds are liquid. The managers are professionals, just as you are in your field, with years of experience, and they can obtain consultants and information unavailable to you. Compared with brokers' commissions, the management costs are a bargain. Since mutual funds deal in large blocks of securities, they carry considerable clout in the market, and their track record over recent years is open for evaluation.

If you decide to invest in mutual funds, you have two options. One option is to walk into any major brokerage house, talk to the manager, have a brief discussion with the broker he assigns you, and sign up in a "load" fund as fast as he can click his ball point. These carry an average sales charge of 8½ per cent. This is deducted in advance, so you have that much less working for you. If you hesitate, the broker may offer you a pseudo no-load fund in which the same sales commission is paid out of high management fees, exit fees, and penalties on early withdrawals.

The second option is a far better one—no-load funds. Write for a list of these funds from the **No-Load Mutual Fund Association,** 11 Pennsylvania Plaza, Suite 2204, New York, NY 10001, or the **Investment Company Institute,** 1775 K Street NW, Washington, D.C. 20006. Subscribe to the *No-Load Fund Investor,* P.O. Box 283, Hastings-on-Hudson, NY 10706 and get their *Handbook for No-Load Fund Investors.* For more information, look in a large public library for reports from Lipper Analytical Services, Weisengerger Investment Companies Service, United Business Service, and for *Standard & Poor's Stock Guide. Forbes* has a good annual review.

Instead of a sales charge, no-load funds have an annual management fee of ½ to 1 per cent. Some are diversified, or you may choose from among those with aggressive growth, moderate long-term growth, and growth with income portfolios, or from specialized funds with portfolios composed exclusively of corporate bonds, tax-exempt bonds, short-term instruments, or almost anything you wish. Select two or three categories that coincide with your investment objectives, obtain several prospectuses in each category, read them carefully, and choose the funds you prefer. If your time is limited, have your spouse do this for you. It is best to invest in three or four with different characteristics. No-load funds do require a little more work at the start, but once you choose the funds you want, the shares are purchased easily by mail. Their performance in the past has been the same as the load funds and should continue to be so.

Sometime during this growth phase, you will want to ask your accountant and attorney about setting up educational trusts for your children. By the time your children get to college it may cost $100,000 per child for the four years. And more students than ever are going on to graduate study. No matter how high your income may be then, these expenses will fracture your financial plan unless you anticipate them now. The standard type is the short-term reversionary or "Clifford" trust, in which the income accrues and compounds tax-free over a period of at least ten years and a day. This kind of trust requires an attorney. Be sure to ask him about gift tax liability. Something you can do yourself under the **Uniform Gift to Minors Act** or a comparable state law is set up custodial accounts which you control. The interest income goes to the child and is taxed at his lower rates.

During Phase II, the first serious attention is paid to your retirement plan. Social security forms its foundation. Contact your local social security office by telephone and ask for the card (SSA-7004 PC) to request a statement of earnings. Send a card in every three years from now on, so any errors can be corrected before it is too late to track them down. You will receive a computerized readout of your earnings and contributions to date. Ask the local office to send you the two pamphlets entitled *Your Social Security* and *Estimating Your Social Security Retirement Check*. With these you can begin to estimate your social security income on retirement. When you are over 60, the office will make the estimate for you.

Continue making IRA contributions early each year. But it is now time to look beyond your IRAs. Read a good reference such as *All You Should Know About IRA, Keogh and Other Retirement Plans* by the J. K. Lasser Tax Institute (Simon & Schuster). One book put out by Medical Economics that I can recommend is *Personal Pension Plan Strategies For Physicians* by C. C. Hardy and H. J. Wiener. Look for other good books on pension plans in your public library.

Basically, there are two types of pension plans, the defined contribution plan and the defined benefit plan. The former is better early in your career when your employees are near your own age. The latter has advantages later and will be discussed under Phase III in the following chapter.

A defined contribution plan permits contributions of up to 25 per cent of net income to a limit of $30,000 a year. This limit will be adjusted after 1988 on a cost-of-living basis. The contributions can be made three ways: (1) with a money purchase plan on a fixed percentage of income; (2) with a profit-sharing plan in which the percentage varies year to year; or (3) with a combination of the two, which allows greater flexibility but carries greater costs than either of the other two plans. Discuss these options with your accountant.

Most physicians start with a profit-sharing plan, although the maximum contribution is limited to 15 per cent of net income. Three-year full vesting of all profit-sharing plan participants is recommended. Integration with social security is also recommended, which reduces proportionate contributions for employees.

The major impetus behind forming individual professional corporations from the late 1960s into the 1970s was the ability of the incorporated physician to establish a tax-sheltered retirement plan. However, the **Tax Equity and Fiscal Responsibility Act** of 1982 (TEFRA) eliminated this major advantage of incorporating by equalizing corporate and noncorporate retirement plans. The only significant advantages of a professional corporation now are (1) deductible health insurance, (2) deductible group life insurance of $50,000, (3) deductible death benefit of $5,000, and (4) deductible disability insurance. These are more than balanced by the disadvantages of incorporation: (1) higher social security taxes, (2) the accountability of the shareholders for corporate debts, (3) the additional federal and state income tax returns that must be filed, (4) the increased likelihood of IRS audits, (5) the requirements to hold corporate meetings and to maintain the minutes, (6) the necessity of submitting the additional financial statements and paying state fees, and (7) the legal and accounting expenses. At the present time, few, if any, physicians are incorporating their practices. In fact, the trend is toward "disincorporation" because of these factors.

Even if you are still at the start of your career as you read this, go on to the next chapter. Although its subtitle is "The Later Years," it contains information you need to know now to form and follow an effective financial plan over your lifetime.

27

Personal Financial Management: The Later Years

PHASE III. THE PEAK INCOME YEARS

Your peak earning years are also the peak income tax years, so a word or two first about tax shelters. In my view, some are benign. These range from owning your home, through IRAs, profit-sharing and money-purchase pension plans, deferred compensation plans, and municipal bond funds, all the way to residential rental real estate investments that you control yourself. The line, at least for me, is drawn just short of the larger real estate investments entered into on a limited partnership basis and controlled by a general partner. These usually involve large commercial properties, undeveloped land or farms. Once over that line, tax shelters become increasingly malignant as they range through equipment leasing and cattle breeding to the more exotic ones such as energy exploration.

Such tax shelters as these "beyond the line" are in highly specialized fields about which the average physician knows little; thus the expertise and reliability of the promoter are critical. The heavy financing of many with negative cash flow due to high interest rates makes them questionable as investments, and all are high-risk and long-term, with limited liquidity.

If you are in the highest marginal tax bracket and invest only income subject to that rate *that you can afford to lose*, then perhaps you can tiptoe across this line if you understand what you are doing. A tax shelter must first of all be a good investment, and most of those past this line are not. Because they are based on tax law, shelters are extremely vulnerable to changes in that law. The IRS recently intensified its scrutiny of those shelters with a tax-to-investment benefit ratio of greater than 2 to 1, required that they be registered, and that this registration number appear on the investor's return. This number often occasions an audit. A subsequent disallowance of a shelter, with taxes, interest, and penalties charged, can be a heavy burden indeed. And this risk is in addition to the risk of the shelter itself.

With that much said, let's go on. At this point in your career, you have accumulated substantial money market mutual funds, broker's certificates of deposit, and treasury bills, and you have put some of your money into carefully selected no-load mutual funds. You have also resisted the temptation to get into the stock and bond markets directly. So far so good.

Time now for some investment philosophy. When we physicians enter the financial world, we find ourselves in somewhat the same position as a patient is in ours. Just as the patient relies upon our counsel in health matters, we have to rely upon professional advice in financial affairs. Accustomed to making independent decisions in our own field, we do not do very well in this role of depending on advisors. And just as patients are often told more about the expected favorable outcome than the risk involved, we are frequently told by financial advisors more about the anticipated rewards than the risks. We understand risk in medicine but too often fail to comprehend it in financial affairs when we are about to make a major investment. Simply stated, in investments, risk and reward are almost always in balance. If a large return is assured, the risk involved may not be mentioned. Always ask. Aim for more modest rewards until you have money you can afford to lose.

Another concept we should be clear on is diversification. This doesn't just mean many kinds of investments chosen at random. It involves making investments that are reliable in inflationary as well as deflationary times. In this context, you should understand the difference between *debt* and *equity investments.* With debt investments you lend your money for a fixed return. The prevailing interest rate usually stays about 3 or 4 per cent ahead of the inflation rate, thus ensuring a modest but reasonably reliable gain. An equity investment means you own a portion of something—real estate or common stock. The effect of inflation on this type of investment is more uncertain, as is the growth or return from the investment itself.

Most of your investment so far has been debt investment. The greatest rewards, however, are on the equity side—but so are the risks. Let's look at the one class of equity investments that, if made carefully, can be the safest. Twenty years ago, Americans had half again as much invested in stocks as in real estate—now it's the reverse. One reason is that the appreciation of good real estate has easily outpaced inflation. Another is that real estate is more easily understood—the average person is capable of selecting and managing certain types of real estate, whereas the arcane language of *puts*, *calls*, and *options* may be beyond him. But the major factor behind the shift has been the tax law. When you purchased your home, you benefited from some of its provisions. Mortgage interest is deductible, and the appreciation when your home is sold is taxed at capital gains rates. You may have some benefits from a home study, and tax-free exchanges are possible. If you purchase a more expensive home and invest your present equity in it, tax on the appreciation is deferred. If you keep your home as your primary residence to age 55, then $125,000 of the appreciation will be tax exempt when it is sold.

These are some of the reasons why it is worthwhile to look beyond the equity in your home to other possibilities in real estate. Because residential rental property receives more lenient treatment by the IRS in terms of depreciation and recapture than other rental property, we should consider the pros and cons of this investment first. If it is well selected, it is relatively risk free.

Another advantage is that it is tangible and familiar. We have lived in similar homes for years. We can predict with some accuracy the trend of neighborhoods we know, and forecast the demand. Unbiased consultants are available for a fee. And most of us can step in and do repairs or obtain tenants if we have to. In short, we can *know* our investment and *control* it.

Residential rental property has certain disadvantages such as slow appreciation (currently), property taxes, high mortgage interest, and realtor's commission—and you need to be careful about rent control legislation. The most important disadvantage is that it is not very liquid, but this is less important now that you have other assets. Balanced against this disadvantage is the major advantage, the power of leverage. If you put only 20 per cent down on a piece of property (ignore such factors as taxes and interest payments), and sell it several years later at twice the price, you do not just double your original investment, you realize a profit of *five times* your original investment!

All of these advantages and disadvantages discussed so far may or may not balance out for you. If they do, the scales are usually tipped toward this type of investment by the three advantages under current tax law. As with your home, the appreciation when the property is sold is taxed at capital gains rates (subject to depreciation recapture), but the sale may be deferred to the most suitable year to minimize this impact. The mortgage interest is deductible, and accelerated depreciation on the structures and equipment (not the land) is available under current law. You are further encouraged by the knowledge that 90 per cent of all millionaires started with this class of investment.

The question is, what *kind* of residential rental property? Houses, duplexes, and apartment buildings are favored by some physicians. Low-income housing attracts others because of its greater tax advantages. But all of these bring with them two major concerns—maintenance and management. Most of us do not have the time or skill to take care of these ourselves. But for those who have talent in these areas and can spare the time, excellent opportunities are to be found in most areas of the country. Maintenance and management can be obtained by the rest of us for a price, but they are expensive and the cost can cancel much of the advantage of this type of investment. Net-lease arrangements can be set up for commercial property, with the lessee handling the maintenance, taxes, and insurance, but this cannot often be done with residential property.

Many physicians find it is easier to invest in vacation condominiums. These come with built-in management and maintenance. If you select an area that you know well, if you have enjoyed the recreational facilities yourself over a number of years, and if you buy the best quality unit available, you can hardly go wrong. The unit you pick must be situated directly *on* the ocean or lake, not 100 yards back, *on* the ski slope so you can ski out and ski in, or *on* the golf course. It must have the finest amenities. No matter how difficult the economic times may be, there are always some in our society who do not deny themselves top-quality vacations and who are able to pay for the best. If you stint in any way on quality, your rentals will fall off sharply in difficult times, and the negative cash flow can hurt. There is also a fringe benefit. You can use your vacation condo up to 14 days a year without losing the tax advantages. Some of the travel and other expenses during your vacation may be deductible if you are attending a homeowners' meeting or supervising your property. If you really like the area and can take more time off, buy two units and enjoy 28 days a year there!

There are many other possibilities in real estate that are beyond the scope of this chapter. My purpose is to present an overview and to point out avenues for further exploration. Among the options you will want to investigate are first and second trust deeds, Ginnie Maes, shared equity arrangements, real estate investment trusts (REITs), and owning your own medical office building. This last option is the subject of Chapter 25. For more information, read *Real Estate Principles and Practices* by Alfred Ring and Jerome Dasso and *Real Estate Investment*

Strategies by Maury Seldin and Richard H. Swesnik. Subscribe to the *Real Estate Investing Letter,* 757 Third Avenue, New York, NY 10017.

I have said nothing about precious metals or collectibles that are a good hedge against inflation. If you wish, put 10 per cent or so of your investment dollars here. Observe a few rules: know and enjoy the items yourself, limit yourself to one or two fields, eliminate middlemen by buying and selling directly, calculate in storage and insurance costs, buy high-quality items, and invest for the long term. For more information read *How to Invest in Diamonds, Metals, and Collectibles* by Arthur C. Simon.

Because you are in your peak income tax years, you will need to be doing more about taxes. This is the time to shift one or more of your no-load mutual funds into those specializing in tax-free local and state bonds, and to increase your investments substantially in them. If you are employed full- or part-time, ask your accountant about a deferred compensation plan under section 401(k) of the Internal Revenue code.

In your retirement planning, you have continued to make maximum IRA contributions early each year and have added a money-purchase plan to your profit-sharing plan. This has increased your annual contribution to the maximum allowed under the combined plans of 25 per cent of your annual net income up to $30,000. (This limit will be adjusted by the cost of living after 1986.) You have also integrated these plans under social security to increase your future benefits proportionate to those of your employees. But if you are chafing at this limit, find out about a *defined benefit plan*. This allows contributions toward a retirement income of up to $90,000 a year. This amount also will be adjusted by the cost of living after 1986. Now that you are older than most of your staff, your own contributions can be proportionately greater. Discuss with your accountant the many variables in defined benefit plans, such as front loading, the effect of different retirement ages, and the target benefit as opposed to fixed benefit approach.

In these peak years, you will continue to review your insurance annually, making only minor adjustments in coverage. These will be reductions for the most part, with one exception that I will mention in the next paragraph. Term life premiums are higher now owing to your age, but so are your assets, and these make possible a reduction in your life insurance coverage. The growing death benefits in your IRA accounts and other retirement plans may allow a further reduction. Cancel your most recent policies first—their cost per dollar protection is the highest. Reductions may be possible in health and disability insurance for the same reasons. If your car is now older and you calculate that you can afford a total loss, you might eliminate collision and comprehensive coverage which are the costliest parts of automobile insurance.

The one item of insurance you might want to *add* at this time is a tax-deferred *annuity policy*. An annuity is a contract with an insurance company to pay a guaranteed income for the remainder of your life, starting at a specified age. If you die before that age, the value is paid as a death benefit to your beneficiary—a provision that further reduces your need for life insurance. If, after that age, you die before your spouse, benefits will continue at the same or a reduced level to your spouse for life. The reason this is worth considering is that the sum of your assets and retirement plans is—and always will be—limited. If you live longer than they last, it is possible that you and yours could be in difficult straits in your later years. There are newer forms of annuities obtainable now with attractive investment portfolios. There is a tax advantage, too: the gain in value is accrued and *compounded* on a tax-sheltered basis.

PHASE IV. THE PRERETIREMENT YEARS

These are the years in which you will be able to travel more and to take time off to pursue hobbies or other interests that have been deferred. At the same time, you have to shift into high gear on your retirement planning. Write the **American Association of Retired Persons** (AARP), 1909 K Street NW, Washington, D.C. 20049 for information, and consider joining their program for those over 50. Browse through *The Complete Retirement Planning Book* by Peter A. Dickinson (Dutton, 1984); *Your Guide to a Financially Secure Retirement* by C. Colburn Hardy (Harper & Row, 1983); *Prime of Your Life* by Joseph Michaels (Little, Brown and Co., 1983); and *The Complete Retirement Handbook* by Forest J. Bowman (Perigee, 1983).

Insurance is simplest in this phase. Let's start with life insurance. By now, your youngest child is through college and all your children are on their own. Your assets plus the death benefits in your retirement plans are probably sufficient to support your spouse for life upon your death. The principal reason for life insurance at this time would be to cover death taxes and burial expenses. The latter are only a few thousand dollars, many states have eliminated death taxes, and federal death taxes have been decreased in recent years. Estimate yours and set aside assets to cover them. Don't rely entirely upon insurance for this purpose—it is much more expensive at your age. Some assets that would otherwise be considered nonliquid are sufficiently liquid for this purpose. Your executor is allowed nine months from the date of death until these taxes must be paid. Most improved property can be sold in that time. If not, mortgages can be taken out or older mortgages refinanced. The two reasons to carry life insurance at this age are if your assets are inadequate to cover expected death taxes or you still have a large mortgage or other major debt. If you decide to continue with a policy, make sure your spouse owns it and pays the premiums herself so the policy will pay her clear of probate and free of death taxes.

The same is true for disability insurance. If your assets can carry you and your spouse at 60 per cent of your current expenses for 10 years beyond your actuarial life spans, you might consider canceling all disability insurance. Remember to figure in your social security disability benefits.

Every three years or so, you have called the local social security office for the card to send in to obtain a statement of earnings. This time, while you have them on the phone, ask for *Your Medicare Handbook*. You may have thought you knew all about Medicare as a physician, but its provisions are quite different from a patient's point of view. Do you know, for example, the limitations on nursing home coverage? It is sometimes surprising what it does not cover and how little it pays on what it does. Only about 40 per cent of all medical expenses incurred by those over 65 are paid for by Medicare. Although the burden of medical expenses may be eased somewhat by professional courtesy, you will need a good supplementary plan, obtained on a group basis if possible. **Blue Cross** and **Blue Shield** offer the best "medigap" policies, but good ones can be obtained through **Reserve Life, New York Life,** and other companies. Some of these do not cover prolonged illnesses, dental work, eyeglasses, or prescription drugs, so be prepared and set aside sufficient funds.

During the last 10 years in practice, refine your retirement planning. Sit down with your accountant and estimate the retirement income that will be available on various dates from social security and your retirement plans. You will need about 60 per cent of your present after-tax income. Be sure to include the assets from the sale of your practice or termination with a group. Make the adjustments in your plans that your accountant recommends.

Insofar as your investments are concerned, as time goes on there will be less need to seek defenses against income tax and more need to search for security with income production. The break-even point for tax-free portfolios in such instruments as municipal bonds is a combined federal and state tax bracket of 35 per cent. When your marginal rate dips below that tax bracket, start shifting to taxable investments that provide a better return. Change your mutual funds to those with lower risk, or add those that favor your changing needs. Selection of longer term government securities is one way to go if interest rates are favorable.

Although you have reviewed your will with your attorney every two or three years (or whenever there was a major change in your financial situation), in the preretirement years this review is increasingly important. Assemble all the data and documents you need, take the time to consider every asset, explore your wishes with him regarding their distribution, try to anticipate possible disputes among your heirs, and reconsider your executor. You may want to select a competent coexecutor to act with your spouse. Reexamine the ability of your attorney in estate planning. Never use for this purpose one who is a family member or close friend. You want the best and most objective advice and should be willing to pay for it. It may be advisable to have at least one consultation with an attorney specializing in estate tax law. Your spouse should accompany you on all of these visits and revise her will at the same time you do yours. Both wills should provide for the possibility of simultaneous death. Each of you should prepare a complete distribution list of all minor personal possessions. Keep these lists where they can be revised frequently. Maintain all your affairs and papers in order from now on. Append notes that would allow a third party to understand all aspects of your finances.

Before you consult an attorney about your will, you have to have some knowledge of estate tax law to be able to understand his advice and to ask intelligent questions. There have been major recent changes in federal law of which you may be unaware.

The **Tax Reform Act** of 1976 adopted a unified estate and gift tax credit to replace the former $30,000 gift tax lifetime exemption and the $60,000 estate tax specific exemption. This is a *credit* against the estate and gift tax otherwise payable, which was later raised substantially by the **Economic Recovery Tax Act** of 1981 **(ERTA).** The unified credit is now increasing in annual increments until 1987, after which it will remain constant. It is possible to calculate the portion of the estate that is made exempt from federal estate tax by this credit for each year to 1987 and thereafter. This is called the *exemption equivalent.* In 1987 and after, assuming no taxable lifetime gifts were made, a person can leave an estate (after deductions) of up to $600,000 to anyone without incurring federal estate tax liability.

Another change brought about by ERTA is the unlimited marital deduction. A married couple is now treated as a taxable unit. Any amount may be left by one spouse to another tax-free, but whatever portion remains at the death of the second spouse, less the exemption equivalent of that spouse, is taxable then. This means that the couple's estate planning must be coordinated.

ERTA continued a provision of the 1976 law regarding gift taxes. Each person may transfer tax free up to $10,000 annually *per recipient*, and payments made for tuition to an educational institution (if not already considered a parental obligation) or for medical care directly to the provider are not included in this limit. You and your spouse together can give up to $20,000 *per recipient* annually. If you would like to know more, read *Die Rich* by Charles Plotnick and Stephan Leimberg (Coward-McCann, 1983).

In view of these major changes and many minor ones, it is important to revise your will if you have not done so since the passage of ERTA. Any unrevised wills and revocable trusts previously executed that refer to a maximum marital deduction will be interpreted under prior law. Don't just add codicils—have a new will drawn up.

Ask your attorney about the plans that have been devised under ERTA to reduce the combined estate taxes of you and your spouse. One is the *bypass trust*. With it, an amount equal to the exemption equivalent of your estate is left in an irrevocable residual trust for your spouse, and the remaining estate qualifies for the marital deduction. Your spouse receives the income from the amount in trust, but it is not taxed either at your death or at the death of your spouse. Upon her death it goes to your children or whomever you wish. A bypass trust may also be used to benefit your grandchildren, but regulations on generation-skipping transfers are stringent, so consult with your attorney.

There is also the *disclaimer plan*, in which all of your estate is left to your spouse with the provision that, to the extent the surviving spouse disclaims the estate, it will be considered to be held in an irrevocable residual trust for your children. Upon your death, your spouse can determine how much to receive and how much to disclaim in accordance with the circumstances and taxes determined at that time. Any amount she disclaims over the exemption equivalent is taxed at your death but not at hers.

Still another option is the *qualified terminable-interest property trust*, or *"Q-tip" trust*. Under such a trust, all of the trust income must go to the surviving spouse at least annually for life. The surviving spouse has a general power of appointment over the trust corpus, and may receive payment of principal under certain circumstances. Upon her death, the remaining assets of the trust are taxed in *her* estate, but distributed in accordance with the provisions of *your* will.

In addition to such plans, there is a lot you and your attorney can do to reduce death taxes. Charitable bequests are deductible in calculating federal estate tax. Transfers between your estate and that of your spouse may be made so that each will be approximately the same size when taxed. This is a considerable advantage, because once the exemption equivalent is exceeded, the federal estate tax is sharply progressive. If a large asset you wish your children to have will appreciate substantially, have a qualified appraiser establish its value, and make the gift now. The estate tax will be based upon the value at the time the gift is made, less the $10,000 exemption for that year—not on the appreciated value at the time of your death. Look again at any short-term reversionary or Clifford trusts that may still be in effect. Both the principal and income accrued will be included in your estate. You may wish to change these to irrevocable trusts in which both are excluded. If you do, a gift tax may be imposed if the annual exemption is exceeded. Most physicians upon retirement sell their larger homes and purchase condominiums or less expensive homes. Those who elect to keep a large home face the prospect that the estate tax on it will be based upon an appraisal made at the time of death. If it will not appreciate substantially, sell it now at its fair market value, take back a large mortgage at standard interest, pay a fair rental to the buyer under a lifetime lease, and thus remove it from your estate entirely. If it will appreciate, have one of your heirs purchase it under the same arrangement.

There are ways in which the costs of administering your estate may be reduced. If your spouse is competent to be the sole executor, her fee of around 5 per cent of the estate is part of the probate cost and will pass to her, free of death taxes, rather than to another party. Attorney fees are approximately the same, and these can be reduced by setting up a revocable lifetime trust in which you are your own trustee. Assets in this trust will be taxable but will not go through probate court proceedings. This eliminates court costs and attorney fees on this portion of your estate. For more information, read *How to Avoid Probate* by Norman F. Dacey (Crown Publishers, 1983).

State death taxes may be either an inheritance tax (on the recipient for receipt of property) or an estate tax (on the decedent's estate for bequeathing property). There is so much variation from state to state that little can be said here. But your state law should be examined. Some states have exemptions for children that can be taken advantage of in both parents' wills, effectively doubling the amount the children will receive tax free. Other states favor jointly owned property so that only one half is taxed no matter which spouse contributed the purchase price. Some do not have death taxes at all.

The intention of this chapter and the one preceding was *not* to tell you all you wanted to know about personal financial planning. It was to stimulate you to form a financial plan at the start of your career and follow it throughout, adjusting it as you go along. If you do this, you will have greater security during your years of greatest risk, accumulate more wealth and enjoy it more, live your retirement years to the fullest, and provide well for your family after you are gone.

28

Constructing A Medical Office Building

Obviously, one chapter can cover only a part of what you need to know in order to carry out a project like this. But I will emphasize certain points that are important in your decision on whether to go ahead or not, and give you some idea of what is involved. There are no good books on the subject to which I can refer you. Instead, you will have to rely upon the advice of the members of the team you will put together. I speak from experience when I advise you that such a project is time-consuming, requires the acquisition of a lot of new knowledge, and has many potential pitfalls.

The first thing to do is reconsider your reasons for wanting to construct your own building. There are valid financial, tax, and other motivations that will be discussed below, but the primary reason in most cases is subjective. These subjective factors can be ranged on a spectrum starting from the understandable and laudable satisfaction in creating a beautiful and functional building all the way to a manifestation of ego that is downright unreasonable. If your subjective reasons are in the latter part of the spectrum, time and again you will make decisions againt the advice of your consultants and the facts themselves. Disaster is a almost always the result. A word to the wise.

Let's look for a moment at some of the objective reasons for constructing your own building:

1. You have greater control over certain aspects of your practice when you build than you do when you lease: some over the selection of the building site, its size, appearance, landscaping,

parking, and the other tenants; more over management and maintenance; and complete over your office space itself, without the usual limitations imposed by a landlord. This includes the inevitable increase in rent at lease renewal time.

2. You can expect a financial return on your investment. The net rental income from a medical office building is usually low, so the principal financial advantage is appreciation of the value of the property. There is also a small increase in equity as the mortgage payments are made, reducing the principal owed. And, if you are the principal organizer, there may be compensation in some form for your time and trouble.
3. The tax advantages are significant. These should be discussed with your accountant, because they depend a great deal upon your personal financial situation. In general, the structure can be depreciated over a long period, whereas equipment such as heating and air conditioning is depreciable more rapidly. First-year expensing and investment credit may apply, and the mortgage interest is deductible.
4. Your practice will be more efficient in space that is designed exactly to your requirements, and your morale—as well as that of your staff—will be higher. These factors often result in a higher net income.

However, there are disadvantages that have to be considered:

1. You will be committed to that building and location for many years. In the future, you may wish to change your specialty or other aspects of your practice, even take on partners or form a group, but your obligations may prevent you. The community can change—in fact, almost certainly will—in terms of economic base, population trends, and other pertinent factors, and you will also change yourself in the years ahead, but your mobility and flexibility will have been curtailed.
2. Unless you are financially able to undertake the project yourself, you will find yourself working with other physicians as partners. At the start, all will be cooperative and enthusiastic and have the capital to invest. But physicians are notoriously independent, and working together over many years may prove to be difficult.
3. More time and trouble are involved than you can now imagine. You must become knowledgeable about construction details, building codes, zoning regulations, legal ramifications of contracts, and many other subjects. Unexpected problems will try your patience. When it is finished, there will be management problems, along with the responsibility of maintenance. For example, a vacancy rate of only 10 or 20 per cent can cause a negative cash flow, so there will be the constant burden of trying to maintain full occupancy.

4. The financial risk is significant. The capital outlay is large and you must calculate the interest or other return that you could realize if your funds were elsewhere. Other medical office buildings may be constructed in the area to compete with yours. You may have located near a hospital that initially welcomed you, but in a few years the hospital itself may construct a medical office building and offer lower rentals to prospective tenants. Future sale is always uncertain. Because of construction requirements, a medical building limits you either to a purchaser who will use the building for the same purpose, or to one who is willing to undertake extensive changes—which would force you to lower your sales price. Either way, you must anticipate a narrow resale market.

Make your own list of advantages and disadvantages, and think about them. Before you decide to go ahead, look at the alternatives available: (1) obtaining a more suitable space in your own or another office building, (2) remodeling your present office, or (3) finding a building in the planning or early construction stage that has space you can design to suit your requirements.

There are attractive aspects to any of these alternatives. You are able to leave at the end of the lease if you wish. Operating and maintenance problems are up to the landlord. Less capital is needed, and less is at risk. There is not as much time and trouble involved in remodeling or setting up a new office as in constructing a building, so that you can devote more attention to your practice. The resale of leasehold improvements is easier than the resale of a building. You will not have to work closely with physician-partners, but can make decisions yourself. And the problems inherent in relocation for patients and staff can be avoided.

These are not the only alternatives open to you. There are others. One is the purchase of an existing multi-office building. Most of the advantages of building your own structure can be obtained this way, and many of the problems avoided.

Another possibility is the purchase of an office condominium. This is a new concept for most physicians, so let's look at it in more depth. You will have title to the suite and be part owner of the common areas: the land on which the building stands, the surrounding landscaped and parking areas, and parts of the stucture such as the foyer and corridors. You will have some of the advantages of constructing your own medical office building: removal of most landlord restrictions, some control (through an elected board of directors) in management of the premises, appreciation in value of your unit, some equity increase, and limited tax advantages. The maintenance and operation are usually done by professionals and will not be a worry to you. Less capital is involved, so less is at risk. You can resell a condominium more easily than an entire medical building. The condominium can also constitute a source of income after retirement if you rent the space to another physician.

But against the advantages of condominium ownership are certain disadvantages. You have less mobility than with a lease, and less control over the premises than if you were to construct or purchase your own medical building. If you are on the board of directors, you will have some involvement in maintenance and operation problems, even with professional management. Property taxes may be high and may increase later. Changes in the community will have greater impact than if you were to lease. The ability to expand your space may be limited, and you are often otherwise restricted from taking in an associate or forming a medical group. Insurance coverage will be more extensive and expensive, and the coordination of your policies with those of the association may be a problem. Diversity of the tenant-practitioners should be maintained to offer a balance, but this may be difficult to achieve unless mandated in your bylaws. Compatibility with other tenant-owners may be a concern. If the builder insists upon continuing the management or has a subsidiary take over, you may be attracted by low monthly assessments at the start, then subjected to unreasonable increases later when all the units are sold. Even the management agent selected by your board of directors can make mistakes, or the accounting procedures may be inadequate, and these will affect you.

Well, don't say I didn't tell you about the problems involved with constructing your own building and the alternatives available. The rest of this chapter assumes that you have weighed the pros and cons, found the alternatives unsatisfactory, and have decided to go ahead. One caveat—the most modest and sensible project can get out of hand toward the end when it comes to interior design, art, and appointments. One more—be sure to reserve space for future expansion beyond what can be foreseen at the present time.

The first major decision is whether to take the conventional or the "turnkey" approach. The latter involves using one of several large companies around the country that will carry out the entire project and hand you the key upon completion. All you have to do is turn the key in the lock and walk in. Such a firm selects the site, handles the financing, uses its own architects and engineers (or contracts for some of the specialized consultation), does the office layouts, interior design and decorating, and even orders the equipment and furniture. Because many of these firms have a great deal of experience, good contacts in the financial world, and can purchase in bulk, they are able to complete the project at 10 to 20 per cent below the cost of the conventional approach. There are only a few disadvantages to using one. You may be dealing with a firm that is headquartered out of state, which would hinder communication. The efficiency, expertise, and array of specialists of a large firm may bewilder you. And, although most of the firms value their reputation and provide high-quality service, occasionally one may take short cuts that are difficult for you to detect. You will have to have your own architect and contractor to guard against this.

Nevertheless, I recommend the turnkey approach unless you have a strong background and talent in this field and can take the time to do it right. The firms that have been suggested to me as both experienced and reliable are:

American Medical Buildings
735 North Water Street
Milwaukee, WI 53202

BBC Health Care
1130 Hampton Avenue
St. Louis, MO 63169

Ellerbe, Inc.
Architects/Engineers/Planners
One Appletree Square
Bloomington, MN 55420

Marshall Erdman and Associates, Inc.
5117 University Avenue
Madison, WI 53705

Nationwide Medical-Dental Building Corp.
797 Market Street
Oregon, WI 53575

Professional Office Buildings
170 Ruggle Street
Fond du Lac, WI 54935

Harold J. Westin and Associates, Inc.
45 East Eighth Street
St. Paul, MN 55101

Although I have had no experience with any of these firms, I received the most favorable reports from the physician clients of Marshall Erdman and Associates. When making your choice, select an architect with considerable knowledge and experience in medical office building construction, and take his advice.

The second approach is the conventional one. This is an extremely complicated undertaking. The most difficult part is *before* ground is broken, and this is what I am going to cover with you. Six steps are involved:

1. The feasibility study
2. Obtaining and organizing your partners
3. Site analysis
4. Selecting your architect
5. Choosing the builder
6. Arranging the financing

This order is not fixed, but it is the usual one. Often there is overlap, and two or more steps can be taken at one time, but I will consider them separately.

STEP ONE. THE FEASIBILITY STUDY

The feasibility study is the most important step of all. It is essential that all factors be considered and included. The hardest part is selecting the person to perform the study. His professional education is not as important as his practical knowledge, experience, and objectivity. An architect who has been in charge of similar projects is the best. A real estate consultant, *not* a real estate broker, is another possibility, but these are rare outside of major urban areas. A practice management consultant who has handled several such projects could be considered. Even a professional business consultant who has performed a similar role in the construction of other medical office buildings would be satisfactory. An accountant who has been involved in prior projects could conceivably do it.

Once you have made the choice, arrange to pay your consultant a fee for the feasibility study. Make it clear that he will not be employed later in the project or in any way derive a benefit therefrom. Objectivity is paramount. You can change your mind if you wish later on, but this should be your stance at the start. Of course, your attorney, accountant, practice management consultant, insurance agent, and even your banker will be involved and work with the consultant. Each will have his own input, but you will be looking to the consultant for information on land values, area growth projections, zoning restrictions, site suitability, site preparation and improvements, traffic patterns, real estate taxes, construction costs, utility connections, operating expenses, required engineering, various permits and licenses, contingencies to be allowed for, and the rental rate.

The feasibility study should follow a standard form. *The first part* is an estimate of total costs, and these include land acquisition, engineering, appraisal fees, the construction loan and mortgage, financing points, interest, building permits, and the fees of various experts, including the architect. *The second part* is an estimate of annual income, expenses, and cash flow once the medical office building has been constructed. It will include the rental rate, salaries for maintenance and management personnel, accounting and insurance costs, repair and replacement expenses for major equipment, debt service including amortization of mortgage principal and interest, supplies, and even depreciation and tax consequences to you figured for your tax bracket. *The third part* is a summary, with an estimate of the total capital required, the amount to be invested by you and each of your partners, the occupancy required for the break-even point, and the net profit at full occupancy.

Once you have the study, *obtain independent opinions on the figures.* Your own accountant may help you or refer you to someone who can. This is a good time to test the top architect in the list already compiled for the fourth step, if you have done this. Discuss the project with him, see how he responds, and listen to his input. If you are not satisfied, move on to the next architect on your list.

STEP TWO. OBTAINING AND ORGANIZING YOUR PARTNERS

By this time, you will have discussed the project with several prospective partners. Having their input and interests in mind, move on to forming the legal vehicle. Consult first with your own attorney, then with whomever he suggests. The organization usually takes the form of a limited partnership, with you as the general partner. Be sure the following points are covered in the agreement:

1. A specific description of the powers exercised by you, the organizer, including your signatory power.
2. A "hold-harmless clause."
3. Your compensation, usually in terms of a greater percentage of equity.
4. The method of arriving at decisions (one vote for each partner or by percentage of equity, with majority vote for all questions, specifying those that require a two-thirds or greater vote).
5. The amount each partner must invest.
6. Provision for assessment in the event of unforeseen expenses.
7. The steps to be taken if a partner fails to pay an assessment.
8. Provision for such eventualities as the death or disability of a partner.
9. The rights and responsibility of each partner in his own office space.

10. How the profits are to be calculated and distributed.
11. Who is to have the responsibility for management when the building is operating and how he is to be compensated.
12. How a partner can withdraw and how a new partner can be added.
13. The duration of the partners' leases, which should match the length of the mortgage obtained for your permanent financing.

With both the feasibility study and the partnership agreement in writing, you are ready to make the final selection of your partners. Choose them carefully—you will be working with them a long time. Lean toward those whose ages, economic status, and sociocultural background are similar to your own. If one should have totally different investment and tax goals than the others, this divergence of views can cause difficulties. Mentally review what you know about their personalities, and how well they have worked in hospital affairs, at the local medical society, and in the community. Then consider their spouses, who could also be sources of conflict. It is best if all investors are occupants, although all occupants need not be investors.

Each partner should review the proposal with his own lawyer and financial advisor, and consult with his accountant regarding the potential tax impact upon him before signing.

The four steps that remain will be done by the partnership as a whole, in accordance with its organization and bylaws. However, the assumption is that you are the general partner and will therefore be the principal motivating force and take most of the action.

STEP THREE. SITE ANALYSIS

Sometimes the site selection is done first so that accurate figures and data can be incorporated into the feasibility study. But unless an option is taken, the owner will learn of your interest and raise the asking price. For this reason, it is usually done third—or even after selecting an architect. It starts with a simple step. Obtain a good map of the community, and circle the area within a 10-minute drive from the hospital you wish to be near. Then go to the local zoning board to obtain a zoning map and to learn of any anticipated changes in zoning that would affect you. Obtain a copy of the area master plan, and, with the attorney for the partnership, study the applicable local ordinances and procedures for obtaining variances.

Don't overlook checking with the hospital to determine its own plans to purchase property and construct a medical office building. Investigate the possibility that the hospital ownership might change, resulting in a dramatic alteration in policies. A wise move is to ask the CEO if the hospital is interested in being involved with you in the project. Whether it is or not, find out about the finances of the hospital.

Leads on property can be obtained several ways. One is to prepare a simple specification sheet and send it to commercial realtors in your area. You will also have noted undeveloped areas on the map that are the suitable size and shape, and the names of the owners can be obtained from the tax assessor. Title companies will offer you possibilities in the hope that they will obtain your business. Advertisements in the local newspapers or suitable journals will provide further leads. Land surveyors are among the first to know of suitable sites that are about to become available. The highway department may be aware of ideal areas near major arterials. You can learn about existing buildings that are due for destruction from the tax assessor. To supplement all of this, drive around and jot down the addresses of what appear to be suitable locations.

In general, it is best to avoid both inner city and rural areas, and concentrate instead on the fringe of the city core, which is a location that can draw from both urban and suburban areas. If there is a nearby high-income residential area, so much the better. Evaluate each potential site in terms of its accessibility by automobile and public transportation. Offsite parking in parking lots and on streets should not be relied upon—these can disappear overnight. Allow adequate space for landscaping. The visibility of the site is important, as is means of traffic entry and exit. The site should be compatible with a medical office building; have at least one bank nearby, some restaurants, and a shopping area. Try to foresee future developments. Eliminate (or make allowances for) those sites with problems in topography—such as low-lying land that accumulates run-off water, soil that is not suitable to support the structure, and rock outcroppings that may be difficult to remove. Utilities to service your structure must be available. The partnership attorney can begin to review the top sites on your list for problems in the deeds such as easements, covenants, and other restrictions. He should look again at local ordinance and zoning restrictions to make certain that the city does not require certain offsite improvements in order to grant a building permit or right-of-way dedication. Ask your accountant to look over the preferred sites for anticipated changes in assessment methods or tax rates. He may be fortunate enough to find an area where a tax break is given for such a building. When you have your suitable sites narrowed down to only a few, it is time to select the architect for the project.

STEP FOUR. SELECTING YOUR ARCHITECT

The care and time that you take in the selection of the architect will be repaid many times over as the project progresses. He *must* have extensive experience in the construction of medical buildings. If you do not know any experienced architects in your area, write the **American Institute of Architects** (AIA), 1735 New York Avenue NW, Washington, DC 20006 for the address of the local chapter. Each maintains listings of members interested in doing various kinds of buildings. Also ask any health professionals you know who have built a similar structure. Look at all the medical office buildings in your area. Go in and inspect those that appeal to you, and talk to the individuals involved in their construction. Ask about their working relationship with the architect—how sensible his suggestions were, how sensitive he was to the originator's goals, and how closely he met his cost estimates. Then talk to the architects who seem to be most suitable. Ask to see models, drawings, and photographs of their work. Get the addresses of buildings you particularly admire and visit them even if they are at some distance. Again, talk to the persons who worked with the architect. Then approach the top two or three architects on your list. Discuss working relationships with each and the method used to determine fees. These should be based on a standard AIA contract. Your final selection from the top two or three will be made after the second interview, based upon compatibility of views and the quality of the working relationship that you feel you will be able to develop.

Your architect will advise the partnership on the final selection of the site, guided by the feasibility study as to the upper price limit and other factors. In all probability, you will be on the committee, and, with a real estate broker, involved in the negotiations with the seller. Be sure to discuss not only the price but the terms and subordination. Consider the cash and tax advantages of leasing rather than purchasing the land. Some sellers are interested in assisting with the financing, or may be induced to provide topographical surveys and maps, soil test, and other services as part of the transaction. Many areas of negotiation are open to you. One is to lower the land price and increase the interest rate of the mortgage the seller takes back if the deductible interest would be favorable to you and your partners in your tax brackets.

STEP FIVE. CHOOSING THE BUILDER

By this time the architect will have developed a site plan and working drawings. He will also advise you and your partners on the fifth step, selection of a builder or general contractor. An architect who has been active in the area is familiar with the ability, reliability, experience, and other attributes of the general contractors who work there. He will suggest the best ones to bid. Once the construction documents and specifications are completed, he will work with you and your partners on the selection of the builder after reviewing the bids. It is then the responsibility of the general contractor to obtain all subcontractors.

STEP SIX. ARRANGING THE FINANCING

Before taking the sixth step, financing the project, look over the advice in Chapter 7 to familiarize yourself and your partners with the terms commonly used, the various types of loans and interest that are available, and the background material to have ready when you discuss the loan with financial institutions. I would suggest that you contact several commercial banks where you and your partners have accounts or have previously done business. Include others that have provided good service in similar projects.

Prepare a package for each. Your architect can have this done for you. The cover should be an artist's color rendering of the building. This is worth the cost. Inside is a cover letter addressed to each institution, summarizing some details and emphasizing others of special interest to the institution that will receive that particular package. The commercial loan officer will use this information in discussing the project with the loan committee. In the cover letter, request a more favorable loan than is currently offered by most lending institutions. In general, banks lend 80 per cent of the *appraised* value, which is the market value of the project as determined by their appraiser, not your estimated or actual cost. If they feel that the loan is somewhat unsafe, this percentage will be lower. Occasionally, they may lend more. It may be wise to have the loan duration as long as possible, at least 20 years, in order to repay the loan with "cheaper" dollars whose value will be reduced by inflation. Request an interest rate of one or two points above prime, and agree to accept variable interest, since this is all that will be offered. Points are calculated at one percent of the *face value* of the mortgage, which reduces the actual amount loaned, so the interest rate you pay will be higher than that stated. Offer to pay the lowest number of points you think you can persuade them to accept.

Other items in your package will be the feasibility study, details of the selected site, a curriculum vitae of your architect, site plans, statements of net worth from each partner, and other information requested by the lending institution in the initial contacts. Each partner will be requested to personally guarantee the loan.

You or the designated representatives of your partnership should then make an appointment with the commercial loan officer at each institution. Discuss the project with him in broad terms, but do not accept any terms he offers or make any other commitments. Instead, thank him for the information he has provided, leave the package with him, and depart. Visit all the institutions this way.

The loan officer at each will have his appraiser review the plans. He will obtain credit rating reports on you and your partners, and then present the package to the loan committee or the board of directors. Their decision will be conveyed to you through him. Reply with a second letter accepting parts of the offer, but requesting more favorable conditions on others. One of your bargaining points might be waiver of the tax escrow account. Banks prefer to collect funds on a regular basis for the payment of taxes which are due only once or twice a year. In the meantime, they earn interest on the impounded funds. The construction holdback is another item to be negotiated and eliminated if possible. This is a portion of the loan that is held by the lender until a certain occupancy level has been reached. After further discussion and comparison of all the offers, the partners will arrive at their decision.

The first loan is a construction loan to pay the builder periodically as each stage of construction is completed and verified by the bank's appraiser. When the project is finished, the construction loan will be converted into a conventional mortgage. In some cases, the mortgage will be obtained from another institution such as a savings and loan association. Don't ever start a project unless the permanent financing is guaranteed in advance. Be prepared for various fees at the time the construction loan is granted, and interest payments on the amount that is advanced at each step.

This chapter has brought you to the start of construction but will not guide you through it. You have learned a lot already and have assembled a good team to help you. Once you have gone this far, the rest will seem simple by comparison.

29

Taking On An Associate

After a number of years, a solo practitioner's thoughts turn toward taking on an associate for several reasons. Let's look at some of the usual ones.

1. Sometimes an older physician feels he may have slipped a bit professionally. He wants to have a sharp younger colleague from a major teaching institution in his office to complement his own knowledge and skill, or perhaps in the hope that by osmosis he might become more current himself. What often happens instead is that he is soon in the younger man's shadow, and within a short time his new colleague uses him as a stepping stone to go on to other opportunities in the community. So this is *not* often a valid reason. It is better for the older man to burn the midnight oil, or hire a *locum tenens* so that he can take a long refresher course.
2. Occasionally, an established physician wants to remodel, move to a larger and more modern office, hire specialized aides, or purchase new expensive equipment, and he wants a colleague to share the expense. The only difficulty is that three physicians operate more efficiently than two, and he will find that he has taken on certain problems with the new associate that are not counterbalanced by the most efficient use of the new facilities. It is usually better if he makes improvements in a limited way while remaining solo for a time, and then proceeds to form a group of three or more with suitable personnel and facilities. Chapter 4 gave some of the reasons why three physicians work together better than two.

   Among the potential problems alluded to that may come with an associate are: personality conflict, loss of some independence, legal responsibility for the professional and business actions of an associate if the association is perceived as a true partnership, less income until the associate can pull his own weight, loss of some desirable patients to the new associate, changes in the practice to accommodate him, conflicts with spouses, and disagreements over different rates of production and division of income. These are the most common ones, but there are other potential problems, so the step should be taken for reasons that will make it worthwhile.

3. Other reasons for taking on an associate that are less frequently given are: to provide better coverage, to provide administrative assistance if the established physician is a poor administrator, and to justify the employment of a professional manager. In my opinion, none of these is valid.
4. Sometimes a physician sees that the community is growing and wants to respond to the growth by offering more service. But this by itself is not a valid reason, either. Other physicians will come to the community on their own and provide the service that is needed. If a nearby area is growing, he may want to set up an associate in a satellite office. However, the adage, "multiplying offices multiplies problems" still holds true, and I would advise this only as a step toward shifting the practice entirely to the other area.
5. Occasionally a physician wants to narrow his specialty and turn over much of what he has been doing to an associate. In theory this is fine, but in actuality it may be difficult finding an associate who will fit in precisely, now and into the future. It is usually better to form a group of three or four in which each concentrates in the area of his primary interest and shoulders an equal share of the other work.
6. Perhaps the most common reason is that a busy physician just wants to reduce his burden. Taking on an associate accomplishes this for a while, but after a year or two the situation may be the same for the two of them. The first physician's overload was caused by one or more demographic factors such as population growth or the ratio of physicians to the population—and these factors are not materially affected by adding an associate. In such cases it would be better to analyze the factors themselves and respond appropriately to them by remaining solo and restricting acceptance of new patients, forming a group designed to meet the needs of the community, or in another way.

Of course, there are other reasons of dubious validity, but these were presented in order to stimulate you into looking again at your own.

Let me suggest the two reasons for taking on an associate that seem to be the best: (1) As a transitional step in forming a group, for which all details have been worked out; (2) as a step preparatory to the purchase of the practice on the retirement of an older physician. As mentioned in Chapter 9, this is an ideal way for a younger physician to acquire an established practice with a furnished and equipped office, trained personnel, and an adequate patient load. The older physician is able to take time off for long-deferred interests, to travel, or to set up his retirement home in another area, and his retirement income can be stabilized through a carefully formulated purchase agreement.

Both of these are transitional, and often involve expense sharing for a period of time. "Permanent" expense-sharing plans are rarely permanent.

Let's assume that yours is one of these two reasons—or another that special circumstances would make as valid. Before you take any action, it is wise to obtain objective evaluation of your motivations, personality, and practice particulars. You really can't do this yourself. Consider employing a practice management consultant just for this purpose. Even a business consultant with some skill in practice management could be of assistance—his opinion would at least be objective. Also, ask your lawyer and accountant for their advice. Listen to what your other advisors have to say. It may well be that some factor of which you are unaware could cause serious problems in an association. If such a factor is foreseen, it can frequently be compensated for. Later may be too late.

The first decision to make is the form the association will take. A salary basis for the first year is customary, followed by a partnership. Later, either a group will be formed or the younger physician will have a solo practice when the older physician retires.

Then start the search for your associate. Almost always his specialty will be the same as yours, so you will know where and how to look. Begin about a year ahead of time, and maximize the market. This means placing ads in journals with nationwide distribution and contacting your colleagues, a number of residency programs, military bases, and employment services. The number of applicants will probably necessitate a telephone screening first, then an initial interview, and the decision will be made at a final interview.

Prepare a list of minimum criteria and another of the questions you want to ask in the telephone screening. These questions will be mostly about professional qualifications, because this is your primary concern at this point. The result of the telephone screening will be the selection of the top five or six candidates. Rank them according to their professional qualifications, and invite each for a personal interview.

For the first interview, don't offer to pay the cost of transportation or lodging. Nor should you invite the prospective associate to your home; instead, take him to lunch or dinner for casual conversation after an office tour. The total time taken need not be more than three or four hours. What you are looking at now are personal characteristics, goals, professional standards, and other such qualities. This is the time for intangibles. Compatibility is the key.

In addition to asking your own, you must be prepared for questions the candidate will ask. Try to anticipate as many as you can and have well-considered answers ready. If an unexpected question comes up, do not be evasive or give careless off-the-cuff answers. Instead, tell him you will get back to him with a definitive answer, and do so.

Here are some items you should be clear on before the first interview: the basic salary, incentive pay or bonuses based upon net income, the time period of the salaried relationship, the relationship that would then be envisioned, the arrangement for paying malpractice insurance premiums and the amount of coverage required, the benefits offered, the on-call schedule, arrangements for continuing medical education, membership requirements in medical societies and hospital staffs, compensation for professional use of the associate's automobile, the division of work responsibility, the process for making decisions on equipment needs and personnel management, and the characteristics of your practice that you will insist upon maintaining, as well as those you would be willing to alter.

Following this interview, contact the references given on the applicant's *curriculum vitae* and additional ones that you requested during the interview. Do this by telephone, peer to peer. Have an idea of what you want to ask before you call. Always include one or two open-ended questions, such as, "Is there anything else I should know about the candidate?" At this point, you can send polite letters of rejection to all but the top two or three candidates.

Before the top two or three are called back for a second interview, prepare a list of the points that will be included in your letter of agreement. Consult with your attorney and clarify all details. If it is to be a pure expense-sharing arrangement, there are suggestions in Chapter 4 for the items to include under those circumstances. The following list presumes that a salary is to be given for a year, after which time another arrangement is to be made:

- The date the employment will start.
- The base compensation for the first year, with an estimate of deductions for unemployment, federal and state income taxes, and FICA.
- Incentive pay or bonuses, and the basis for awarding them.
- Benefits, which might include life insurance, professional liability insurance, disability insurance, workers' compensation coverage, retirement plan contributions, automobile expenses when used for professional purposes, and expenses of continuing medical edu-

cation. An approximate annual cost to you of these benefits should be given.

- Time off—vacation, sick leave, continuing medical education, and other such as emergency leave. If needed, provide for religious holidays, recall by the military, or reserve military obligations.
- Work responsibilities and decision-making processes should be spelled out: the space and facilities the associate will use, the on-call schedule, required emergency room coverage, methods of resolving disputes, authority over office personnel, how decisions will be made on equipment, fees, collection policies, patient care, and other matters. Specify the input that the associate will have in these decisions.
- Provision for the disability or death of either. Your associate may want to purchase a life insurance policy on you to cover purchase of the practice.
- Activities expected of the associate in the local medical society, hospital staff committees, speaking engagements and other practice promotion, and restrictions on outside employment.
- Details on dissolution. Include the notice required by either party, disposition of patients, medical records, and accounts receivable, any continuing benefits, and a restrictive covenant. This last agreement is particularly important. Protect yourself by specifying that the telephone number, office, office contents, and staff will remain with you unless other arrangements are agreed upon.
- Expenses that will be the associate's responsibility, such as professional dues, journal subscriptions, and business entertainment.
- An outline of the conditions, date, and details of the relationship that will be established at the end of the salaried period. Include its legal form, the method of evaluation of the assets, goodwill, and accounts receivable, their apportionment, and the method of payment. This will form the basis of the paragraph of intent in your letter of agreement.

Invite the preferred two or three candidates for a second interview about a week apart. Start with the top one. Offer to pay all travel and lodging expenses. Invite the spouses, and involve yours as appropriate. Plan to take at least a full working day, that evening, and one day of a weekend with each candidate. Have a list of the questions that were unanswered in the first interview and those that arose from your reference checks. Request each candidate to bring evidence of licensure, board certification, experience in certain procedures, and current DEA registration. Toward the end of the second day with the top candidate, try to make a decision on the spot and inform him. If you accept the first, and the two of you come to an agreement, cancel the interviews with the second and third.

Whichever one you decide on, have your attorney prepare a letter of agreement in the next day or two according to the terms and conditions discussed and agreed upon. Sign the original and a copy, and send both to your new associate. He will sign the original, return it, and retain his copy.

Let the word out to hospital administrators and nurses, to colleagues, and to patients as soon as your decision is made. Start scheduling patients for him when this is appropriate. Have your receptionist give all patients requesting appointments the choice of a *later* appointment with you or an *earlier* one with him.

Prepare your office for his arrival. Make necessary alterations in the space, and add the furniture and equipment agreed upon. Hire additional personnel if this is also part of the agreement. Change your office manual and the appropriate job descriptions.

When he arrives, help him adjust. Introduce him to all patients, yours and his. Include him in staff conferences and decisions. Treat him as an equal. Work with your staff to smooth out any wrinkles.

When he has caught on, the best thing you can do is take that vacation you have been putting off for so long.

30

Forming Your Own Group

This chapter will be brief. It is not that there is so little to say on the subject, but that there is so much. The standard reference produced by the **Center for Research in Ambulatory Health Care Administration,** *The Organization and Development of a Medical Group Practice,* is 700 pages long, plus 30 more of notes and bibliography. Out of curiosity, I ran a computer search for other publications by that same organization whose titles indicated that they supplemented or amplified the basic reference. The total came to 13! In the medical library I use for research, two long shelves are filled with books on the subject. Beyond these, the relevant brochures, pamphlets, and periodicals are almost past counting.

With so much information available, my role here is better limited to offering a few tips from personal experience, pointing out the individuals and organizations that can assist you in forming a group, and guiding you to the best references for further information.

Let's assume you are a solo practitioner, that you are about to take on an associate or have done so, and that you are looking ahead to the possible formation of a group of three or more. As with any major venture, it is important to first understand your motivations. They are usually multiple, and fall into three categories.

1. **Benefits to the members**. These consist of better coverage, worry-free vacations, more time for continuing medical education, availability of consultations on complex cases, stimulation from peer contact, the maintenance of a better library with subscriptions to more journals, in-house journal clubs, ability to practice more intensively in a specialty or subspecialty, increased time available

for teaching or for medical society and hospital staff activities, better and fewer hours with a more regular schedule, a stable income throughout a career, and a better retirement plan.

2. **Improvements in practice management**. These include employment of more specialized or highly skilled personnel, such as a nurse practitioner, physician's assistant, or professional manager; the ability to purchase and better utilize more advanced or specialized equipment; more efficient use of existing personnel and equipment; better use of present space through staggered office hours; the ability to move to larger and more suitable facilities; greater economy by ordering supplies in bulk; and other advantages that depend upon the particular circumstances.
3. **Benefits to the patients**. Patient care is improved by many of the factors already listed, but there are additional benefits: the introduction of new physicians and specialties to the community; less costly care by allied health personnel; more resources located on site; new diagnostic and therapeutic procedures heretofore unavailable in the area; improved continuity of care with medical records available when one member is off call or on vacation; establishing a satellite clinic in a nearby underserved area; and others.

Once your reasons are understood, set them down and define them as clearly as possible. Some may be complementary, others internally inconsistent. Write the **Department of Practice Management** of the AMA, 535 North Dearborn Street, Chicago, IL 60610 for information and their booklet, *Group Practice: Guidelines to Forming or Joining a Group*. Reflect again on the definition of a group practice. One by the AMA was given in Chapter 4. One by the **Medical Group Management Association** is "a formally organized group of at least three licensed physicians who are engaged in the practice of medicine as a legally recognized entity, sharing business management, facilities, records, and personnel."

This is one of those times to use a practice management consultant. You need one who is knowledgeable and experienced in setting up groups. Contact the **Society of Professional Business Consultants,** 221 North LaSalle Street, Chicago, IL 60601 and the **Society of Medical/Dental Management Consultants,** 4959 Olson Memorial Highway, Minneapolis, MN 55422.

There is a good section on planning in the reference I cited at the start of this chapter. Study that section and, if possible, read the entire book.

Start thinking about the legal structure the group will have. Two major factors are involved: tax implications and liability. These two factors are gradually causing a shift in the usual organization of groups from partnerships to corporations. Although a small percentage (about 5 per cent) of groups are either sole proprietorships, foundations, or associations, 27 per cent are partnerships, and 68 per cent are now corporations. Competent legal counsel will be required before you come to any conclusions, but some aspects of the latter two organizations can be considered here.

A partnership is defined as "a legal relationship which is created by an oral or written agreement between two or more persons who combine their capital and labor to engage in business or the practice of a profession." Some advantages of a partnership are:

1. Financial and professional risks are shared.
2. The partners have an equal voice in management.
3. No new partners can be admitted without the consent of all other partners.
4. The partners have the right to a formal accounting of partnership affairs.
5. Legal and accounting matters are usually somewhat simpler than in a corporation.

Some disadvantages are:

1. All partners are liable for each individual partner's acts in the partnership.
2. Individual partners are also liable for acts of the partnership as a whole. The partnership can neither sue nor be sued as such; however, individual partners are liable if a suit against a partner concerns the principal business activity of the partnership.
3. The partnership is dissolved when any one partner withdraws or dies.

The dictionary defines a corporation as "a body formed and authorized by law to act as a single person although constituted by one or more persons and legally endowed with various rights and duties." This brief and general statement does not fully capture the concept of a corporation, however. That of Chief Justice Marshall is more informative: "A corporation is an artificial being, invisible, intangible, and existing in contemplation of law. Being the mere creature of law it possesses only those properties (i.e., powers or characteristics) which the charter of its creation confers upon it."

The point in common of these two definitions is that a corporation is a separate legal entity distinct from its individual members. The members are employed by the corporation, which owns the equipment, supplies, and real property, if there is any. The corporation pays expenses and corporation taxes. Profits are distributed to the member-shareholders as dividends.

The main advantage of a corporation over a partnership is that the nonprofessional liability of each physician is limited to the extent of his investment, and the individual physician is entirely liable for his professional acts. Other advantages include the continuity of life of a corporation, that the operation may be less cumbersome in that it is formalized under the articles of incorporation and bylaws, and that transferability of interest may be an advantage under some circumstances.

The principal disadvantage of a corporation is the potential double taxation. Corporate income tax rates are first levied on its profits, then dividends to the shareholders are taxed again to those individuals. This loss can be minimized three ways.

Section 351 of the Internal Revenue code permits retention of corporate profits up to a limit of $150,000 without taxation. Dividends can be declared from this at a time that is most advantageous to the shareholders. Earnings can be retained over that limit if a reasonable business need is demonstrated.

The corporation can pay income tax on small amounts of the accumulated earnings at a 15 per cent rate. If the remaining 85 per cent of the profit is used to purchase high-quality, high-yield utility stocks, the corporation then receives dividends on these shares of stock and utilizes the 85 per cent corporate dividend exclusion to accumulate further income.

Or the corporation can pay out all of the income of the corporation in the form of bonuses to the shareholders. When this is done, the corporation pays no income tax—only the shareholders do.

A fourth method, not often elected, is to organize the corporation under Subchapter S of the Internal Revenue code. This permits the corporation to receive the same tax treatment as a partnership, and all income is passed through to the shareholders. However, this method often brings with it more problems than it solves.

A few tips:

- Be especially careful to avoid structuring your corporation as a personal holding company under Section 531 of the Internal Revenue code.
- Consider the ages, personalities, and goals of all prospective members carefully, and either adapt the structure to fit them, or exclude them.

- The medical records system is frequently an unexpected cause of conflict. Decide this in detail early on.
- Be sure your attorney is cognizant of all possible constraints, such as state anti-trust statutes and certificate-of-need laws.
- Work out the formula for distribution of income at an early date, and have all prospective members agree to it.
- Avoid purchasing a building at the outset. There are advantages to leasing first and owning a facility later as the group matures.
- When you do buy a building, set up *another* legal entity to own it and all physical assets.
- Visit other well-run groups and learn from them. Books, articles, and advisors cannot cover all points.

But read all you can. Start in your medical library. Some of the directories there that will be of value are *American Group Practice Association Directory, The American Medical Directory,* and *The International Directory of the Medical Group Management Association.* Two of the best textbooks there are John W. Field, *Group Practice Development* (Aspen Systems, 1976), and Seth B. Goldsmith, *Ambulatory Care* (Aspen Systems, 1978). Browse through articles that are appropriate.

There are three organizations that can help you. One that will probably be of most assistance to you is the **Medical Group Management Association** (MGMA), 1355 South Colorado Boulevard, Suite 900, Denver, CO 80222. This is an organization of group administrators and managers. It maintains the most complete library on group practice in the country. Its information service will answer questions from their library and other data bases, and has prepared "search summaries" on selected topics, such as capital financing and cost containment. It will provide extensive bibliographies on a wide variety of subjects, for example, forming a group practice and medical group governance.

The MGMA has a consulting service covering several areas of expertise and maintains a placement service for physicians. It publishes a bimonthly journal *Medical Group Management* and a monthly newsletter. The organization also holds annual conferences and more frequent sectional meetings. It publishes an extensive list of books and brochures on its own. Typical book titles are *Practical Financial Management for Medical Groups,* and *Personnel Administration Handbook for Medical Group Practice Administrators.* Two helpful brochures from the same source are *Digest of Bylaws and Buy/Sell Agreements,* and *Digest of Medical Group Employment Contracts and Income Distribution Plans.*

Another organization that may be of assistance is the **American Group Practice Association,** 1422 Duke Street, Alexandria, VA 22314. It represents physicians in group practice. Like the MGMA, it has a consulting service and a placement service, publishes a monthly journal *Group Practice*, and holds a national annual meeting.

The **Group Health Association of America,** 1717 Massachusetts Avenue NW, Suite 203, Washington, DC 20036 is an organization of *prepaid* group practices. It publishes some educational materials and *Group Health and Welfare News*, a monthly newsletter.

This chapter is short, as I said it would be. I have not set out a step-by-step course of action as I did in many other chapters, for a reason. Most of the serious problems that occur in forming a group happen when a group gets started almost by accident. The usual story is that a busy solo practitioner takes in an associate, and when both are busy, takes in a third. Then the problems begin—and they may last for years. A step-by-step approach is not nearly as important as the suggestions I have offered to avoid this.

31

Computers In Office Practice

A chapter on this subject could easily become obsolete as it is being written, so I will touch lightly on details and instead emphasize general principles and guidelines that should remain of value for some years. Fortunately, this approach makes the subject easier to understand for those who are new to the field. I make one assumption that also simplifies the subject. Larger groups of physicians require complicated multi-user set-ups and employ consultants, so they do not need a chapter such as this. However, an individual practitioner or small group can effectively employ a single desktop microcomputer. The assumption of this chapter is that your interest is in this area. Nothing will be said about service bureaus. Their expense (without equity or tax advantages), lack of flexibility, inadequate data analysis, and limited services made them obsolete years ago.

Although computers have been used in the health field for over two decades, most physicians in private practice have not yet entered the computer era. Only 10 per cent of private practitioners utilize computers today, but it is estimated that 60 per cent will by 1990. In the years ahead, this number will probably include you and your practice. In truth, there *is* a computer in your future. So you owe it to yourself, your staff, and your patients to learn the fundamental facts now and to keep up with them as they change.

What can a computer do for you? First, a few things one cannot do. It can't magically make your office more efficient or solve a particular problem. Your office organization must be operating effectively already, and then a computer can be used to enhance efficiency at one or more steps. Nor will it replace an employee, although it might allow you to postpone hiring the next one.

For example, let's say your appointment system is not working well. Putting in a computer to solve this problem will actually set you back, at least at first. Changing your system, training your receptionist, and entering a data base all take time and cause difficulties. Personnel resistance may be encountered. So stop and look at your system again. Actually, the time and labor of making entries in an appointment book are approximately the same as they would be with a computer. Reminders and recalls are not all that cumbersome. Even such changes as cancellations and work-ins are simple for a receptionist with a sharp mind and a sharp pencil. Instead of acquiring a computer for this purpose, you might be thinking of ways you could make your present appointment system work better. However, if a computer is to be installed for another purpose, it would be well to have this capability.

A similar argument can be made against the installation of a computer for handling accounts payable and payroll. These are simple tasks that can be done manually. But, again, a system installed for another purpose should have the capability to take on these tasks as well.

The same is true *at present* for clinical applications. But here the potential for future use is much greater, for several reasons. Computer clinical entries are less time-consuming and always legible. The detection and correction of errors is much simpler, as is access to the information. Diagnostic programs are being developed. Correlation of data for such purposes as differential diagnosis and drug interaction is possible today. And treatment options can be explored more completely. However, the maintenance of a written record is required by law, so the use of a computer to record clinical data is not at present justifiable in most circumstances. In the future, when hard copy printouts are accepted and as data banks are developed, clinical record-keeping may constitute a valid reason by itself to have a computer.

There are four principal reasons now to consider installing a computer in a medical office. First and foremost is in the area of billing and collections, with the maintenance of associated financial records. Two advantages are particularly important: (1) ease in information processing and analysis, and (2) rapid production of statements, insurance claim forms, and collection letters. Data are entered easily, there is greater facility in detecting and correcting errors, the information is readily accessible and can be analyzed many ways (e.g., for account aging and for demographic data). Peak-load production of statements is eased, and insurance claim forms can be prepared in seconds. Most third-party payers hope in the future to eliminate the insurance claim form entirely and use electronic claims submission, with data being transferred directly from an office computer to their own mainframe.

Word processing is a second valid use of a computer in many offices, when much repetition and revision of letters and forms are required and a great deal of correspondence is generated—at least ten letters or the equivalent per week. Many word processing systems merge with your data base, so that recall letters can be sent to all patients who have not had a physical examination in three years, a Pap smear in two years, and so on.

A third reason for a computer today is in the area of data retrieval. At this writing there are seven data bases, starting with the well-known **Medline** of the **National Library of Medicine.** All together, they contain approximately 12 million references from the medical literature. Summaries are obtainable directly, and copies of entire articles can be ordered by mail.

A fourth reason would be to utilize the nonmedical information sources such as *Delphi*, *Compuserve*, *The Source*, *Dialog*, and various news, financial, and travel services. More of these are coming on line all the time.

Those are the things a computer can do for you today. Now let's look at the equipment itself. You have heard the terms *hardware* and *software*. The hardware consists of the physical parts of the computer, and the software contains the instructions and information upon which the hardware operates. At any one price range, the hardware is remarkably similar from manufacturer to manufacturer and is a much less important consideration than the software. In fact, a computer should be thought of not as a machine, but in terms of the functions it performs under the control of the software. Accordingly, when selecting your system you will be looking at software first. However, it is simpler here to start with a description of the hardware.

The most important element of the hardware is the box-like *central processing unit* (CPU). It contains the working memory and mass storage.

The working memory is what the computer is currently working on, and consists of two portions. One is the *read only memory* (ROM), which is permanently stored in the computer and not erased when the machine is turned off. It is here that language interpretation from English to machine language takes place. The second part of the working memory is known as *random access memory*, or RAM. This is the main part of the working memory. Data are entered into the RAM when the computer is on, can be changed during operation, and are lost when the computer is turned off. The RAM data are kept in the mass storage while the computer is in operation. The RAM capacity is an important feature of a computer and is measured in *kilobytes*. One K or kilobyte equals 1,024 *bytes* of information. Older microcomputers had a RAM capacity of 64K to 128K, but 256K is the present standard, with 512K and 640K available.

Mass storage contains the main data base on either a magnetized "floppy" disk (also called a diskette) or a hard disk. Most programs designed for medical offices operate with floppy disks, but a hard disk may be required. The latter has ten times the speed and 20 times the storage capacity of a floppy disk. If you have over 100 patient contacts a week, your program may require a hard disk. The newer floppy disks are 5¼ inches in diameter, double-sided, and double-density. Their capacity is expressed in megabytes. As typically employed in a medical office, a double disk drive would have one floppy disk containing the main program in constant use in one drive, with other floppy disks inserted in the second drive as required for special tasks.

Features to look for in a CPU are at least four expansion slots, three ports (monitor, serial, and parallel), double disk drive, and the provision for adding memory to the motherboard. The latest CPUs use 16 bits at once (i.e., they handle "words" of 16 characters) for greater speed and memory, but most programs are written for 8-bit computers, so the latter is preferable at present. Most of the time delay in a medical office is in data entry, so the faster processing of a 16-bit machine is not needed.

The second element of the hardware is the keyboard. This is attached to the CPU with a cord. The keyboard is similar to that of a typewriter, with an auxiliary numeric key pad to make the entry of numbers more convenient. Key surfaces should be sculptured, not flat. Tactile or sound feedback when they are pressed is desirable. Automatic repeat, rollover, and special function keys controlled by software are all valuable features.

The third element is the cathode ray tube (CRT), which is a video display much like a television screen. It is important to select an adequate screen size (at least 12 inches diagonally) to avoid eye strain, and to have nonglare glass for the same reason. The display must be at least 80 characters per line and 24 lines of text. Green phosphor is preferable, but amber is satisfactory. Resolution of the characters is better if only one color is used. For this reason, you may not want to have color graphics capability. Swivel and tilt features are advantageous.

The fourth piece of necessary hardware is the printer. There are three types. The dot-matrix printer is most common because of its high speed of up to 3000 characters per second, and lower cost. The most readable of these produce characters seven dots wide by nine dots high, with letter descenders (the tail on letters such as y and g) below the line. However, dot-matrix printers are not recommended for a medical office for two reasons: the characters are not finished in appearance, and many of the forms used in a medical office require an impact to carry through to several copies. Making photocopies can be a nuisance. The second type is a laser printer which prints letter quality at 8 to 12 *pages* per second. But its cost is prohibitively high. A letter-quality or formed-character printer is slower (15 to 55 characters per second), noisier, and more expensive than a dot matrix. It works like a daisy wheel electronic typewriter, produces similar formed characters, and does carry through to copies beneath, so this is the type you want. The continuous forms used in a medical office have detachable strips with holes on each side so that the tractor drive with sprocket wheels will align entries properly in the appropriate spaces and feed the paper as your program commands it to. Be sure you get this type of feeder and not a cut-sheet feeder designed to use ordinary typing paper.

The last item of hardware is the *modem*. This term is an acronym formed from the words *mo*dulate and *dem*odulate. Originally, these were devices that translated the computer code to musical tones so they could be carried over telephone lines, with another device in use at the other end to convert these tones back into computer codes. The type of modem now in use is electronic, is installed as a board in one of the expansion slots in the CPU, transmits and receives at much higher speed (1200 impulses per second, or *bauds*, instead of the earlier 300), and operates with far fewer errors. With a modem, your computer can "talk" to large mainframe computers and other microcomputers.

With this description of the hardware as a basis, the software is more understandable. Think of the software as the information and instructions that make the computer intelligent. It can be divided into three categories: *operating systems*, *languages*, and *applications programs*.

The *operating system* gives operating instructions to the computer. It coordinates and controls the information flow and provides certain "housekeeping" functions. It is loaded into the computer from a floppy disk automatically when the computer is turned on, or it may be part of the permanent memory. It loads programs, runs them, controls input from the keyboard and output to the CRT, and sends instructions and data to the printer. It controls the disk drives and is in charge of other peripherals such as the modem. Each computer has its particular operating system. One is the type used by Apple computers, another is used in Radio Shack computers, and still another is common to several manufacturers such as IBM and Xerox. The most widely used system for business programs is DOS, which stands for *disk operating system*. Programs written to run under this operating system can be used in several types of computers, so it will probably be your choice.

It is important to keep in mind that the operating system of your computer determines the applications programs you can run.

The second category of software is the *language interpreter*. A computer operates only on its own machine language. Communicating with a computer using this machine language directly would be extremely cumbersome. For this reason, several higher level languages have been developed to enable the operator to use English. The most common of these is called BASIC, which stands for *beginners' all-purpose symbolic instructional code*. The largest amount of software is in BASIC. Others such as MUMPS, FORTRAN, and PASCAL are for more specialized uses with a narrower range of software. You will be selecting your program primarily for what it can do for you, and although the one you select will probably be in BASIC, the language your program uses will not be important to you.

The third category of software consists of the *applications programs*. Each application program is designed to perform a specific function, such as handling accounts receivable. They are written in a higher level language, utilize the language interpreter software to translate English into machine language, and are under the control of the operating system.

Once again, I should emphasize that a computer is best thought of not as a mechanical device with its several components, but in terms of its *functions*. Therefore, the first consideration in the selection of a computer is the suitability of its available software for the functions you wish it to perform. It is here that your criteria are most critical. In selecting your software, try to look ahead at least three years to other potential uses of your computer.

If there *is* a computer in your future, you have to start learning some of the technical details. By far the best practical guide is *How to Buy: A Comprehensive Guide for Computerizing the Medical Office*, available from Articulate Publications, 402 North Larchmont Boulevard, Los Angeles, CA 90004. A good book is *Microcomputers and the Private Practitioner* by Robert M. Pressman, published by Dow-Jones/Irwin. Two trade paperback books that are less complete and also somewhat dated are *The Role of Computers in Medical Practice Management* by Ann Ehrlich, obtainable from Colwell Systems, and *The Physician's Guide to Desktop Computers* by Mark Spohr, M.D., available from Reston Publishing Company, Reston, Virginia 22090.

Good sources of background information are *Computers for Medical Office and Patient Management* by Stacey B. Day and Jan F. Brandeis (Van Nostrand Reinhold Co.), *Artificial Intelligence in Medicine* edited by Peter Szolovits (Westview Press), and *Information Systems for Patient Care* by Bruce I. Blum (Springer-Verlag). You might also subscribe to two journals: *Medical Computer Journal*, 42 East High Street, East Hampton, CT 06424, and *Computers and Medicine*, AMA Subscriber Services, 535 North Dearborn Street, Chicago, IL 60610. Drop by your local vendors, browse, ask questions, and pick up the literature there. Attend seminars held in your area. Talk to colleagues who have put in computers.

Once you are conversant with the terminology and are clear on what a computer can do in your practice, put it down in writing. This will help you organize your thoughts, make it easier for a vendor to understand and respond to your needs, and help you compare vendors and prices. There are three options in regard to vendors:

1. The local outlet of a national manufacturer like IBM or NCR. The prices will be a bit higher, but the firms are reliable and will provide training for your staff. You will be limited in software options, however.
2. A turnkey-systems house that buys computer components and software from manufacturers and assembles them into a workable system. Most of these also provide training.
3. A retail store that sells computer components. These can be independently owned, part of a chain, or backed by a major manufacturer. Reliability and services vary.

It is usually advisable, unless you have extensive experience in the computer field, to purchase all hardware and software from a systems house even though the cost may be up to 50 per cent more than if you did it yourself. Select one that has performed well for other physicians. Ask your accountant and the local medical society for their recommendations. Be sure you have more than one hardware manufacturer to choose from, that you can get the best for your purpose, and that the software is appropriate. A "request for proposal," used in obtaining bids on large computer installations, is not necessary. Ask about training, problem-solving on site, repair, and other support. Prompt service is extremely important. So is service and support several years down the line. Inquire about programs still under development. Ask the provider if he will train future staff in the event of turnover.

There are about 1200 applications programs for the health care field. It is better to select the one "off the shelf" that most closely approximates your requirements and adapt your practice to it, rather than have custom software developed for you. The latter is prohibitively expensive, usually full of bugs, and will cause you no end of trouble.

Assuming that your principal purpose is to handle accounts receivable, here are some things to look for:

- The program should be for your specialty. An internist can develop a dozen line items in a complete physical examination, while a surgeon may have only one per patient.

- The system should provide for future upgrading by adding boards or changing components.
- It should have menus that are easy to follow.
- Security is important. A user password (one for each person) to access each main system option is advisable, with several levels of control.
- Report generators appropriate to your practice.
- Screen-oriented programs, with on-screen help and error messages.
- Most medical software systems provide activity analysis, by procedure and diagnosis. Most also can send out messages with statements and recalls. Just be sure you have these capabilities.
- Flexibility is important, to change fees, make adjustments, use new forms, add new codes, and so forth.
- Alpha search capability. This means that an account can be located quickly by name, even if the name is misspelled or only part of it is known.
- The system should also be able to handle patients who have different last names from the person who is financially responsible, and different addresses. You also need to be able to use the new nine-digit zip codes.
- A safeguard to prevent accidentally deleting any account with a balance outstanding is a feature you should look for.
- Diagnostic and procedure codes that fit your practice must be included. Payment codes, that is, by cash, check, or insurance, are essential. All code descriptions should allow for at least 25 characters, and it should be borne in mind that computers count spaces and punctuation as characters. It should be easy to enter several diagnostic procedures linked to a single diagnostic code. One "user friendly" feature is a complete description of a procedure when the procedure code is entered, which enables your aide to check for accuracy. Your software system should be able to cross-reference facility modifiers, diagnostic codes, and service codes.
- The system you select should automatically post fees according to the procedure code entered. It should generate sequentially numbered charge slips for each patient, and a rapid "walk-out" statement. This serves as a receipt, bears enough information to be used as a superbill, and facilitates collection at the time of service.
- If your practice accepts Medicaid or workers' compensation, for which the universal claim form cannot be used, be sure that your system can produce the required forms. Also, those patients who have coverage under more than one plan should be handled easily by your system. It should be able to track, age, amend, and resubmit claim forms, and generate insurance status reports.
- It is important to have a readily produced accounts receivable record, with aging and other management information such as daily proof and trial balance. You may want account aging to appear on your statements with appropriate messages.
- Other desirable features include a built-in training program and the capacity for remote diagnostics and correction through your modem.

Before you make your decision, have a few long conversations with the assistant who will be operating the computer. Be sure she has no "computer block" and is motivated. Be cautious if she requires strong reading glasses. These focus at 15 inches, and the CRT is most comfortably viewed at 20 to 25 inches. Have her take the tasks to be performed to the vendor and perform them on the computer. Go with her and watch her reaction and facial expressions. Both of you should look at the manual to see if it is thorough, complete, spells out procedures step by step, and is free of computer jargon.

Be sure you have sufficient and appropriate space for the use of a computer in your office. Then consult with your accountant regarding the tax ramifications of the purchase. Ask about investment tax credit and the depreciation schedule. Estimate the amount of time that will be required for staff training and data base entry—usually about 90 days—and allow for this overlap. Arrange courses for your personnel. Consider the items that have to be changed: your patient information book, the patient registration form, and the office procedures manual.

Computer hardware is usually warranted for 30 to 90 days. After this time, service contracts are advisable. The best is a full-service contract for the first year or two, and then you might want to pay for each service provided, travel time *not* included. A "carry-in" contract is not advisable, unless a loaner is readily available.

Because of the rapid advances in both hardware and software, there may be a temptation to wait for a further improvement that is just around the corner. Remember that both will constantly be improving, so in theory you could wait forever. If the hardware and software perform the tasks that you need them to do now, they will continue to be capable of doing so.

32

Medicolegal Aspects

with WILLIAM W. HUSS, J.D.

Throughout the course of his professional career, a physician is faced with legal situations for which he is ill-prepared by his education. Some of them may be complex and some are subtle. The simpler ones were covered when we were discussing such topics as legal requirements relating to employees and office leases. This chapter will go beyond these to legal aspects of the physician-patient relationship.

It will stop short of ethical considerations, however. Over the course of history, ethics have always preceded formal law. They derive from a wide variety of philosophical and religious viewpoints. Each physician is himself a product of one set of societal ethics, so the subject is more suitable for a book than a single chapter. Three of the best references are *Clinical Ethics: A Practical Approach to Ethical Decisions in Clinical Medicine* by Albert R. Jonsen, Mark Siegler, and William J. Winslade (Macmillan Publishing Company); *Medical Ethics: A Clinical Textbook and Reference for the Health Care Professions,* edited by Natalie Abrams and Michael D. Buckner (The MIT Press); and *American College of Physicians Ethics Manual* by the Ad Hoc Committee on Medical Ethics, American College of Physicians, available from Subscriber Service Division, American College of Physicians, 4200 Pine Street, Philadelphia, PA 19104.

Society's concerns about physicians and their care of patients were expressed in the earliest civilizations. Some appeared in the laws written by the ancient Sumerians and in the famous Code of Hammurabi. Similar concerns were shown in the later Egyptian papyri. In some instances, severe punishments were prescribed for physicians who treated their patients improperly.

Other admonitions are found in the writings of Aesculapius and Hippocrates, and in our heritage of Judeo-Christian ethics. They permeate both English common law and the Napoleonic Code, which form the foundations of our legal system.

We will look at the medicolegal aspects under six headings. This is not intended to be a primer on law or a "do-it-yourself" guide. You should consult your lawyer in any particular situation, and go by his advice.

I. THE PHYSICIAN-PATIENT RELATIONSHIP

The general rule is that this relationship begins when a physician accepts a request to provide his medical services. This request from a patient (or his guardian) may be either expressed or implied. It has been held in some states that the relationship begins when your aide (who is considered your extension) makes an appointment in response to a telephone request. There are certain specific exceptions to this general rule. The rendering of first aid in an emergency does not usually establish the relationship, and in states with "Good Samaritan" laws it never does. A single office visit for a purpose that is accomplished at that visit does not, either, provided that there is mutual agreement that the relationship has not been established. The same is usually true for a single emergency room visit if it requires no follow-up treatment, or if the patient is specifically referred to another source for the follow-up treatment.

Once the physician-patient relationship has been established, the physician must provide continuing care to that patient as long as the patient's condition requires it. He also must keep the patient informed of the nature of his condition and all aspects of his treatment. On his part, the patient is expected to participate responsibly in his own care.

The physician-patient relationship can be terminated in various ways. The most common is when the condition reaches a clinical end-point and no longer requires the physician's services. The physician then must make it clear that there is no need for the patient to return, and the patient must understand and accept this. The relationship can also be terminated unilaterally by either party. The physician always bears a certain responsibility because of his knowledge of the medical circumstances. He also must be alert for nebulous situations, such as the patient who follows some advice but not all, or one who misses an appointment and then keeps one, and continues in this pattern. Or when a patient is sent for consultation and continuing care, but it is not clear to the patient or consultant whether the referring physician has ceased to assume responsibility.

Whenever the relationship is terminated, the physician must make an effort to ensure that competent care is continued from another source and that pertinent records in his possession are made available to the new provider of care. He also must formalize the termination. A letter of termination should be very specific in setting out the reasons, and be phrased so as to avoid creating any antagonism or animosity. There are many ways to draft a termination letter, and the *Medicolegal Forms* produced by the **Office of the General Counsel** of the AMA provides sample letters. A copy is retained in the patient's medical record. The original is sent certified mail, return receipt requested. The signed receipt is attached to the copy of the letter in the medical record.

II. PRIVILEGED COMMUNICATIONS

The physician-patient relationship generates a special privilege in the eyes of the law. The basis for this privilege is that the physician must possess as much information as possible in order for the proper treatment to be provided. The patient must feel free to divulge this information and confident that it will not be revealed to another party. The privilege rests with the patient, and may not be released except by the patient, with certain exceptions. One of these exceptions is when release of the information is required by law, as in cases of certain communicable diseases, gunshot or stab wounds, and suspected child abuse. In some states, this extends to situations in which the patient threatens the health of another person or appears to be suicidal. Another common exception is disclosing the limited information requested by medical care providers. This has been held to be authorized by implied consent when the patient requests the third party to compensate the physician for the medical services rendered. Still another is if the patient reveals information to a third party not assisting in his care, in which case implied consent is assumed.

The privileged communication protection is waived automatically in many jurisdictions when a lawsuit for personal injury is filed. This waiver enables the defendants to examine the medical history and background of the plaintiff. Nonetheless, a signed release authorization should be presented or a subpoena served with respect to the records.

Physicians are most often caught on one of four points. One is that just mentioned. The physician may be told that the release of information is legal because a lawsuit has been filed, when it may not be legal for any number of reasons. The second point is that it is not just the information given him by the patient that is privileged, but all information he has learned from *any source* about the patient. The third point physicians trip up on is that information may not be disclosed to the patient's spouse or other close relative *unless* the patient himself is unable to comprehend, or if, because of his condition or emotional state, disclosing the information to the patient would be detrimental. The fourth point is that the privileged status of the information continues after the patient's death.

In every case, you should obtain a signed release, specifically referring to the information in question. If you have any doubts, ask your attorney.

III. RIGHT TO PRIVACY

In addition to this privilege, a patient continues to have the same constitutional right of privacy as does any other person. Although a patient may submit to an examination or other procedure, he retains the right not to have anyone except those necessary present and not to have a picture taken. His written consent to have observers present, even medical students and residents who are not directly concerned with his care, or to have pictures taken (photographs, television, or motion pictures), must be obtained. A broad consent to invasion of privacy is usually obtained on hospital admission. Read it over to be sure it covers what you intend to do, and in your office use the standard AMA form.

IV. INFORMED CONSENT

The "consent" part of this term is easy. It means that the permission of the patient is given to proceed with a treatment or procedure. It's the "informed" part that presents problems. The patient must be mentally competent—sufficiently so to understand the explanation. Then the nature of his illness, the procedure or treatment itself, its probable benefits and major risks, as well as the alternative means of treatment with their benefits and risks, must all be explained clearly so that the patient can make a choice. If the patient is unconscious, under the influence of drugs, or emotionally disturbed, the method of obtaining consent should be that set forth in your state law. This is also your guide if the patient has not attained majority. The exceptions to obtaining informed consent are few, and these are also specified in the laws of each state. The only one common to all states is an emergency situation threatening the patient's life, when obtaining an informed consent would be inappropriate. Bear in mind that all of these situations are subject to scrutiny after the fact.

In deciding what information to include in the explanation, the physician is guided by the principle of what is best for the patient.

All of the remote risks or consequences of a treatment or procedure need not be given. Those that are *reasonable* to disclose in view of the patient's emotional and physical state are all that are required. If either his mental or physical condition seriously limits the information that can be given the patient, a reasonable disclosure should be given to the patient's spouse or to the nearest relative if there is no spouse.

The consent should be worded specifically for each situation, and obtained for a wide variety of treatments and procedures. Some of these may surprise you: disposal of amputated limbs and removed organs, the spouse's consent for abortion and sterilization, procedures that could be considered experimental, use of drugs under clinical investigation, blood transfusions, and treadmill stress tests. Never use general consent forms, not even those provided by your hospital—they are designed to protect the hospital, not you. Be careful never to give any express or implied guarantee of results during your explanation, or on the consent form itself.

V. THE PHYSICIAN AS A WITNESS

A physician may be a witness under three sets of circumstances: (1) as one who participated in providing medical care for a patient testifying as to the facts in that treatment; (2) as an expert witness, having never treated the patient; and (3) as a defendant in a malpractice lawsuit.

The last circumstance will be covered when we discuss malpractice. The first is common for traumatologists, those who cover emergency rooms, and those who handle workers' compensation cases. As these physicians well know, the most important thing is to keep accurate medical records and to be sure that others involved in the patient's care do also. In such cases a physician will be advised about being a witness by the receipt of a subpoena for the production of his medical records, often with the requirement that he appear for a deposition or hearing as well.

A subpoena serves notice to a prospective witness that the court is exercising its jurisdiction over him to require that he perform in accordance with it, under penalty for failure to comply. The power that is exercised in the issuance of the subpoena is pervasive and will be enforced by courts without exception.

As a consequence, attempting to avoid a subpoena is futile. It is wisest to accept it, then to seek some agreement on the time and place of the appearance to accommodate your schedule. If this cannot be done, videotaping a deposition may be possible. This is accomplished by stipulation among the parties.

Whenever you are subpoenaed as a witness, consult your lawyer. Be sure your records are accurate and complete, and do not alter them. Ask your lawyer if a release from the patient is required. Have the details of your credentials in mind, including dates.

In the second situation, a physician may be a witness when his testimony is given as expert opinion. Most jurisdictions provide that an expert witness be given a fee in advance. These arrangements are made between the physician and the lawyer who is seeking his testimony. Experts' fees vary widely. Ask the local medical association or bar association what the prevailing fee is in your area for your specialty.

You may be called as an expert witness regardless of your level of experience as a physician. Most often, however, those called are recognized authorities in their fields.

Expert opinion evidence is *weighed* by the jury, which means that they assign relative importance to it. They do not regard it in the same light as they do objective, direct evidence, but oftentimes expert opinion is the only way certain evidence can be given to the jury. Also, it may be the only way the jury can understand the basic issues in a case, particularly in those involving personal injury or medical malpractice.

Your duty as an expert in a malpractice case is to testify as to the standard of care for that particular kind of medical procedure under the same or similar circumstances. First, it will be established that you know the standard of care and have a foundational knowledge enabling you to express an opinion on the standard of care. Second, you will testify with respect to the facts in the particular case and how they comply, or do not comply, with that standard. Third, in casting the facts in relief against the standard of care, you will be expected to express an opinion as to whether or not the conduct of the physician, or other health care practitioner, is within that standard.

In any of the three circumstances, when you are on the stand:

1. Tell the truth. This goes without saying, but more is meant than not telling a falsehood. State all that is pertinent in a succinct and accurate way without bias.
2. If you don't know the answer, admit that you do not.
3. Be sure you understand the question before answering it. If you don't understand it, say so. The lawyer questioning you will rephrase it or ask the court reporter to read it back.
4. Take the time you need to think about the question and to formulate your answer before responding. Don't be rushed.

5. Answer the question that is asked and then stop. Don't volunteer information.
6. Speak loudly enough so everybody can hear you, and keep your hands away from your mouth. Always give an audible answer so the court reporter can record it. Don't nod your head yes or no.
7. Never look at your lawyer when you're on the stand. You are on your own. You won't get any help from the judge either.
8. If you have to make an estimate, be sure that everyone understands that you are estimating.
9. Don't argue with the lawyer on the other side. He has a right to question you within the limits of propriety set by the court. Try to remain calm and not lose your temper no matter how you are provoked.
10. Always be courteous yourself. Answer "Yes, sir," and "No, sir," and address the judge as "Your Honor." A soft answer turneth away wrath.
11. If asked whether you have talked to the lawyer on your side, or to an investigator, admit it freely.
12. Make no attempts at humor. A lawsuit is a serious matter, and all concerned are serious.
13. Look jury members in the eye when you testify.
14. Don't let the lawyer on the other side catch you by asking you whether you are willing to swear to what you have said. You were sworn to tell the truth when you took the stand.
15. Your demeanor should reflect a search for the truth. It is not a theater, nor a place to manifest your ego, nor to demean an attorney who apparently doesn't know as much about medicine as you do. He may know just enough.
16. Bear in mind that the known may be asked as if it were unknown, and the unknown as if it were known.

VI. MALPRACTICE

In the 1980s we are caught in another mounting crisis in malpractice claims, when we thought the worst was behind us after the 1970s. Three times as many actions are being filed today, compared with a few years ago. *Twenty per cent* of all physicians now have one or more suits pending against them. It is not just the number of suits, but the size of the awards, that has precipitated the present crisis. In 1984 nearly 300 were for more than one million dollars.

The reasons for this situation are multiple, and only the major ones can be mentioned here. Many individuals have become more litigious, as indicated by the same trend in product liability and personal injury litigation. One of the chapter authors disagrees, but the other believes that the increasing number of attorneys is another factor, and that the contingency fee system is another. The doctrine of strict liability as applied to all connected with the case, whether responsible or not, as long as they have "deep pockets," is another. Still another is the tendency of judges and juries to grant astronomical awards, which in turn encourages more litigation.

Some underlying societal factors are at work, too. The population of the United States has shifted from the rural areas to the cities, and this has weakened the personal relationship between physicians and their patients that often existed in the smaller communities and rural areas. Patients now depersonalize the physician somewhat, and the physician may do the same to his patients. Litigation thus becomes a more acceptable means of resolving disputes. This increase has resulted in an increased demand for lawyers who specialize in medicolegal matters. There is now a large number who are more sophisticated in medical matters and who are eager to pursue litigation in this area.

Because of rapid advances in communications, the standards of practice are no longer limited to the local community. Standards of practice now are national, or even international.

There are other factors in the medical field. The increasing sophistication of medicine means undertaking treatment or procedures that carry high risk, and it also means utilizing those that are not in themselves risky on patients who are in much more serious condition.

Few contend that physicians are contributing to the current crisis through decreasing competence. In fact, the indications are that physicians are becoming increasingly competent. In Florida, where there are now more complaints of malpractice than in perhaps any other state in the Union, the State Board of Medical Examiners reports that fewer than 10 per cent of the cases it reviews involve substandard medical care. Still, physicians must do more to keep their own house in order and eliminate incompetence wherever it is encountered.

Whatever the causes, the result for physicians is higher malpractice premiums and a diminishing number of carriers willing to write professional liability policies. Premiums have risen over the past ten years by more than 600 per cent. In some parts of the country, for specialties such as neurosurgery, obstetrics, and orthopedics, the annual premium is over $100,000, and could be twice that by 1990.

Before we get into what you should do if you are sued, and how to reduce the likelihood of a suit, a few other points need to be mentioned. Review your carrier to make sure it is the best available. It should have the largest reserve per policy and the best reinsurance provisions. Try to get contract (occurrence) coverage. If it is not available, see if you can buy a "tail" now at the going rate and at each renewal to have, in effect, occurrence coverage. Review the amount of your coverage in view of recent decisions. Be sure your policy allows you to retain your own counsel. In some jurisdictions, if there is conflict between the insurer and the insured, the insurance company must pay reasonable fees for your own attorney. Have a talk with your lawyer now about your exposure. Look over your assets together. Consider items that could be put in trust, property that could be changed to joint tenancy, or set up under a gift-leaseback arrangement. Ask if there is a homestead act in your state to protect your home. Think about getting a license for a possible move later to another state where there is lower risk.

If you are sued, the first thing to do is notify your insurance company by telephone and follow up in writing. Then call your own lawyer. If you are served with process, don't try to avoid it. Service may be made by publication when a defendant is clearly attempting to avoid it. Review the records. Make sure they are complete, including all lab and x-ray reports. Under no circumstances make any changes or alterations in the records. This can lose the whole case for you even if you did nothing wrong. Make no oral or written statements to anyone about the case without talking to the lawyer appointed for you by your insurance carrier and your own lawyer. Make a copy of your records and keep it in your safe deposit box. Keep the original in your office under lock and key.

The complaint filed by the plaintiff requires a written pleading, which is filed on your behalf by the insurance company lawyer. After the basic facts of the case are known, you can expect the plaintiff to take your deposition.

A deposition is testimony *under oath* of a witness or party to a lawsuit. It is like testimony in the court itself, although the deposition is held outside of the court for the purpose of discovering facts about the case and preserving testimony.

You have the right to schedule depositions to suit your convenience, subject to mutual agreement of counsel or court approval.

You also have the right to see all medical records involving the case ahead of time to prepare for your deposition. Review the case thoroughly in conference with both your lawyer and the lawyer assigned to you by the insurance company before you appear for the deposition itself. Never be deposed without both of your lawyers there, and don't be misled by the informality. Your testimony may come back to haunt you in court.

Both the plaintiff and defendant have the right to be present at the deposition. Attorneys for both sides are always there, and so is a court recorder. The opposing party is entitled to copies of all documents which a witness uses to refresh his recollection. If you plan to use any, show them to your lawyers and discuss them ahead of time. You will have an opportunity at a later date to review the deposition after it has been typed and to make minor corrections.

Testifying as a defendant in your own malpractice case has to be the most trying situation you, as a physician, can be in. Your intelligence, education, judgment, and skill—most of what is *you*—are being called into question. It helps if you can be present during the entire trial, from the selection of the jury, through opening statements, the presentation of evidence, the arguments of counsel, to the instruction of the jury. It not only helps *you* in preparing for your own testimony, but your presence may help your case.

Remain the calm observer. Any expressions of anger or disbelief will only interfere with the due process and hurt your case. The key words are objectivity and equanimity—try to appear serene and detached even though you don't feel that way.

There is a lot you can do to avoid being there in the first place. Without doubt, the most fundamental factor is the quality of your relationship with your patients. In many cases it is the physician's arrogant attitude that is the chief cause for the action. This has no place in the practice of medicine. Let patients know you care, treat them as human beings, be interested in their personal lives, take enough time with them, answer their questions, and explain your diagnosis and treatment plan.

Render quality care. Keep up with advances in your field. Sharpen your medical skills constantly.

Obtain informed consent when required. Indicate in the chart that the consent was obtained after giving sufficient information to the patient (or his guardian or conservator).

Follow up on all referrals. If the patient is badly treated (or merely feels badly treated), is abandoned (or feels abandoned), you may be the one whom the patient holds responsible.

Communicate with the physicians who cover for you and those you cover for, or the same thing can happen.

Settle misunderstandings over fees as amicably as possible.

Use the best diagnostic methods and procedures available. Document the differential diagnosis and indicate your reasons for discarding all but the primary one.

Reduce the number of procedures that increase both your risk and your insurance rates. For example, if you are in general or family practice, consider giving up certain surgical procedures or all of them. If you are in Ob-Gyn, think about discontinuing obstetrics. If you are near retirement, change your practice to Class I status now.

Always have an assistant with you when you examine patients of the opposite sex.

Be especially careful never to guarantee results, implicitly or explicitly.

Be attentive to the legal rights of patients as described in this chapter.

Whenever the possibility exists that your competence may be exceeded, obtain consultation without delay.

Keep good records. This does not mean writing long notes, just ones that clearly show what your findings and actions were. Remember that in court, the medical records speak for themselves. They should be clearly legible, and any error is corrected by a single line through it with the correct entry, your initials, and the date of the correction.

Pay particular attention to hospital records, because these patients are more seriously ill and have more procedures performed. Your initial history and physical examination should be accurate and complete, properly corrected as described earlier, with your signature on each page. Be careful to use consent forms correctly, your own in addition to those of the hospital, and document all explanations given the patient in the progress notes. Review all laboratory and x-ray reports, and comment upon them in your notes. Any suggested diagnoses or treatments that appear there must be reflected in your notes. Review the nurse's charting daily, and comment upon it. Review your "op" reports and discharge summary carefully when typed, and make corrections properly before signing them.

In your office, set up standard procedures in your manual, train your assistants properly, and supervise them as required. The law holds you responsible for everything they do or say.

Participate in your hospital staff functions and quality assurance system. You can be held accountable if you participated in the care of a patient even when the error itself was committed by an employee of the hospital.

Try not to treat patients over the telephone. Although limited follow-up advice may be given if the patient was recently seen and is reliable, no new diagnoses should be made or treatment instituted. Document all telephone calls in the chart.

Make sure that your office is accident-proof, and that all the equipment in your office is functioning properly. Go through it from time to time and imagine "worst case scenarios" such as falls against sharp corners, furniture tipping over, or infirm patients slipping. Correct any hazardous conditions. Have your assistants routinely help patients on and off examining tables.

Be certain that you have adequate emergency procedures established in your manual, that your emergency equipment is up to date and complete, and that your staff holds regular drills.

Always advise your patients of both the intended effect and any side reactions that may occur from the medications you prescribe. Package inserts go far beyond any such reasonable advice, yet you may be held to them in court. The best course of action is to use the AMA drug information sheets, or photocopies of the pertinent pages of patient information books, as suggested in Chapter 14. Explain the side reactions to the patient as you make notes upon the form, then hand it to him. Document that you did so in the chart. Then be alert for side effects and care for them properly when they occur.

Note that the above list does not include practicing "defensive medicine"—ordering unnecessary laboratory work, x-rays, or other procedures. This only increases the expense, not the defense.

Many states have attempted to alter their laws in the area of tort reform over the last decade. One of the changes suggested is that that the statute of limitations run from the date of injury, not of discovery. Another is to require summary judgments in cases where there is no material disagreement on the facts. In this way, a judge could decide a case without a lengthy hearing and expensive attorney fees on both sides. Another is doing away with the doctrine of joint-and-several liability, so that a physician would be held liable only for the portion of damages attributed to his actions. Still another is a mandatory limit on the contingency fee of plaintiff's attorneys. One so far sustained on appeal in California is a cap on the awards for noneconomic losses such as "pain and suffering." These account for approximately 60 per cent of the large awards at the present time. In addition to these changes in tort law, there has been legislative effort in several states to establish a no-fault system resembling workers' compensation. However, the outlook for most of these attempts at reform is bleak over the long run because of opposition by trial lawyers.

33

Stress and the Physician

with BERNARD VIRSHUP, M.D.

The popular image of a physician—or perhaps what we would like to *think* of as the popular image—is that of a tower of strength caring for all with compassion. How strong is that "tower"? The AMA tells us that 10 per cent of physicians cease practice prematurely for one or more stress-related causes. What about the 90 per cent who hang in there? The data may be mixed, but the message is clear—stress takes its toll on all of us.

We are well aware of some of the sources of stress that are similar to those of other professionals and executives in industry—long hours, limited leisure that is frequently interrupted, time constraints, personnel problems, and all the frustrations, forms, and regulations. We may not be as aware of conflicts and causes of tension that lie just beneath the surface. Medicine is more than an art, but it is not quite a science. All diagnoses are uncertain or incomplete in some way. So are most therapeutic modalities. Outcomes are always problematic. We stand helpless in the face of incurable illnesses. The selflessness of our calling is in conflict with the selfishness of having to make a living. We work in a society that has medicalized all sorts of aberrant behavior, that makes it advantageous for many to remain sick or disabled when we want to make them well. We deal with topics that are taboo, and with intimacy in thought and person. Our concern with the cost to our patients is sometimes in conflict with our desire to do the best we can for them.

There are many other sources of stress that affect us. Through them all we have to keep in mind that our physical and mental health are important, not only to us, but to our families *and* our patients.

During your education and training you acquired a great deal of knowledge and skill to use in caring for others. Nowhere along the line were you taught the skills to cope with the responsibilities, the frustrations, and all the feelings and fears that you experience in practice. What we should have acquired then, and need to develop in practice, are the abilities (1) to recognize and meet our own needs, (2) to develop methods to cope with the special stresses inherent in medicine, and (3) to allow ourselves to be comfortable with and to express our own emotions.

We may have learned something about these abilities since graduation, but let's look at them in more detail to see if we can learn more now.

THE ABILITY TO RECOGNIZE AND MEET OUR OWN BASIC NEEDS

The needs of a physician are the same as those of his patients or anyone else. Yet the thrust of our preparation and practice is to concentrate on the needs of our patients and to ignore or neglect our own.

What *are* they? Let's suggest some of the most essential. You have physical and physiological needs for exercise, rest, good nutrition, and recreation. You need good, warm, intimate, supportive relationships. You need to be able to define yourself and have a sense of purpose. You need a solidly based feeling of self-esteem. And you need to establish a sense of security.

Most basic are the physical and physiological needs. Of course, as physicians, we are well aware of their importance, and there is no need to belabor this point. Or *are* we as aware as we might be? Look back at your medical education. The demands on your time made little or no allowance for *your* physical or mental health, nor did the subject appear anywhere in your curriculum. A message may have been transmitted to you then that your own health was not important. Did you on some level accept this message, so that ever since you have minimized your own need for regular exercise, a low-calorie, low-fat diet, and regular periods of relaxation and rest? We override these needs at our peril.

The same may be true of our supportive relationships. Many physicians in practice are too busy to develop good, warm, close relationships with their peers—or with their families. Some find it difficult even when they have the time. The physician with such constricted relationships may try to satisfy his emotional needs through his patients, leading to a vicious circle in which longer hours increase estrangement from family and peers.

It is a sad paradox that the intensity of medical practice tends to isolate the caring physician from a caring and compassionate world, and to hinder the physician in receiving the revitalizing support he requires. The demands allow little time or opportunity to heal the healer.

A quality personal support network does not happen by chance. It must be created. One must *take the time* to cultivate friends. One has to *learn* candor, congruence, and openness; nothing less will do. This is risky; you will be offering something of value—yourself—and rejection is always possible. If this gives you pause, consider making your first efforts in a group of colleagues or friends selected for that purpose. Look around for a few other physicians with whom you can safely share your problems, fears, tensions, and successes, and who might want to share theirs with you. Form your own group and select a compatible professional facilitator. Then it will be much easier in the real world.

Self-definition is equally important. Your professionalization began in medical school. Most physicians graduate with pride in their new identity and with a sense of purpose, but some emerge confused, angry, and depressed. If you are in the latter group, take the time to sort yourself out, to understand your motivations and goals, and to define yourself accurately. One way is to make a list of all your important qualities, a list that will answer the question, "Who am I?" When you have finished, cross out those qualities that are less important to you. Then look at the others. As Socrates said, "Know thyself."

Self-esteem is not the same as self-definition. Most physicians set their personal and professional expectations—their standards, if you will—higher than can be met realistically, and then feel inadequate, often imagining they are the only ones who feel so. Low self-esteem is common in physicians in spite of the image they project. Many are not in touch with the basis of their feelings and tie their self-esteem to symbols, such as status or economic display. Symbols are no cure for an ailing self-esteem.

What does give a sense of self-worth? It is composed of two separate and distinct elements. There is the *unconditional*, "no matter what" part, and the *conditional*, "I'm okay *if*" element.

The *unconditional* part of self-esteem characterizes those fortunate "invulnerables" who grow up feeling good about themselves through the worst possible circumstances. It is in others who are able to survive repeated catastrophes without throwing in the towel. Perhaps it is the result of a decision they made about themselves as children. Or the decision may have been made for them earlier in their genes.

We can do more about the *conditional* part. It has two loci: external and internal. The external locus begins with our parents and our acceptance of their estimate of our worth. This estimate too often depends on what we do, how we behave, what we say, and perhaps even what we think. As time goes on, we substitute peers, authority figures, and others as the external locus of our self-esteem, and their evaluation becomes increasingly important to us. Throughout, we internalize a portion of the external locus and use it to develop our inner locus of control and self-evaluation.

These three—the unconditional and the two parts of the conditional—must be in balance. If you, like many physicians, have too large a conditional *if* to your self-esteem, if you have this large need to prove to yourself and others that you are a good person, then you will be vulnerable in the practice of medicine. Try to shift some of your dependency on external sources to inner ones. It is less important what others think than what *you* think about what you have done. Competent counseling can allow you to see that no matter how you perform, you are still a good, worthwhile person.

The last basic need on our list is a feeling of security. Much of this is achieved early in life, when a parent was there for protection and reassurance in times of danger. But it is added to by experience in coping successfully with a variety of situations. Security does not mean the absence of storms, but the confidence that when a storm comes, your house will stand. If we lack security, we spend much energy erecting symbolic defenses, establishing rigid codes of behavior for ourselves and others, and attempting to control the uncontrollable. This search for safety can lead to constricted, dull, unspontaneous behavior in our personal lives, and in our profession to interminable lists of differential diagnoses, innumerable laboratory tests, and procrastination. Too often, we begin to think in terms of the mistakes we may make and lose the intellectual excitement of new ideas. Without security, you cannot practice good medicine. Again, counseling can help reinforce your sense of security.

THE ABILITY TO COPE WITH THE SPECIAL STRESSES INHERENT IN THE PRACTICE OF MEDICINE

Many physicians live with a chronic, low-grade anxiety that on occasion is distressing, even disabling. Physicians often have to work at levels of anxiety that would incapacitate other people. And we must do this with a "competent face" and genial professionalism.

Much of this anxiety arises from the stresses that are unique to medicine. Some were mentioned at the start of this chapter. No other profession deals so intimately with life and death on a daily basis. We must cope with our own fears and emotions while maintaining scientific objectivity, balance empathy with clinical detachment, and somehow embrace both the highest idealism and rectal examinations. We keep trying to treat incurable illnesses, patients who won't help themselves, and those who are self-destructive. Our clinical judgment often conflicts with politics or economics. We must remain calm with those who are anxious, fearful, irritable, and angry. And, dealing with the possibility of death for our patients, we must face our own fear of it.

Still, stress, like Janus, has two faces. In physics, stress is defined as the force impinging on an object, and the deformation the object undergoes is called strain. Although the forces affecting us are stressful, the degree to which we are "bent out of shape" is determined largely by our own inner critics. Our level of anxiety depends directly on these critics. We all carry within ourselves a voice or voices that tell us no matter how much we do, it should have been more, and no matter how well we do, it could have been better. These inner voices evoke feelings of guilt, embarrassment, and inadequacy and our fear of these emotions is experienced as anxiety. We can reduce excessive internal criticism relatively easily through several techniques. An especially effective way is in an assertiveness training group.

Overwork is an occupational hazard for physicians. Some are unable to set limits for themselves. As in all addictions, the causes are complex. Overwork may help the physician reduce feelings of guilt or anxiety about his self-worth. It can be an escape from domestic or personal stress in the short run, but aggravates it in the long run. It may help him discharge a never-ending sense of obligation, while increasing his resentment at the lack of recognition or compensation received.

We are all human and limited by human frailties; none of us has endless personal resources. Limits must be set and they must be realistic ones. Your resources of time, energy, health, even of knowledge and skill, are finite. It is not realistic, for example, to expect to challenge death and win consistently. What patients need to see, and to hear from you, is that you care—then they are more able to accept the vagaries of fate even when they are cruel. Our responsibility lies not in the product but in the process. Our *goal* may be health, or cure, or warding off death, but our *responsibility* is to be competent and do our best, to indicate that we care, and to help the patient cope with his illness. If you accept the burden of these three responsibilities, you have assumed enough.

THE ABILITY TO BE COMFORTABLE WITH AND TO EXPRESS OUR FEELINGS

Physicians are subject to many painful and uncomfortable feelings in the course of their work, and many have not learned to handle these feelings well. For example, some have difficulty dealing with a dying patient and withdraw. Some have unresolved feelings about anxious, cranky, fat, demanding, or noncompliant patients. Many find sexual feelings, either in themselves or expressed by patients, disconcerting. When we are frustrated we then feel anger, resentment, hostility, or even alienation and depression. When we are prodded by our internal critics we may feel guilt, shame, embarrassment, and humiliation. When our self-esteem is low we often feel inadequate, inferior, unworthy, and ineffectual.

If resolution of such feelings is to occur, it will not happen behind the shell that many physicians erect to defend themselves from them and from the patients who arouse them. Most of us try to avoid these feelings, but this just avoids their resolution. We have many positive emotions during the course of our work when it is fulfilling and satisfying: pleasure, interest, joy, affection, love, exuberance. These are what make the practice of medicine rich and rewarding. However, if we are to be open to *these* emotions, we must be open to *all* our emotions; we cannot pick and choose. If you are to lead a full, rich life and interact deeply and completely with others, you have to allow, accept, and deal with all the emotions involved—those in yourself as well as those in others.

The negative emotion most frequently experienced by physicians is anger. In the course of a typical day, we encounter many situations that produce anger. If we suppress or deny our anger, we only replace it with chronic resentment or worse. We may repress it, producing psychosomatic ailments. Or displace it to innocent people or unrelated issues. Worst of all, we may turn the anger inward and express it self-destructively.

We are, of course, descendants of predators and almost the only species lacking a built-in biological imperative not to kill its own kind. Instead, we have social, moral, and religious injunctions, which are at best superable barriers. We must accept that anger is, for better or worse, a normal human emotion, and that people who feel it are still good people. We may have been taught that anger is bad or that we are bad for having anger. The social reasons for this view are understandable, but the individual cannot blame himself for a characteristic of the species.

Sometimes we want to make ourselves feel better about being angry, and try to justify it by blaming the person who made us angry. Blaming others is, in the long run, counterproductive. It is better to accept the anger along with whatever caused it, and start thinking about our next step. Or we may believe that we should attack or in some atavistic way act out our anger. This is also nonsense; we may not be in charge of experiencing the feeling, but we are certainly in charge of what we do about it.

There are better ways to handle anger. The next time you feel it, try these three steps.

First, allow the feeling of anger to exist without denying, rationalizing, or justifying it. Accept it as normal and natural under the circumstances and yourself as normal and natural for having it. Just experience it.

Second, express the anger in nondestructive ways. Don't "act out" against other people or use it to get your way. Do something physical, even if you have to leave the room to do it: take a walk, pound a pillow, slam a door. Allow some time to pass until the peak of the physiological reaction subsides.

Third, get down to the serious business of examining the situation. It is your responsibility to use and interpret your anger as a message that *some important basic need was not met* or that its satisfaction was somehow threatened. It is very easy to jump from this to the conclusion that another person or the world should be different or better. Instead, explore alternate ways of satisfying this need. Anger usually includes the message that there is no other way. This is almost never true. In the last analysis, it is you who must take charge of fulfilling your own needs; you cannot assign this job to anyone else.

Depression is another negative emotion we must learn to deal with. It is closely linked to anger. In essence, depression means that you have given up because you see no way to meet some basic needs. Physicians are especially vulnerable. After years of deprivation and trying to do the right thing, we may encounter a series of frustrations. When surmounting them seems hopeless, depression frequently follows. There are often other factors involved. Among these may be low self-esteem, an emotionally impoverished childhood, present needs that are not being met, losses that are difficult to handle, or an inability to deal with some of the stresses of practice.

If one were to draw up the perfect plan for producing depression in an otherwise normal person, a medical career would fit that plan well. Teach him to be conscientious; tell him that if he meets the needs of others and defers his own long enough, he will eventually be happy. Constrict his life until medicine is almost all he knows, and keep deferring satisfactions and rewards indefinitely. Make personal intimacy suspect. Tell him to repress or deny his feelings, then remove most of the channels that he would use to express them. Place him daily in situations that arouse intense feelings. Alienate him from those who would support him. Make his self-esteem depend on being mistake-free in a world where mistakes are inevitable, and on saving lives when death is inescapable.

The best way to prevent impairment is by developing the ability to enjoy your practice, to find it worthwhile and satisfying. A sense of purpose and of value goes a long way. Make sure your working conditions fit *you*. Don't rely for your happiness solely on helping other people. Take responsibility for your own well-being. If you will not, who will? And start right now, for if not now, when?

34

Discontinuing A Private Practice

There is a tendency for physicians today to discontinue practice abruptly, rather than taper off over several years as they did in the past. The reasons for this shift are several. One is the rapid progress in medical knowledge. If a physician lets up in his daily schedule and begins to take longer vacations, he will soon fall behind. Another is the more intense competition. Now, when a physician begins to taper, he may find his practice plummeting as his patients transfer to physicians who they know will be there for a number of years. Another is the cost of malpractice insurance. Many carriers do not reduce rates for part-time or limited practice. Even the cost of maintaining a medical license has become a factor in some states. Many hospitals now limit surgical or other privileges at a certain age. The high cost of personnel salaries, rent, and other expenses at the present time also tends to make a part-time practice less practicable.

Another major difference today, due to the increased competition in the medical marketplace, is that most established practices have a substantial goodwill value. In the past, discontinuance for many physicians merely meant paying attention to the future employment of personnel, to the notification of patients, and to the disposition of records and accounts receivable. Today the emphasis in most cases is upon the sale of the practice.

The first half of this chapter will be primarily for those who will sell their practices, and the second for those who, like the old soldier, will just fade away.

SELLING A PRACTICE

If you are going to sell, decide on the date you would like to leave as far ahead as possible—at least one year, preferably two. At the next lease renewal time, lock up the location for a purchasing physician and include a clause to let you out. Much of the value of your practice depends upon the physician who takes over being able to occupy the same premises for a year or more after you leave. At the next performance review, probe each employee's long-term plans. But don't hint at your own. It is too soon to tell them. Look for any evidence of discontent. Make salary and other adjustments as necessary. You would like to turn over a happy team.

Then look over Chapter 9, "Purchasing a Practice," for the information it gives from the point of view of the purchaser. I will not cover the same ground here from a seller's perspective, but you have to know how the components of a practice are valued and the tax consequences to you upon sale.

The next step is to perform an analysis of your practice. Use some of the suggestions in Chapters 5 and 17 to study your patient drawing area. Note any demographic or socioeconomic trends. Be alert for any positive factors that may be worth emphasizing to prospective purchasers. Summarize this information on paper in a paragraph or two.

Extend this analysis to your patients along the lines suggested in Chapter 17. Note the same demographic data and socioeconomic background for your patients as you did for your drawing area. Determine the proportion covered by commercial insurance, Medicare, and Medicaid. Note the number of active, inactive, and new patients with their sources of referral. Summarize this information in another paragraph or two.

Then describe your competition in a few sentences.

The last part of your analysis is a summary of the financial aspects of your practice. Start with your fees for key services and procedures. State the charges for these by month over the preceding year, total charges each month and for the year, collection rates, and the status of your accounts receivable. Follow this with expenses by category for the same periods, and total overhead. Describe income from other sources and indicate if this would continue for the incoming physician. The net profit for these periods is the final item. Get out the quarterly reports from your accountant for the last four years, make copies, and attach these to your notes.

As you assemble these data, be alert for any improvements you can make. From now on, you must make extra efforts rather than slack off. Favorable recent trends will enhance the value of your practice—and downturns discourage potential purchasers.

This is most of the information you need to prepare a practice description. This description is the basis for your ads, answering the questions of prospective purchasers, preparing a proposal for sale, and drawing up the sales agreement. The description itself starts with your specialty, location, information about your building, distance to hospitals and other medical resources, the size and layout of your office, the number and qualifications of your employees, and specifics on the equipment. Then all you have to do is add the results of your practice analysis, and you have it.

The proposal for sale requires only a few more items. Determine the asking price of each component with the help of your accountant (adjusted in accordance with its tax implications for you), and add these with the total to the description. Then decide, again in consultation with your accountant, the payout period, interest to be charged, and the form your security should take. Be sure to charge an acceptable interest rate. If it is lower than prevailing rates, the IRS may impute an interest of 10 per cent and tax you for this income even though you did not receive it. It is time then to go over your proposal with your attorney, to add a covenant not to compete, an exact description of what is included in the sale, and the statement describing the introduction you will give the purchasing physician. Add anything else your attorney suggests, and this is your proposal. Have it typed up in a presentable form, and it will be the basis for negotiation and the subsequent sales agreement.

Now you can begin to let the word out that you are looking for an associate—*not* that you will discontinue practice. Chapter 29 sets out guidelines for taking on an associate. In addition, you might consider having confidential conversations with selected colleagues in the community who would find it advantageous to purchase your practice. Groups, and even hospitals, might be in the market. Be discreet. If it became widely known that you were interested in selling, it could have an adverse effect on your practice.

In addition to the suggestions in Chapter 29, two or three more are pertinent when you plan to turn your practice over to the associate. His professional interests, personality, and style of practice must be similar to yours so that your patients will stay. Check into his financial resources more thoroughly than you would otherwise. Make sure he is competent. Go back a little further in checking his references. As you talk to him look for any factor that might cause him problems in retaining your patients. You want to *discontinue* practice, not step in again and pick up the pieces.

The time to notify your employees and determine if they will stay is best decided upon by you in accordance with your circumstances. In most cases they can be advised of your plans just before you begin to look for your associate. Ask that they keep this information confidential.

Your attorney and his will draft the sales agreement, so I will make only a couple of suggestions here. The covenant must be worded so as to allow you to take back the practice in the event of default. Agree on how overlapping obligations for personnel salaries and taxes will be handled, and on related matters such as accrued vacation time or other benefits. Make sure the buyer will keep—and that you will have access to—the charts for as long as your attorney advises. If he is to use your name in the practice in any way, restrict this use to a year or less after you leave. Some remaining expenses (such as telephone and utilities) should be covered in the agreement, even though you will settle all bills payable before leaving. A life insurance policy on the buyer covering the balance owed, as well as adequate disability insurance, are *essential*. You should be the beneficiary of both and pay the premiums.

Before he joins you, inform your patients, colleagues, hospitals, and others that you are taking on an associate. Schedule him heavily. Use one agreed-upon fee schedule when he starts. Introduce him to patients—those you see, too—and to colleagues and hospital personnel.

About a month before you leave, notify your patients, colleagues, and others by letter, stating that the practice "will continue as usual" at the same address.

During the last month, get out your professional liability insurance policy and read it over. If you have maintained occurrence coverage, your policy covers you after you leave practice, no matter when the claim is made. However, if your policy is on a "claims made" basis, you will have to pay a premium now to cover any claim that may be filed within the term of the statute of limitations for your state after you discontinue practice. Write the carrier for clarification on any points and tell them your intentions. When you do, ask if part-time practice is covered at a reduced premium. Request a premium adjustment for the period of time the policy runs after you quit practice. Keep the policy for later reference.

If you decide to retain your state license, remember to advise the State Board of your new address, which will now be your home, not your office. Notify the DEA of your intentions, and request instructions as to disposition of scheduled drugs, order forms, and narcotics records under your name. If you have an equivalent state agency, do the same with them. It is advisable to destroy all your unused prescription pads when you leave.

Your medical societies—local, state, and the AMA—should be advised that you are discontinuing practice. You will probably cancel your membership, but inquire of the AMA about their special dues-exempt membership category for retired physicians. This permits subscription to *JAMA* and specialty journals at half price. Also notify your specialty societies.

Your insurance carriers, Medicare, Medicaid, and Blue Shield should be notified that you are discontinuing practice and informed of your new address.

Review all your professional insurance coverage with your insurance agents. Arrange for the policies to be transferred to your successor. The premium adjustments are included in the sales agreement if they are substantial.

The hospitals at which you practice should be notified, and any position on a hospital staff must be passed on to another as the Chief of Staff directs under the bylaws.

If you find that you are unable to sell your practice, it may be possible to structure its donation to a hospital as a charitable contribution. Almost always your furniture and equipment can be sold. If you cannot get what they are worth, consider having them appraised and donating them for the tax deduction. Your medical books can usually be donated to a medical society or hospital library.

LEAVING PRACTICE WITHOUT A SALE

The rest of this chapter offers guidelines for leaving practice when, for whatever reason, you will not be selling it. Again, decide on the date at least a year ahead.

In this case the first action to take is the insertion of an escape clause in your lease at the next renewal time. Alternatively, you can time your discontinuance to coincide with the expiration of the lease.

Then, look over the personnel section of your office manual, and discuss both payroll records and benefits with your accountant. It may be that your health insurance plan is transferable. Unused sick and vacation time must be compensated for according to the terms in your manual. Look over all personnel records carefully, paying special attention to the attendance record. A disgruntled employee sometimes selects this time to put in a claim with the Labor Relations Board for overtime over the past several years. Sit down with your employees four to six months before you intend to leave and inform them of your plans. Offer to assist them in obtaining other positions. Ask them not to inform patients of your decision. Get your accountant's advice about your employee retirement plans and how to handle them once you have discontinued practice. In general, you are required to keep accurate and complete records on retirement plans for at least ten years. If you terminate a retirement plan you need to go back ten years and give all of the employment data, including the number of people originally in the plan, number of new people entered, number of payouts, and so forth, in order to terminate the plan. Select one key employee and offer her an incentive to remain for a month or two after the last patient has been seen. There will be a number of details to take care of after your office door is closed.

A more stringent collection policy must be instituted as soon as your staff has been notified. Many patients become reluctant to pay once they know you are leaving practice. Emphasize time-of-service payment and send a letter to your patients if doing so represents a substantial change in policy. A copy should be sent to all active patients, and you may wish to post a copy in the office as well. Then tighten up your collection procedures. Age your accounts receivable monthly. Intensify your collection efforts on delinquent accounts. Contact insurance carriers that have shown themselves to be slow payers. The accounts receivable still remaining when you leave practice may be turned over to an ethical collection agency.

Your medical records will have to be reviewed, starting three or four months before you close your doors. The guiding principle is that medical records must be accessible to you past the statute of limitations in your state. Some can be purged, however. Those of patients you have seen for only one visit and those you saw a few times for minor matters several years ago can usually be discarded. Those of patients who are deceased can be disposed of after the statute of limitations has expired. The remainder of your charts must be stored in an accessible location. Ask your local medical society if it has storage facilities. If not, then look around your home for a dry and safe area. If you are planning to move, consider a storage company. Microfilming is a possibility. The actual cost is low, but the labor involved in selecting the appropriate material and preparing it for microfilming can be substantial. Whatever your decision on medical record storage, advise your local medical society.

About two months before leaving, cancel office magazine subscriptions and ask for refunds. Consider which medical journals you wish to continue and notify them of your change of address. Cancel the others and request refunds. Have your assistant write "Return to Sender" on all junk mail for at least a month before you close your office.

Your patients should be advised by letter approximately two months before you discontinue practice. The letter is sent to all patients considered to be active. An example of a legally correct form can be found in the AMA publication *Medical Forms and Legal Analysis*. Enclose a release form. Address each patient by name and retain a copy of each letter. The last sentence or two should be a personal farewell to each patient. The letters to certain selected patients—those whose condition or care is complicated or those who may be inclined to cause difficulties—are best sent by registered mail, return receipt requested.

Your accountant will continue to be responsible for filing tax returns and unemployment returns, preparing W-2 forms for the employees, and other tasks for up to a year after you leave practice.

He and your attorney will advise you on the retention of office records. A suggested retention schedule acceptable in most states is:

Accounting Records	**Retention Period**
Accounts payable, invoices, and credits (assumes no pending audits)	3–5 years
Accounts receivable ledger cards (inactive, and equivalent computer reports)	3–5 years
Appointment book	3–5 years
Bank statements, reconciliations, and cancelled checks	3–5 years
Capital asset records	3 years after disposal of the assets
Cash receipt books or vouchers	3–5 years
Deposit books and slips	3–5 years
Employee travel and expense reports	3 years
Financial statements	3 years
General books of account	Permanent

Medical Records	**Retention Period**
Records of adults	10–15 years
Records of minors	The period of local state statute of limitations after the patient reaches majority
X-rays of adults	5–8 years
X-rays of minors	The period of local state statute of limitations after the patient reaches majority

Payroll and Related Records	**Retention Period**
Employees' deduction authorizations	2 years after termination
Individual personnel files	4 years after termination
Payroll register	10 years
Records of payments and reports to government	4 years
W-2's returned by Post Office, addressee has no forwarding address	4 years

During the last month, have your assistants look over the supplies on hand to see if any unopened stock can be returned for credit. Request final statements from all your suppliers. Unused supplies may be given to colleagues.

Notify the utility companies of the date you wish to have service terminated. Your telephone and answering service will be coordinated and terminated at a date decided by you.

The practice checking account is usually maintained for approximately three months after discontinuing practice. Thereafter, any receipts can be deposited in your personal checking account and professional bills paid from it if you maintain adequate records. Consult your accountant about this.

During the last month or so, send letters of farewell or appreciation to your colleagues. Advise all correspondents of your change of address. Notify the local post office of your forwarding address the last day. Then take down your shingle, bring it home with you, and treasure it.

35

What Lies Ahead?

with MARLENE COLEMAN, M.D.,
and DIANE WILNER LAIRD, M.P.H.

A book on medical practice management must be applicable not only when it is written, but for at least a few years into the future. This is especially true in the 1980s, when more changes are taking place in our field than at any other time in modern memory. And still greater changes lie just over the horizon.

Without doubt, most of these will have the greatest influence on physicians who are just now starting their careers, and more on those in private practice than others. Because this book has endeavored to supply the fullest information where the need is the greatest, it has inevitably acquired an orientation toward the physician who is starting a career in private practice. Although some future trends were alluded to where appropriate, this last chapter will look more carefully at them taken together and try to estimate their effect upon the private practitioner.

Futurists generally base their projections on extrapolation of recent trends, making minor adjustments for the most current data available. This technique has its limitations in the health care field. Only factors having a major impact can be considered because the degree of accuracy of an overall prediction is so limited. Even two or three minor factors acting in concert would have less effect than the inaccuracy that is inherent in the methodology itself. And it should be borne in mind that a single significant technological breakthrough or legislative act could make most if not all predictions valueless.

The first task then is to sort through the hundreds of operant factors and try to decide which are "major" and should be incorporated into our predictions, and which are "minor" and are best ignored.

The obvious factor to start with is the population itself, its characteristics, and the demographic shifts that are expected over the next 10 to 15 years. The Census Bureau projects a continued increase in the total population—249,731,000 by 1990 and 267,990,000 by the year 2000. By itself, this growth would have only a minor impact, and is one of the factors to set aside in making predictions. Those who make up the largest "bump" in the demographic curve, the baby-boom generation, will not reach their maximum utilization of health services until the years 2000 to 2025. But the elderly will continue to be the fastest growing segment of our population before that surge comes. Combine this fact with others: their susceptibility to injury and chronic diseases, our increased capacity to care for these conditions, and the greater affluence and political potency of this age group, and we do have a factor that is significant and should be included. Other population shifts, such as continuing migration from the Northeast "Rust Belt" states to the Southwest and West "Sun Belt," will only have a minor impact.

More important than this is the physician-to-population ratio, which brings us to the number of physicians that will be practicing medicine over the next 10 to 15 years.

Responding to a perceived shortage of physicians in the 1950s, Congress passed the Health Professions Educational Assistance Act in 1963, which expanded the size and number of medical schools. The totals of 89 allopathic and 5 osteopathic schools of 1950 became 127 and 15, respectively, by 1980. The Health Manpower Act of 1968 provided financial assistance to medical students, along with capitation grants to the schools designed to increase class size. Immigration regulations were also eased during this same period, increasing the influx of foreign medical graduates (FMGs). Oddly, these and other actions of the federal government, such as encouraging the Fifth Pathway Program, were taken without clearly defining the nation's health care needs or setting specific goals in relation to them.

As a consequence of these actions, the number of medical school graduates was approximately doubled by 1980, and nearly 5000 FMGs per year have set up practice here since 1960. Although the Health Professions Educational Assistance Act of 1976 restricted the influx of FMGs somewhat, the number of U.S. citizens studying medicine abroad, especially in the "offshore" Caribbean medical schools, more than made up for this decline. The overall result is that between 1960 and the present time there has been an approximate doubling of the number of physicians in practice. Because this shifted the mean age of the physician pool downward, additions will exceed attrition for the rest of this century, even if medical schools respond to the recently decreased federal support by leveling off the number of graduates. But there is little indication so far that they will do so, or that licensure of FMGs will be prohibited.

The Graduate Medical Education National Advisory Committee of the Department of Health and Human Services projects a total physician population in 1990 of 596,840, which represents by its definition a surplus of 35,000 to 85,000. By 2000, the surplus will be 130,000. A more somber prediction is that of the Congressional Office of Technology Assessment—a surplus of 185,000 physicians by 1990. Neither estimate takes into consideration such factors as physician maldistribution or the decreasing utilization of physicians' services, a trend that has been evident since 1977.

The physician-to-population ratio averaged about 140 per 100,000 for the decade prior to 1960. It rose to 152 by 1970 and will increase to 215 by 1990. By the year 2000 it will reach 240, which will almost certainly be the highest in the world. This factor will be a major one.

In looking at such figures, physicians tend to regard themselves as the only providers of health care services. But we must also include such ethical allied health professionals as podiatrists, optometrists, clinical psychologists, nurse practitioners (including anesthetists and midwives), and physician's assistants. Most of these offer less costly care, and many provide more personalized attention. Nevertheless, the projected numbers of such professionals based upon the present education and training programs mean that they will have only a minor effect, at least through 1990.

Patients are becoming more interested in alternatives to traditional science-based health care. All sorts of self-styled nutritionists, stress counselors, acupuncturists, chiropractors, and "naturopaths" are addressing this need with increasing success. Of these, chiropractors are the most adept at using the media and in lobbying for political and legislative action. The number of chiropractic graduates has quadrupled over the last decade. Their median age is now a young 37. Medicare and workers' compensation pay them in all 50 states, and Medicaid does in most. So we will probably experience a significant influence from this quarter before 1990, and after that date chiropractors may be joined by one or more other alternative care providers in having a major impact from then until the end of the century.

The rising cost of medical care is certainly a major factor. Over $400 billion per year is being expended today, and the best estimate is that $754 billion per year will be spent by 1990, despite efforts to control this cost. This figure is so large that it has little meaning for most of us. But it is clearer as a percentage of the gross national product, where the exponential rise is easily seen: 1970—7 per cent of GNP; 1980—9 per cent of GNP; 1990 (projected)—12 per cent of GNP; 2000 (projected)—17 per cent of GNP. And bear in mind that the inflation-adjusted GNP has increased each year and most likely will continue to do so. At somewhere around 10 per cent of GNP these costs begin to encroach on support for other social needs. It is a hard truth that, although the resources are limited, the demand for medical services is virtually without limit. Increased medical knowledge and technology applied to a population whose mean age is increasing will further extend the average life span. In a sense, a vicious circle of rising costs will be set up. Modern medicine has almost ensured that most of those alive today will die after years of chronic care or a lingering terminal illness. Already, 70 per cent of Medicare's money goes to fewer than 10 per cent of the beneficiaries. Added to this will be the effect of medical and technological advances for all age groups: in perinatology, correction of genetic disorders by genetic engineering, organ transplantation, artificial organs, and the like. Society in the future will have no choice but to accept the rationing of medical care in principle as well as fact.

Under the present retrospective fee-for-service system, with most patients having medical insurance in some form, there is a lack of incentive for those involved to be concerned with cost control. Although physicians' fees represent only 20% of health care costs, his decisions affect 70 to 80 per cent of the total. With the physician's focus on providing the best for his patient while paying only secondary attention to the cost, the latter can get out of control. Hospitals try to please both the physician and the patient, emphasizing equipment and facilities for the former, and service and amenities for the latter, with only secondary regard for the cost. The patient himself is thus satisfied with both the physician and hospital, and in most cases, is able to pass along the expense through the insurance intermediary to the taxpayer or corporate employer. The most strenuous efforts toward cost containiment can therefore be expected to come from government and corporate action.

The federal government pays the greatest portion, about 40 per cent, of the nation's medical bills, so it is not surprising the first action came from this quarter. The Medicare system of hospital payment by diagnosis-related group (DRGs) is the most dramatic change to date. But it is probably only a "first generation" mechanism, beginning a movement toward prospective capitation payment without regard to diagnosis.

In 1975, researchers at the Yale School of Medicine developed the case classification system on which it is based. They found 467 clinically coherent groups of diagnoses that consumed reasonably comparable medical resources. A federally sponsored trial then took place in New Jersey starting in 1978, in which all but three of the 116 acute care hospitals in that state participated. These hospitals were compensated for each patient according to the diagnostic group in which the patient was placed, by discharge diagnosis, and the trial was found to be reasonably successful. The Health Care Financing Administration (HCFA) then modified the classification to fit elderly Medicare beneficiaries, and this resulted in a list of 356 DRGs. This list was used in preparing a case-mix index for every hospital in the country that accepts Medicare patients.

The use of diagnosis-related groups was mandated as the basis of hospital compensation for Medicare beneficiaries in the 1982 Tax Equity and Fiscal Responsibility Act (TEFRA). The system was phased in over three years, starting October 1, 1983. Reimbursed on the cost-per-discharge diagnosis, hospitals were given incentive to minimize ancillary services and length of stay. Medicare represents a substantial portion of any hospital's business—from 30 to 80 per cent. The previous decline in average length of stay due to improved technology and treatment was accelerated sharply with the institution of this system. Cost constraints are now felt severely during each stay, and even the total number of admissions has declined.

TEFRA also directed the federal government to contract with peer review organizations (PROs), the successor agencies of the professional standards review organizations (PSROs), and targets were set for minimizing Medicare utilization (in many states, Medicaid was included as well), and for shifting surgeries and treatments to a less costly outpatient setting. It also mandated a future report by the HCFA on applying DRGs to physician payment for hospital services under Medicare.

In 1984, Congress imposed a fee freeze on physician services to Medicare beneficiaries, created the Medicare participating-physician program, and moved up the due date on the physician DRG report. Also under active consideration is the application of DRGs to payment for Medicare patients in skilled nursing facilities, rehabilitation and other programs, and for home health care.

It is almost certain that the fee freeze will be extended and that the next step will be the institution of some form of DRG-based payment of physicians' fees for their hospitalized Medicare patients. It is possible that the "service window" will be widened to include related pre- and post-admission service to encourage outpatient care. Some serious problems will be encountered if payments are made directly to the physician. The limited number of patients each physician has in any one DRG will not permit effective averaging. Some physicians may avoid the care of seriously ill patients, and specialists who care for them may be undercompensated. For these and other reasons, there will most likely be some form of contractual payment to the hospital staff on an Individual Practice Association (IPA) model. This, too, has problems but would be preferable to paying the hospital directly on an HMO model. These payment problems will prevent the effective implementation of a DRG-based system so that a fee schedule will be substituted until a capitation program can be set up.

Because only 61 per cent of Medicare payments to physicians are for inpatient services, it is almost inevitable that the same steps will follow for physician outpatient treatment under Medicare. Before this happens, and sooner rather than later, our choice of accepting assignment on a case-by-case basis will be eliminated, and the deductible and copayment portions payable by the patient will be raised repeatedly. Most state Medicaid programs will, to a greater or lesser degree, follow the lead of Medicare. And the medical insurance carriers are just waiting in the wings and watching.

Hospital cost-shifting to privately paying and insured patients is currently approaching the limits of tolerance. When the hospital DRG-based remuneration system has been fully phased in for a few years, and hospitals are hurting even more than now, cost-shifting will probably pass that limit. Physicians by then may be forced to do some cost-shifting too. In response, corporations will change their health benefit plans to the less expensive capitation payment types, and privately paying patients may almost disappear as most obtain individual insurance or join prepaid programs.

To date, the federal government has been in the forefront of cost containment. In our opinion, corporations will soon assume the more active role. Health benefits now cost industry over $100 billion a year, and this is rising. The cost now amounts to about 60 per cent of after-tax profits. At the present rate of increase, profits would be eliminated entirely in the early 1990s without corrective action before then. Foreign competition is growing greater, and the trade deficit has become the most serious in history.

In the last two years, studies have shown that most employers have made significant changes in their health benefit package to make the employees more responsible for their health care expenditures. Many companies are hiring physicians and nurses as advisors, requiring second surgical opinions, increasing outpatient coverage, and providing financial incentives for the employee to be prudent with the health care dollar.

These are only stopgap measures. The catalyst for more decisive action by employers may be the decision of the federal government at some time in the future to tax both medical insurance contributions and benefits. Business, with its "management by objectives" approach, will then focus on the objective of cost-containment. By then the rather inefficient government programs will have had some success in controlling costs for the poor and elderly. Corporations will set about containing costs for the employed middle class more efficiently, and the government may adopt some of their methods. A three-level health care system will then emerge. Government programs will provide the first-level minimum care to the poor and elderly. Corporations will offer better care to the employed. Those individuals who can afford it will purchase insurance or pay directly for their medical care. The most capable physicians will compete intensely for the third-level patients. Those who do not succeed there will participate in plans at the lower two levels.

Recently, articles have appeared in medical journals decrying the "monetarization" of medical care. In reality, this began to occur soon after World War II. The really significant factor has been the entry of big business into the health care field. This brought innovative ideas, trained management, marketing skills, economies of bulk purchasing, and greater ability to develop capital in the equity markets. The entry of big business started slowly during the 1960s with nursing homes. During the 1970s, about 77 per cent of these became for-profit, and over half are now owned by large corporations. In that same decade, business interests began to build or acquire smaller hospitals in carefully selected areas. They were often able to increase charges, and through cost efficiencies and selecting private patients who could pay or were insured, these proprietary hospitals flourished. Chains were formed by purchasing nonprofit rural hospitals, independent physican-owned hospitals, and by building their own. In the 1980s these chains began to purchase or merge with the larger prestigious non-profits.

Prior to then, most hospitals were both nonprofit and independent. Some were linked loosely together or operated under the centralized management of a religious or other nonprofit organization. To meet this threat hospitals in the non-profit sector began forming alliances and merging to form multihospital systems.

Just over the horizon lies more extensive horizontal integration. Ours is the finest health care system in the world, and it will be marketed overseas much like any other product. The multicentered corporations will become multinational.

Vertical integration has also begun to take place. Both individual hospitals and chains have acquired nursing homes, rehabilitation centers, central and satellite ambulatory care centers, home health care programs, diagnostic facilities, health promotion ("wellness") centers, medical supply houses, and even medical insurance companies.

The age of conglomerates in the health field has arrived, and this is undoubtedly a major factor. Some strange terminology is now being heard. We are no longer physicians, but "providers." Caring for the patient has become "health care delivery." Patients are not patients, but "consumers." The traditional emphasis on providing the best care possible has given way to more attention to the figure on the bottom line. Caring for the patient is becoming more of a means than an end.

This has altered the hospital environment in which we work. Historically, hospitals were established for the social good. Physicians determined which patients were to be admitted and were in charge of the care provided. The goals and role of the physician were in harmony with those of the hospital. This is not as true today. Management is often now at odds with medicine. A subtle shift is taking place whereby physicians are coming under the control of the hospitals they once, to some degree, controlled. Medicare payment by diagnosis-related groups has resulted in shorter hospital stays and cost-cutting measures that often adversely affect quality of care. Corporate regulations and algorithms emanating from computer software and statisticians are less susceptible to the influence of physicians. More and more decisions are made at a distance in corporate headquarters.

There is some danger that, ultimately, hospitals and physicians may assume an antagonistic rather than the traditional synergistic relationship. As physicians are gradually edged out of administrative functions, hospital staffs will lose much of their influence. Some larger chains and even individual hospitals pursuing vigorous business and marketing policies are already carrying the conflict into the community with satellite clinics and other outreach programs in direct competition with physicians.

Big business hasn't been the only thing to hit hospitals. The effects of Medicare's prospective payment system was mentioned.

At the same time, there has been a shift to outpatient services and home health care. In many areas, recession and unemployment have increased bad debt service. Federal eligibility restrictions on Medicaid have increased charity care in city and county hospitals. State Medicaid cost-containment programs, especially in Rhode Island, California, Massachusetts, and Maine, have further limited hospital income. Although certificate-of-need regulations have helped hold down new construction, in most areas today there is an excess of hospital beds. Many hospitals are trying to operate with a patient census under 50 per cent. Most of these, despite cost-cutting measures, require more than that to cover their expenses.

The result of all this is that the smaller hospital, unless it is the only hospital in the area or has some other unique feature that allows it to survive, today has only three choices: merge with a larger chain, convert to a skilled nursing facility, or close.

Most mid-size hospitals, especially those in suburban areas, are weathering the storm. Parochial pricing, physician support, and community and patient backing all help to sustain them.

The larger teaching hospitals are affected more significantly. Teaching hospitals are 18 to 33 per cent more costly to operate than nonteaching hospitals. They are more dependent on Medicare and Medicaid, care for more complex cases, and have more expensive equipment and sophisticated personnel. Their salaried physicians spend time teaching instead of on patient care. Medicare has made some allowance for these and other differences, but this is due to phase out in 1987.

Inner-city municipal hospitals face the most severe problems. Most are already underfunded and have higher bad debt costs. Their clientele often fails to practice adequate preventive care and post-care regimens. Serious accidents and trauma are much more common, and the intensity and complexity of care tend to be greater. As costs continue to increase, public support on a tax basis will decline. At first, those public hospitals that are the hardest hit will try altered patterns of financing from local and state governments. When this fails, federal funds will be sought. With the anticipated efforts to control the federal budget deficit, this source of support is not likely to be substantial. Some will then resort to management contracts with conglomerates. But even the most efficient management will prove to have its limits.

There have been three significant efforts toward cost containment in recent years— HMOs, PPOs, and IPAs—that, with other acronymic alternatives to come, will constitute major factors affecting medical practice.

The first of these to appear, the Health Maintenance Organization or HMO, received its unfortunate name from the 1973 federal lesiglation assisting such plans. The prototype was the Kaiser-Permanente Plan instituted during World War II, and in reality this and subsequent HMOs came into being, not to *maintain* health as their primary purpose, but to provide medical care in a more cost-effective way. An HMO is essentially a combination of group practice and a medical insurance company. The term "prepaid health plan" is more appropriate. An insurance premium is paid by an employer or individual to the health plan, and, in return, individuals are guaranteed access to all the health care services they need under the defined coverage. For the most part, the covered services are free to the individual—without deductible, coinsurance, or added expenses. However, patients are restricted to the use of specified physicians and hospitals. If they go outside the system, they usually have to pay for the services they receive. In the past, these programs had limited appeal owing to this lack of freedom and the lower quality of care received in many.

However, as health care costs and standards of care in HMOs have risen, employees have become less concerned with freedom of choice and employers more concerned with saving money.

Initially, the lower costs were attributed to two factors: (1) the selection of employees only as members, thus avoiding the poor, the elderly, and the chronically ill; (2) the limitation of expensive diagnostic and therapeutic modalities, including hospitalization. More recently, savings have been realized more through lower rates of hospitalization than any other single factor.

At first, these prepaid plans grew slowly. Then the number of enrollees began increasing at a rate of about 10 per cent a year in the early 1980s. Since 1983, they have grown more rapidly. According to Interstudy, the total number of subscribers was 12.5 million in 1983, 15 million in 1984, and 16.7 million in 1985. If this rate of growth continues, HMOs will achieve a market penetration of about 15 per cent of the population by 1990.

An even greater rate of growth may lie ahead because of the new Medicare regulations that allow and encourage extension of prepaid health benefits to the elderly. Pilot programs have already demonstrated the potential for Medicare HMO programs. The lower and more predictable expense appeals to the bureaucrats. The elderly, who are often on fixed incomes, are offered reasonably comprehensive health benefits with little out-of-pocket expense, which appeals to them. Physicians and hospitals alike face the prospect that a large portion of their Medicare patients may soon be opting for these plans.

At first, out of a concern for the quality of care rendered by HMOs, and later because of the economic threat they posed, physicians in private practice formed Individual Practice Associations (IPAs) in many parts of the country. The typical IPA consists of a group of physicians organized in a common health plan. They continue to practice in their own offices and see other patients. The IPA accepts capitation payment for all subscribers, who have free choice among the panel of affiliated physicians. The latter are paid on a fee-for-service basis by the IPA according to an agreed-upon fee schedule, less a percentage retained as a reserve for contingencies.

According to an article in the July 22, 1985, issue of *Medical Economics*, IPAs are growing even more rapidly than HMOs. In 1980, only about 5 per cent of physicians belonged to one. In 1985 nearly 25 per cent did. By 1990, perhaps half of all physicians in private practice will. It is anticipated that chains of IPAs, consisting of both groups and independent practitioners, will form in the years ahead.

One unique feature being used by some IPAs that may spread to other types of plans is the physician "gatekeeper." The primary-care physician chosen by the patient decides upon diagnostic and other procedures, hospitalization, and even consultations. In many cases, the gatekeeper physician is given a set fee out of which all costs come, to add incentive for cost control. So far, it appears to be effective.

Also, partially in response to HMOs, insurance companies and employers developed preferred-provider organizations (PPOs). Conceptually, they fall somewhere between an HMO and a standard indemnity (fee-for-service) insurance plan. The health care plans offered by PPOs are less costly for the employer than traditional indemnity plans, yet more freedom of choice is available to the employee than in an HMO. The PPO negotiates discounted fees from physicians and hospitals, and in return provides employees with financial incentive to select the "preferred" providers. The premise for these negotiations with providers is that they will receive an increased volume of patients to justify their discounts.

The major growth of PPOs has occurred since 1983. According to the Institute for International Health Initiatives, there were 334 operational PPOs as of June, 1985, with approximately 176,000 physicians and 2750 hospitals participating.

Because a PPO must offer volume to a hospital, it typically contracts with full-service hospitals. Hospitals without obstetric services rarely get contracts, and those with comprehensive services, such as cardiovascular surgery, neonatal intensive care, dialysis, and psychiatric care are preferred. PPOs initially offered contracts to all the physicians on staff at a contract hospital; however, it was later found to be more effective to contract organized groups of physicians in the community.

If Medicare HMOs are as successful as expected, and the present rate of increase in IPAs and PPOs continues, the solo private practitioner will be hard pressed to maintain a traditional practice much past 1990. By then, as much as three fourths of a typical physician's practice will be from one or more of these plans.

We have decribed a dozen factors that, in our opinion, will be the major ones to affect medical practice over the next 10 to 15 years. Of course, there are and will be many others, and the position of each physician in regard to them will be unique. Some minor ones may be major for any one physician, and vice versa.

Let's mention a few more that are considered to be major factors by some, with reasons why we think they will be minor.

Third-party payers currently affect us all, and it might be anticipated that their influence will grow in the future. But look at the dynamics and economic realities. Most of their costs are passed on. Third parties that are intermediaries between the physician and one or more levels of government will yield to the policies of the latter. Those that represent employers will be slower to organize than the employers themselves and become allied with these new centers of power. Some third-party carriers may band together to carry out studies and pilot projects, but otherwise their influence will not be a major one in the future.

Conventional fee-for-service groups will grow in both size and number. But in any one geographical area there is an inherent limit to the size even of a multispeciality group. The largest are unable to extend effectively into rural areas with a low population, but smaller ones will. Profit considerations also restrict group growth in the inner city. Chains of groups may develop, but even so, their influence will be minor.

The threat of malpractice actions and the increasing cost of insurance are serious concerns now and are becoming more so. But much of the cost, if not the threat, can be passed on to the patient, and thus becomes part of what truly is a major factor, the rising cost of medical care. This type of litigation is becoming a burden under which all of us must labor, as taxpayers shouldering the rising cost of municipal liability protection and as consumers paying the expense of increasing product liability insurance with each purchase we make. This is a social change that certainly does and will affect the way we practice medicine and live our lives. But it is a minor factor compared to the major ones set forth.

The "convenience clinic" or "Doc-in-a-box" got its start in 1973, and they have sprouted like mushrooms everywhere since then. This growth is attributable to the fact that they provide medical care at convenient hours, without waiting, and at lower cost than either the private practitioner or hospital emergency room. They are also able to avoid the gory M*A*S*H atmosphere of the latter. They will continue to sprout up over the next few years, and in some areas their impact will be major. However, their growth will be limited by several mechanisms, so that in the long run their overall effect will be minor.

Physicians in the vicinity tend to alter their practice styles to offer much of what the convenience clinic does. And physicians offer such traditional advantages as long-term continuity of care, more personalized attention, and the formation of a strong patient-physician relationship. There is also a growing concern over the quality of care offered by some of these clinics. Many states are looking into their licensure, and some third-party payers have already taken the stance that they will require such licensure before paying hospital emergency room rates. The Accreditation Association for Ambulatory Health Care of the Joint Commission on Accreditation of Hospitals has a pilot program underway that may lead to accreditation requirements for convenience clinics. The Health Systems Agency is contemplating imposing the same requirements on them as it maintains for hospitals. Even sectors of the public have become disaffected with those that have "emergency" as part of their name, because few are open 24 hours a day, seven days a week, or are able to handle critical care cases and major trauma. Tertiary care hospitals are already moving into the field with satellite emergency care centers that do provide these services.

What will the effect of all these factors taken together be on the average physician in private practice? Some doomsday prophets have predicted that those factors categorized as major, along with an assortment of minor ones, will make private practice obsolete. We see no evidence of this. In our opinion, such prophets will join a long line of their predecessors, among which is William Mayo, who, upon forming the first group practice in 1910, declared, "Individualism in American medicine is dead." Analogies are inherently inaccurate, but look back on your own experience. Forty or fifty years ago, the consensus was that all small grocery stores would soon be replaced by larger and more efficient chains. Many were. But those that had unique locations, or carried specialty items, or provided personal service, continued to exist and, in some areas, flourish. The same was said of department stores, and the same thing happened. There are many other examples one can look to for reassurance.

But the character of private practice *will* be changed. Physicians leaving training will not have unlimited choice of where they will locate. Some established practitioners will have to move to rural and other underserved areas. Recent graduates will seek residency training in those specialties that are most in demand—psychiatry, geriatrics, anesthesiology, physiatry—rather than those they would personally prefer. A number will enter the business arena as medical managers. Some specialists will have to offer more primary care, or even change specialties. All will have fewer patients and lower incomes. Most physicians will have to reorient their philosophy of practice away from the correction of abnormalities to preventive measures and to the enhancement of patient well-being. The physician-patient relationship will be redefined in view of the multiple obligations of the former instead of the single obligation to the patient alone. More young physicians will join groups or seek the security of salaried positions. A 1983 survey by the Association of American Medical Colleges indicates that the percentage of graduates planning to enter private practice had already fallen to 61.7 per cent by that year.

All physicians in practice will have to adjust to some loss of autonomy. The traditional two-party physician-patient arrangement that changed with the entry of third-party payers will move back to two parties. But this time one party will be the government or business purchaser of health plans, and the other will be the megacorporate health care provider. The influence of the patient and physician will approach the vanishing point.

The style of patient care will be changed. Office hours will be held at times more convenient for patients. Scheduling will be improved so that patients are seen promptly. More time will be spent with each patient and more on providing patient education and nonmedical services. Physicians will become more cost-conscious on behalf of the patient, who will participate more in discussions and decisions regarding his own care.

Most of us, relating more to both corporation and computer, will have to manage our practices more efficiently. Marketing and public relations will take a higher place in the scale of priorities of all. Those whose practices are largely procedure based will suffer the most drastic cuts in income, as plans hire recently trained physicians and require that a certain number of procedures be performed for a stipulated salary. Surgeons and others in private practice who perform procedures will not be able to withstand this competition.

These and other changes will have less impact on the physician who is in the last ten years or so of his practice. A large roster of affluent or well-insured and satisfied patients will serve as a buffer for the remainder of his time in practice. The effect will be most dramatic on those just starting their careers. Already younger physicians are demonstrating an acceptance of lower incomes and less autonomy. Many are more interested in freedom *from* their job than freedom *in* their job.

In summary, we believe that private practice will survive—even thrive. But it will be altered significantly in these and other ways. Throughout the changes to come, physicians should not lose sight of one goal: the retention of their automony in making medical decisions. This may well be the battleground of the future.